Healthy Dining
in Los Angeles
Fourth Edition

Restaurant Nutrition Guide

Featuring Healthy Entrees from
Popular Los Angeles Restaurants

Including:
- ✓ **Calories**
- ✓ **Fat**
- ✓ **Cholesterol**
- ✓ **Sodium**

Diabetic Food Exchanges, Fruit & Vegetable Servings,
Protein, Carbohydrate & Fiber Information

by

Accents On Health, Inc.

Authors and Contributors:
Anita Jones-Mueller, M.P.H.
Esther Hill, Ph.D.
Erica Bohm, M.S.
Susan Goldstein
Mikah Felago

Healthy Dining in Los Angeles

Healthy Dining
in Los Angeles

Fourth Edition, Revised September 2003

Restaurant Nutrition Guide
by
Accents On Health, Inc.

<u>**Authors and Contributors:**</u>
**Anita Jones-Mueller, M.P.H., Esther Hill, Ph.D.,
Erica Bohm, M.S., Susan Goldstein, & Mikah Felago**

<u>**Published by:**</u>

**Healthy Dining Publications
Accents On Health, Inc.
8305 Vickers Street, Suite 106
San Diego, CA 92111**

**(858) 541-2049
(800) 953-DINE
www.healthy-dining.com**

Cover graphics by Andrew Curl, logo by Ramon Hutson, staff photos by Michael Ross.

Library of Congress Cataloging in Publication Data
Jones, Anita
Healthy Dining in Los Angeles
1, Nutrition.
2, Diet.
3, Restaurant Food
91-71724
ISBN 1-879754-23-1

Table of Contents

Preface by
Dr. Ilena J. Blicker, M.D.
President, Los Angeles County
Medical Association

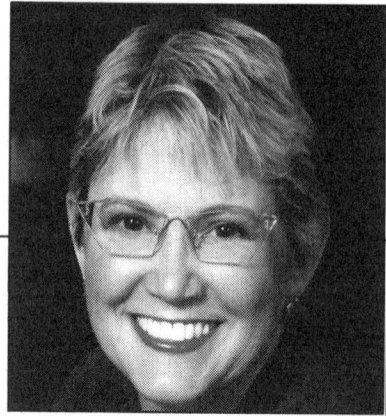

Los Angeles County
Medical
Association

Leadership and Excellence in Health Care

523
West
Sixth Street

10th Floor

Los Angeles,
California
90014-1220

Mailing Address:

P.O. Box 513465

Los Angeles,
California
90051-1465

Telephone:
(213) 683-9900

Fax:
(213) 630-1150

One of the great pleasures in life is eating well. We have usually not associated "fine" dining with "healthy" dining, but it is time to change that concept. Fine dining — even gourmet dining — can be synonymous with healthy. A diet low in fat, cholesterol and sodium can be not only nutritious but also tasty and intriguing. Using *Healthy Dining in Los Angeles* will guide you in making wiser choices in your selection of a menu.

All of us, even if we don't have any significant diseases that would necessitate specific diets, can benefit by being more selective in what we choose to eat. If you have a family history of high blood pressure, diabetes, high cholesterol, etc., learning to eat healthfully now will help you later.

In addition to learning where to eat and what to order, this book can give you ideas of dishes to make at home. So whether you eat out or at home:

ENJOY! EAT WELL and BE HEALTHY!

Ilena J. Blicker, M.D.
President, Los Angeles County Medical Association

A Message from Marilu Henner

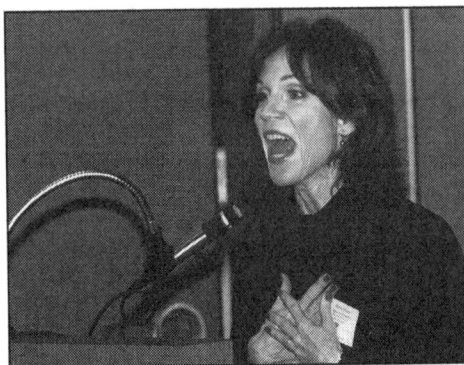

Marilu speaks passionately about the importance of nutrition and health.

With good health, you can do it all. And without health, what do you really have? Health is the single most important factor in your life. It's the basis from which every aspect of your life stems. You can have all the money in the world, you can have all the power in the world, but if you do not have your health, you have nothing. You have been dealt a certain hand in life, and you have been given all the opportunity to play that hand the best you can. Disease doesn't discriminate.

Everything you need to live a longer, happier, healthier life is literally at your fingertips. And, **what you eat makes all the difference**! Whole, natural, high-quality foods will get -- and keep -- you in top form. Lots of fresh fruits and vegetables, whole grains and lean proteins will bring you health and vitality and add years to your life.

Congratulations to the chefs and restaurants participating in the *Healthy Dining* program. They truly have your health and tastebuds in mind. Enjoy the delicious dishes featured in this book. And, best wishes for a very happy, healthy and balanced life!

Sincerely,

Marilu Henner

Marilu Henner

"With good health you can do it all." And "do it all," she does. Marilu Henner is a celebrated television and film actress, best known for her role as Elaine Nardo on *Taxi* and her role opposite Burt Reynolds in *Evening Shade*. She recently starred in the smash Broadway musical *Chicago* and the first national tour of *Annie Get Your Gun*. Marilu is the author of several *New York Times* best-selling nutrition books: *Total Health Makeover, The 30-Day Total Health Makeover, Healthy Life Kitchen* and *Healthy Kids*. Marilu is the mother of two young boys and is also the author of a parenting book, *I Refuse to Raise a Brat*.

About **Healthy Dining** and Accents On Health

Healthy Dining's team of highly qualified nutrition and health professionals is committed to an ambitious and exciting vision: to foster an ever-expanding trend toward healthier menu selections in restaurants. The *Healthy Dining* project began in San Diego in 1990 and expanded to Orange County and Los Angeles. The team has worked with hundreds of restaurants throughout Southern California and has analyzed over 7,000 menu items for nutrition content. *Healthy Dining* is earning respect from all corners -- health professionals, the media, the restaurant industry, and tens of thousands of consumers, many of whom write and call, expressing appreciation for the impact that *Healthy Dining* continues to make in Southern California. In 1998, *Healthy Dining* won the Meritorious Service Award from the California Dietetic Association. In 1999, Accents On Health, Inc. was awarded a three-year research grant from the California Department of Health Services, resulting in the landmark study/campaign called **TrEAT Yourself Well**.

Anita Jones-Mueller, M.P.H. – Director

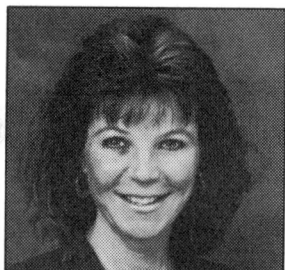

Anita earned her Master's Degree in Public Health from San Diego State University. Her background includes extensive work in the health and nutrition fields, both with individuals and with community group education and support sessions. Anita is one of the founders of the *Healthy Dining* program and the lead author of the book series. She has directed the *Healthy Dining* project from its inception into a growing community program. Anita oversees the nutrition analysis, directs marketing and public relations, and speaks frequently to health professionals and community groups.

Esther Hill, Ph.D. – Editor/Publisher

Esther Hill, a physiologist with a Ph.D. in Biomathematics, worked for over 15 years in medical research at the University of California at San Diego. Her motivation for being involved in this project comes largely from dealing with her son's unstable diabetes. Dr. Hill's family has found traveling and restaurant dining difficult, and she understands why nutrition information is so important to those with dietary restrictions. Dr. Hill is one of the founders of the *Healthy Dining* program. She assists with editing and publishing and was the Principal Investigator of the **TrEAT Yourself Well** research study.

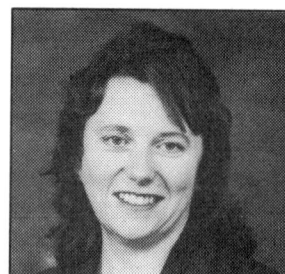

Erica Bohm, M.S. – San Diego Regional Director

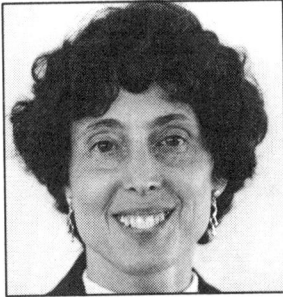

Erica Bohm earned her Master's Degree in Community Health Sciences from New York City's Hunter College. Her experience includes nutrition education, cholesterol reduction, weight control and smoking cessation. During her 20+ years in the health field, Erica has worked for the American Red Cross, the American Health Foundation, and other health organizations, research projects and businesses. Her roles in *Healthy Dining* include seminars, program promotion, and networking with the restaurants, health professionals and organizations, community groups, businesses and the media. Erica also served as Campaign Manager for the **TrEAT Yourself Well** campaign.

Susan Goldstein – Orange County Regional Director

Susan Goldstein earned her Bachelor of Science Degree with distinction in Human Development from Cornell University. She has a strong background and knowledge in nutrition, health promotion, human resources and fundraising, with over 15 years professional and volunteer experience in small and large corporations. Susan works directly with restaurants to create the *Healthy Dining* books and expand participation in the community. Through ongoing projects and activities, Susan promotes *Healthy Dining* with health professionals, the media, corporate and retail partners, special events, marketing, sales and community relations.

Mikah Felago - Projects and Communications Manager

Mikah Felago earned her Bachelor of Science Degree in Foods and Nutrition from San Diego State University. Mikah manages the publication and distribution of the *Healthy Dining* book series, the website and *Healthy Dining's* Cuisine Connection newsletter. She is involved in the sales, marketing and promotion of the *Healthy Dining* books and events. She works closely with restaurants, health professionals and the general public providing health and nutritional education in the context of restaurant dining.

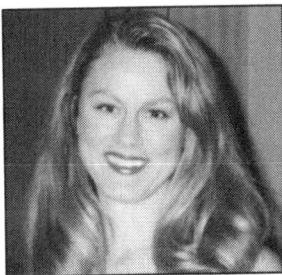

Healthy Dining,
Recipient of the 1998
Meritorious Service Award
of the California Dietetic Association

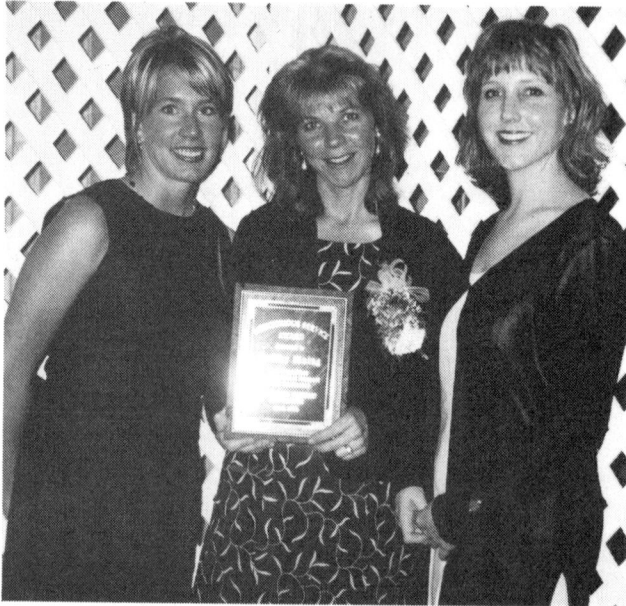

Healthy Dining Director Anita Jones-Mueller (center), dietitian Sherri Corey (right) and Publishing Coordinator Amy Sturm (left) accept the 1998 Meritorious Service Award from the California Dietetic Association at its annual meeting in May, 1998. This award was presented to *Healthy Dining* in recognition of exceptional service to and support of the profession of dietetics.

California Dietetic Association

7740 Manchester Ave., Suite 102, Playa del Rey, CA 90293-8499
Tel. (310) 822-0177 • Fax (310) 823-0264 • E-mail: CDAEP @aol.com • WebSite: www.dietitian.org

Eating out is no longer the "special occasion" treat that it used to be. It is now a way of life in California. A recent survey of eating habits found that over 40% of California adults consumed at least one meal from a restaurant or cafeteria on the previous day. This survey also reported that the rates of obesity for California adults has risen 25% since 1990 (survey conducted by the Cancer Prevention and Nutrition Section of the California Department of Health Services and the Public Health Institute).

People who dine out frequently have diets higher in fat and sodium and lower in fruits and vegetables, but it doesn't have to be that way. Thanks to Healthy Dining's work with chefs and restaurants, you can enjoy delicious and healthy selections when dining out. This book serves as an excellent tool for Los Angeles residents working on improving their eating habits. It is wonderful to have such a useful resource to recommend to patients and clients.

Congratulations to Healthy Dining and the participating restaurants for doing their part to improve the health of Californians.

Sincerely,

Lisa Gibson, MS, RD
Executive Director

People Are Talking About *Healthy Dining...*

"What you eat makes all the difference! Lots of fresh fruits and vegetables, whole grains and lean proteins will bring you health and vitality and add years to your life. Congratulations to the chefs and restaurants participating in the Healthy Dining Program. They truly have your health and tastebuds in mind."
- *Marilu Henner, Nutrition Author and Television & Film Actress*

"Your involvement with the American Heart Association is very special since you are doing exactly what we believe in...I am so glad there is Healthy Dining."
- *Sally Fenton, Executive Director of the American Heart Association and President of the Women's Health Initiative (WHI) Community Advisory Board for Orange County*

"Most of our nation's leading causes of death are related to what we eat; therefore, it is crucial to establish healthy eating habits early in life...Along with other physicians, dietitians and health professionals, I am grateful for Healthy Dining as a resource."
Alan M. Heilpern, M.D., Medical Director,
The Center for Health Enhancement at Saint John's Health Center,
Past President, Los Angeles County Medical Association

"I encourage patients to use the book whenever they dine out. It's great that there is finally a 'nutrition label' for restaurant dining. That's exactly what Healthy Dining provides for health-conscious Americans."
- *Mary Felando, M.S., R.D., Cardiac Rehab Nutritionist*

"I always applaud any effort to bring nutritional information to the community. You've done an outstanding job."
- *Jeanne Jones, cookbook author and internationally syndicated columnist*

"It is a rewarding challenge to please our customers with healthy, innovative and creative dishes which are not loaded with butter and fat."
- *Joachim Splichal, chef and proprietor, Patina and Pinot Restaurants*

"The guidelines developed in this book closely correspond to those I've used in my books and with my clients. This resource will make my job as a nutrition counselor much easier and more effective."
- *Mary Donkersloot, R.D., Dietitian and author of* Fast Food Diet: Quick and Healthy Eating at Home and On the Go *and* Everyday Diabetes Gourmet Cookbook

"This is something very near and dear to my heart. I think every restaurant should have a Healthy Dining section on their menu."
- *Tom Feltenstein, Chairman & Founder, Neighborhood Marketing Institute*

"I love this book! In the perpetual battle of the bulge, it arms me with the knowledge to finally win the war."
- *Rieva Lesonsky*

Distinguished *Healthy Dining* Advisory Board

The following individuals serve on *Healthy Dining's* Advisory Board. Each advisor completes a comprehensive review of one of our publications -- the San Diego, Orange County, or Los Angeles edition -- and provides feedback and suggestions. The *Healthy Dining* team is proud, honored, and fortunate to gain the input of such a distinguished group. We thank every Advisory Board member for his or her commitment to this important community health program.

Margot J. Aiken, MD, FRCPC, FACE. Dr. Aiken is a board certified internist and endocrinologist in clinical practice with Scripps Health and XIMED Medical Group. Dr. Aiken is involved in education programs and professional societies related to infertility, menopause and endocrinology. She is a member of numerous professional organizations including The Am. Assoc. of Clinical Endocrinology, The Am. Soc. of Reproductive Medicine, The Pacific Coast Reproductive and Endocrine Society and The International. Menopause Society.

Robert Ashley, Director Hospitality Services/Executive Chef - UCSD Medical Center, Thorton Hospital. As a world traveler with 102 countries visited, Chef Robert's exposure to the cuisines of the world has driven him to develop authentic regional food creations that have won national and international acclaim. By using indigenous ingredients, Chef Robert improves the nutritional profile of his dishes. A television show evolved from "Chef Robert's Healthy and Exotic Cuisines of the World" brunches that are open to the public at Thorton Hospital. Chef also lectures, consults and conducts cooking classes with numerous government and private organizations in California.

Marilyn Biggica, Instructor of Foods & Nutrition, San Diego Comm. College. Marilyn teaches low-fat cooking at San Diego Community College and is active in the Community College District, where she serves on the Curriculum Council and Advisory Committee. Marilyn also advises restaurants about healthier alternatives on their menus. She teaches that healthy food can taste good, as reflected in her cookbook *"101 Ways to Eat for Health and Pleasure."*

Antonio Cagnolo, Owner/Operator, Antonello Ristorante. A native of northwestern Italy, Antonio has emerged as a dynamic force in the field of dining, having received honor after honor for his many contributions both in and out of culinary circles. He has earned national acclaim for the award-winning Italian cuisine served at Antonello Ristorante in Santa Ana. Antonio has been the recipient of the prestigious Golden Scepter Award several times and has been named "Restaurateur of the Year" by the Southern California Restaurant Writers.

Marie Connors, Special Services Manager, Weight Watchers of San Diego and the Inland Empire, Inc. Marie has been with Weight Watchers since 1984, lecturing on weight management and nutrition. She coordinates and supervises Weight Watchers' involvement in health fairs, sports expos, charitable events, Wellness at the Worksite as well as their annual participation in the Del Mar Fair.

Danna Demetre, RN, Founder and Director, Lifestyle Dimensions. Danna has been actively involved in the health and fitness industry for over 20 years as a registered nurse, fitness professional, corporate marketing manager and professional trainer. Her company, Lifestyle Dimensions, offers a comprehensive program designed to equip and empower women to meet their long-term health and fitness goals.

Mary Donkersloot, RD, Nutrition Therapist. Mary is a Beverly Hills-based consulting nutritionist who treats clients dealing with diabetes, weight control, eating disorders, and fitness and nutrition issues. She is the author of *The Simply Gourmet Diabetes Cookbook* and *Fast-Food Diet, Quick and Healthy Eating.* Mary is also the nutrition consultant for numerous national food corporations.

Lisa Dougherty, President, Orange County Nutrition and Fitness Council Inc. Lisa oversees all aspects of the Orange County Nutrition and Fitness Council; from business planning, membership recruitment, fundraising, workplace programs, speakers bureau to website and newsletter production. Lisa has an extensive background in nutrition and fitness. She graduated from the Fitness Instructor Program at UC Irvine, is a certified ACE personal trainer and Lifestyle and Weight Management Consultant. She designed a unique 6-week lifestyle weight management program that includes a comprehensive approach to weight management and nutrition education which she used in her own business, Whole Body Fitness.

Karen C. Duester, MS, RD, Owner, Nutritionist, The Food Consulting Co. Karen provides nutrition analysis services and custom food labels to restaurants, cookbook authors, publishers and food manufacturers through her company The Food Consulting Co., which she founded in 1993. Karen was named "Recognized Young Dietitian of the Year" in 1987 and has been listed in *Two Thousand Notable American Women, Who's Who in Young Professionals, Who's Who in Emerging Leaders* and *Who's Who in American Women.*

Judith Ewing, Adult Education Instructor, San Diego Community College District. With a Bachelor's degree in Home Economics, Judith is involved in a variety of projects and programs related to health. For the past 27 years, she has been an Instructor at the San Diego Community College, where she teaches cooking classes. Judy is also a consultant in menu and recipe development for Creative Culinary Concepts, and also does appliance demonstrations.

Mary Felando, MS, RD, Cardiac Rehab Dietitian. With a Master's degree in Human Nutrition from Cornell University, Mary has worked in the nutrition field for 23 years. Currently employed as a Cardiovascular nutrition specialist in the Los Angeles area, she is responsible for the development and implementation of the nutrition component of one of the largest cardiac rehabilitation programs in the country.

Tom Feltenstein, CEO, Feltenstein Partners; Chairman & Founder, Neighborhood Marketing Institute. Tom's energetic, dynamic style and proven marketing strategies have gained him celebrity status for 20+ years with restaurant and hospitality associations and corporations worldwide. His successful career stems from his association with powerhouse corporations such as McDonald's and Burger King, plus owning a chain of 14 restaurants. Tom's high-level executive training and hands-on, "in the trenches" experience provide him credibility as the most respected and highly sought after marketing consultant in the foodservice industry.

Sally Fenton, Executive Director, American Heart Association. Sally has over fifteen years of professional experience in the areas of management and fundraising, in which she combines creative and analytical abilities to reach targeted goals. Sally has also been very active in professional organizations and community activities including the American Cancer Society, Directors of Volunteers in Agencies (DOVIA), and the Women's Health Initiative, where she currently serves as the President of the Orange County Advisory Board.

Evelyne Fleury-Milfort, MSN, C-NP, CDE, Nurse Practitioner USC Center for Diabetes, Instructor in Clinical Medicine Keck School of Medicine as USC. Evelyne practices as a diabetes educator and a nurse practitioner. She has over 15 years experience in diabetes care. She is very active in the diabetes community doing professional and public education and served as president of the Diabetes Teaching Nurses of Southern California and the Greater Los Angeles Association of Diabetes Educators. Her clinical interest focuses on intensive management of both type 1 and type 2 diabetes.

Gail C. Frank, DrPH, RD, CHES, Professor of Nutrition, Cal. State University Long Beach. Gail has been active in the fields of nutrition and health for over 30 years. Along with directing many programs at Cal State Univ. Long Beach, Gail is an Adjunct Professor of Primary Care and Internal Medicine at Univ. of Cal., Irvine, and Co-Principal Investigator for the Women's Health Initiative. She is active in many professional organizations, and has served as the Media Spokesperson for the American Dietetic Association for 15 years. Gail has had over 650 media interviews including the LA Times, CNN, NPR, KABC, US News & World Report and USA Today.

Annette Globits, R.D., Nutrition Educator and Counselor. Annette graduated from Cornell University, completed her internship at the University of Michigan Medical Center, and has worked as a dietitian at the UCLA Medical Center and the Los Alamitos Medical Center. She teaches classes on various subjects from weight reduction to nutrition during pregnancy, and has lectured extensively throughout the community. She now operates a private practice in nutrition and believes "What you eat can make a difference."

Robyn L. Goldberg, R.D., Private Practice. Robyn began her career at Cedars-Sinai Medical Center in Los Angeles as the inpatient dietitian in the Department of Cardiology. She currently has her own private practice in Beverly Hills, CA, where she specializes in medical conditions, disordered eating, preventative nutrition and athletes maximizing optimal nutrition. Robyn promotes opportunity to excel in personal health and fitness maintenance through a lecture series in association with several medical groups. She serves as a Nutrition Consultant for the Celiac Disease Foundation, and is the nutritionist for the Susan Krevoy Eating Disorders Program.

Michelle Heilpern, President, Heilpern & Associates. Michelle has over 15 years of professional experience in the health care field. Her company specializes in strategic planning, marketing, public affairs and fund-raising for health care and non-profit organizations. She is the winner of nearly a dozen national awards for communications excellence.

Connie Hippensteel, Manager, San Diego Tech Center/Fitness Center. With a Master's degree in Exercise Physiology, Connie manages one of the most unique and modern fitness centers in San Diego. The Tech Center leases office space to 30 different companies and provides them with a state-of-the-art gym where over 2500 employees have the opportunity to get fit.

Elizabeth James, MPH, RD, President, Elizabeth James & Associates, Inc. With an educational background in nutrition and dietetics, Elizabeth has over 20 years experience in food styling, design, journalism and nutrition consulting. She has contributed articles and presentations to publications such as *Bon Appetit*, *NFL Properties*, *Valley Magazine* and *The Los Angeles Times*. As a Food Stylist and Consultant, some of her clients include Del Monte Foods, Healthy Choice, General Foods, McDonald's and Proctor and Gamble.

Jeanne Jones, President, Jeanne Jones, Inc. Jeanne is a prolific author, having completed 30 popular cookbooks. Her most recent book is *Healthy Cooking for People Who Don't Have Time to Cook* (Rodale Press, January 1997). Her internationally syndicated column "Cook It Light" is eagerly anticipated by millions each week. She regularly speaks to medical and lay audiences and has appeared on radio and TV shows such as "Donahue" and "Good Morning America." Jeanne's consulting services have been sought by such varied clients as the Pritikin Longevity Center, Canyon Ranch Fitness Resorts, Windstar Cruises and The Golden Door.

Cindy Stack Keer, RD, MPH, Senior Health Educator, Kaiser Permanente Medical Center. As an educator and trainer, Cindy works as a consultant in developing, coordinating, implementing, evaluating and teaching educational programs. She manages a variety of projects such as a Latino Diabetes Education Program, where she utilizes her fluency in Spanish. Cindy works closely with physicians, nurses, managers and other health professionals in facilitating multi-disciplinary groups to improve the continuity of care for Kaiser members.

Kay Kimball, RN, MSN, Coordinator of Cancer Wellness Programs, Palomar Medical Center. Kay is an oncology certified nurse. She maintains the Cancer Resource Centers at Palomar Medical Center and Pomerado Hospital in North San Diego County. Through these centers she coordinates patient education classes addressing the prevention, detection, diagnosis and treatment of cancer. Information on nutrition is always offered as part of a 6-wk cancer wellness program presented several times yearly. She facilitates 3 cancer support groups and collaborates with the American Cancer Society to provide other services as well.

Shirley Klein, Personal Trainer. As a Certified Personal Trainer and Weight Management Consultant in Leucadia, California, Shirley is committed to helping others get in shape and live a healthy lifestyle. Current positions include San Diego Regional Training Instructor for Secure Horizons and Senior Fitness Instructor at the YMCA. She is associated with the Am. Council on Exercise and the International Dance & Exercise Association.

Jeffrey Krebs, MD, FACP. Dr. Krebs has been practicing Internal Medicine in San Diego County since 1989. He is an Associate Clinical Professor of Medicine at the UCSD School of Medicine. Dr. Krebs has served on the Council of the San Diego County Medical Society and is past Chair of the California Medical Association's Young Physician Section. As a former competitive athlete, Dr. Krebs has always had an interest in nutrition.

Rieva Lesonsky, Senior Vice President/Editorial Director, Entrepreneur Media, Inc. Rieva has over 18 years experience at Entrepreneur media, currently serving as VP/Editorial Director of *Entrepreneur and Business Start-Ups* magazines. Rieva served on the Small Business Administration's (SBA) National Advisory Council from 1994 - 2000. The SBA has also honored her as a Small Business Media Advocate and a Woman in Business Advocate. For five years, Business News Reporter has named her one of the Top 100 Most Influential Journalists.

Phyllis Ann Marshall, FCSI, Principal, FoodPower. Phyllis is a foodservice industry consultant specializing in concept development and strategic plans to increase sales and profits of full-service restaurants and foodcourts. She holds a B.A. degree from Cornell University and has extensive experience in the areas of market positioning, menu development, merchandising and four-walls marketing. Phyllis develops growth strategies with an eye to adding new profit centers and establishing brands. She assists shopping centers with the development of new foodcourts and the retrofitting of existing properties in order to create destination restaurant locations.

Barbara Mallman, RD. Since 1977, Barbara has been guiding her clients, readers and audiences to a healthier lifestyle. She has been in private practice since 1985 and is currently a Registered Dietitian for Clinical Research Studies. Prior to 1985, Barbara was the head spa dietitian at La Costa Health Spa in Carlsbad, California and chief nutritionist at Cardio-Fitness Centers in New York City. Barbara has reached thousands of people through her lectures, interviews on *Hour Magazine* and Channel 10's "Staying Fit" program.

Cindy Maynard MS, RD. Cindy is a health and medical writer and a registered dietitian with a Masters degree in health and nutrition. She has been a freelance writer for over 10 years and her articles have appeared in *WebRN, www.barnesandnobleuniversity.com, Prime Health & Fitness, Idea Inc., Benning's Health and Fitness Journal, Current Health, Delicious! magazine, Sea Kayaker* and *Fitness Management.* Media experience includes television appearances and radio interviews. Cindy, has a private practice specializing in eating disorders and sports medicine and is currently the sports nutritionist for the San Diego State University athletic department. She is working on her first novel entitled, *Un-Diet Your Way Into a Healthy Body Size* and can be reached at clmaynard@earthlink.net

Agnes McGlone, Senior Vice President, Youth Market Programs, American Heart Association. Agnes has been in the non-profit industry since 1989. Her work with the AHA began in the Inland Empire as a fundraiser. She then transferred to LA as Director of Special Events, fundraising for many large events. Agnes then became the Executive Director in Orange County where the office experienced a 30% increase in income in two years. Currently, she oversees all aspects of the AHA programs serving the youth of California, Nevada and Utah.

Patti Tveit Milligan, MS, RD, Registered Dietitian, Henry's Marketplace. As Corporate Dietitian at Henry's Marketplace, Patti is responsible for customer education and nutrition updates to staff. In her previous position as Director of Nutrition and Marketing for Daily's Fit & Fresh Restaurants, she assisted with the development of the restaurant and provided nutritional expertise to the foodservice operation. Patti is also the Sports Team Nutritionist at San Diego State University's Aztec Gymnastics Club and lectures throughout San Diego.

April Morgan, V.P. of Sports and Fitness, The Sports Club Company. April has over 20 years experience in the fitness industry and holds a Bachelor's degree in Commercial Recreation. In her current position, she oversees all member programs such as private training, group exercise, nutrition, sports and children's programs for The Sports Club Company which operates upscale health and fitness clubs throughout the country under The Sports Club/LA name.

Victoria Pepper, MS, RD, Marketing and Promotions Coordinator, Kaiser Permanente Preventive Medicine. Victoria has worked for Kaiser Permanente's Positive Choice Wellness Center since 1987. She teaches nutrition, weight loss and stress management for the wellness center. In addition, she coordinates the marketing and promotion for the Department of Preventive Medicine, which includes the Positive Choice Wellness Center and Health Appraisal.

Patricia Perrault-Mattison, Writer and Designer, Write to Design. Patricia's professional career includes more than 10 years of experience as a writer and editor and 8 years in graphic design. In fact, Patricia designed the covers of several editions of *Healthy Dining*. She has a Bachelor's degree in English from the University of Oregon and has been employed in the public relations field for the last ten years.

Susan Plese, Public Information Specialist, San Diego County Sheriff's Department. Susan has extensive experience in marketing, communications, public relations, desktop publishing and special event management. She has a Bachelor's degree in Journalism.

Diane Powers, Owner, Bazaar del Mundo. Diane is the founder, owner and operator of Bazaar del Mundo, the landmark San Diego tourist destination that helps attract over 5 million visitors to Old Town State Historic Park each year. She received the "Entrepreneur of the Year" Award from the California Travel Industry Association and the "San Diego Woman of Achievement" Award from the League of Women Voters, along with numerous honors for her achievements in design, recycling/environment, marketing and management.

David Priver, MD, Past President, San Diego County Medical Society. Dr. Priver served as the president of the San Diego County Medical Society in 1996 and 1997. He has been in private practice as an OB/GYN since 1974 and is on the staff of several prestigious hospitals in San Diego, including Sharp Memorial Hospital and UCSD Medical Center. He is a member of the American Medical Association and the California Medical Association. His special interests include a healthy diet approach to good prenatal care and menopause.

Elyse Resch, MS, RD, FADA, Nutrition Therapist. Elyse has been in private practice in Beverly Hills for 20 years, specializing in eating disorders, intuitive eating and preventative nutrition. She is the co-author of "Intuitive Eating" and does regular speaking engagements. She is a certified child and adolescent obesity expert and was the treatment team nutritionist on the Eating Disorder Unit at Beverly Hills Medical Center. She participates in a variety of organizations and activities including the Sports, Cardiovascular and Wellness Nutrition Practice Group of the American Dietetic Association.

Paul Rosengard, Executive Director, SPARK Program. Paul is the Executive Director of the SPARK Programs of San Diego State University (SDSU); Co-Director of the Physical Education Intervention for Project TAAG (Trial of Activity for Adolescent Girls) at SDSU; and was the Director of the Physical Activity Intervention for Project M-SPAN (Middle School Physical Activity and Nutrition) at SDSU. Mr Rosengard instructs physical education methods for future teachers at the University of California, San Diego, and is the former Deputy Director of the California Governor's Council on Physical Fitness and Sports. He is nationally known as a consultant and for his work in curriculum and staff development.

Joan W. Rupp, MS, RD, Director, Project LEAN (Leaders Encouraging Activity & Nutrition) and Assistant Clinical Professor, University of California San Diego. Joan is an Assistant Clinical Professor in the Department of Family and Preventative Medicine at the University of California San Diego and a Lecturer in the Department of Exercise and Nutritional Sciences at San Diego State University. She is also the Director of the Southern Coast Region of Project LEAN, a state-wide nutrition education program involving restaurants, chefs, grocery stores, schools and the media promoting the healthy eating message.

John Ryan, General Manager, Walt's Wharf. John has been in the food industry business for over 20 years. He is a firm believer in healthy dining and its counterpart, physical fitness. His position at Walt's Wharf has been a perfect fit, with a menu emphasizing freshness and healthy choices. John, wife Dana and two sons have many fitness accomplishments that currently include swimming and triathlon competition.

Mary Ryzner, MS, RD, Clinical Dietitian, Palomar Medical Center. Since receiving her Master's Degree in Nutrition in 1988 from California State University, Northridge, Mary has worked as a Clinical Dietitian for various hospitals and care centers. Mary is active in the San Diego Dietetic Association and is the event coordinator for the Nutrition Fuels Fitness 5K/10K Run/Walk. She also has her own business specializing in weight regulation. Mary contributes monthly nutrition articles for the Heart-To-Heart Volunteers newsletter.

Clarice M. Schickling, RD, CDE, Diabetes Wisdom, Inc. Clarice has been a Certified Diabetes Educator since 1986 and is a past President of Orange County Chapter of the American Association of Diabetes Educators. Trained at the Univ. of Minnesota, Clarice has since worked in California as a therapeutic, teaching, administrative and consulting dietitian, college teacher and administrator. She is a member of the American Dietetic Association, American Diabetes Association and the American Association of Diabetes Educators.

Jamie Steele, President & Fitness Director, Steele Bodies. Jamie has been in the health and fitness industry for over 20 years. His company, Steele Bodies, a personalized fitness, wellness and nutrition program, specializes in high-intensity training principles. Jamie has owned and operated 10 health and fitness facilities in California and Arizona and worked in upper level management and business development for a large California health and fitness chain.

Stacy Steinberg, MS, RD, Associate Executive Director, Cedars-Sinai Comprehensive Cancer Center. Stacy is the past President of the LA Dietetic Association and recipient of the Young Dietitian of the Year Award by the American Dietetic Association. She has served as the National Nutrition Services Coordinator for Salick Health Care and is now responsible for the associate management and direction of operations at the Cedars-Sinai Comprehensive Cancer Center.

Debra L. Tindle, RD, Clinical Dietitian, Garden Grove Hospital & Medical Center. Debra received her Bachelor's degree in Dietetics & Food Admin. from Cal. State Univ., Long Beach and has over 20 years experience as a health educator in areas of nutrition, internal medicine and weight management. She served as a reviewer for the *Journal of Nutrition Education* and the *National Weight Control Resources Directory*. Debra presently manages clinical nutrition, food service and community education at the Garden Grove Hospital & Medical Center.

Christopher Trela, Journalist, *OC Metro Magazine*/"Metro Menus." Christopher is the restaurant writer for Metro Menus and the theatre critic for the *OC Metro Magazine*. He also writes a Health & Fitness column for the *OC Metro Magazine*, and is a freelance writer and photographer for many local magazines, a public relations consultant, and the President and owner of Paradise West Creative Services.

Evelyn Tribole, MS, RD, Nutrition Editor, *Shape Magazine*. Evelyn is an award-winning registered dietitian with a counseling practice in Beverly Hills. She reaches over 3 million readers with her monthly column in *Shape Magazine*, "Recipe Makeovers." Evelyn has served as the "Good Morning America" Nutritionist and is author of several books including *Healthy Homestyle Cooking*, *Eating on the Run* and *Intuitive Eating*.

Patricia Van Donck, CVT, ADN, Clinical Research Associate, Advanced Tissue Sciences, Inc. Patricia spent 10 years in the Navy, specializing in cardiovascular medicine. She earned an Associate's degree in Nursing and is certified as a Clinical Research Associate.

Gene Warneke, Freelance Tour Director & Commercial Photographer. Gene has a special interest in food and dining. In his prior position as Executive Director of the American Institute of Wine and Food (San Diego Chapter), Gene administered and planned the organization's food and wine events. Gene now works as a freelance tour director for a destination management company and as a commercial photographer specializing in food.

Terry Zierenberg, BS, RN, CDE, Education Manager, Marketing Dept. at Medtronic MiniMed. Terry has spent many years educating health care professionals, patients and the community about diabetes. Previously, she was a Diabetes Nurse Clinician for the Diabetes Treatment Centers of America, Tarzana, Ca. and the Program Coordinator for the Diabetes Care Center at Encino-Tarzana Regional Medical Center. Her affiliations include the American Association of Diabetes Educators, the American Diabetes Association and the Juvenile Diabetes Foundation.

Disclaimer:

The purpose of this book is to provide nutrition information for selected menu items from restaurants that have chosen to participate in the *Healthy Dining* program. Please note that the items listed in this book are not necessarily appropriate or healthful for all individuals. Some people need to be more careful about certain items such as salt or sugar, or have food allergies which put additional restrictions on their food choices. Each individual is responsible, in cooperation with his or her physician, dietitian or other health consultant, for making personal dietary decisions. We have not included all the restaurants that serve healthy food, nor are we recommending all entrees from restaurants that are included in this book.

It is also important to note that the numerical values for the nutrition information included in this book are approximations only, and that the categories "Good Choice" and "Excellent Choice" give a better overall indication of the nutrition content of the menu items.

The nutrition information provided is based on the United States Department of Agriculture (USDA) nutrition information database, the source most commonly used for estimating nutritional content of foods. Participating restaurants supplied their recipes for the computerized analysis. The analyses were completed using the Nutritionist IV Computer program. Research shows the Nutritionist IV program to be one of the most current and reliable nutrition analysis programs available. If values for recipe ingredients were not available from the USDA database, the manufacturer was contacted for the nutrition information. If the manufacturer did not have nutrition information, ingredients were closely matched to a similar product's nutrition information. Data were rounded as follows: for calories, cholesterol and sodium, to the nearest 5 (mg). For fat, protein and carbohydrates, to the nearest whole number, and for diabetic exchanges to the nearest ¼ exchange.

All information contained in this book has been carefully compiled and reviewed by qualified health professionals. Nutrition information is based on recipes supplied by the restaurants. Participating restaurants have agreed to prepare food according to the recipes submitted for a period of one year, or to clearly notify customers otherwise.

The authors are not responsible for maintaining quality control over the food that is prepared by the restaurants. The restaurants are ultimately responsible for the quality of the food they serve.

A Message from the
Healthy Dining Team

Welcome to the *Healthy Dining* "family." This program has grown from San Diego to Orange County to Los Angeles. More than 1000 individuals have participated in this effort, including restaurant chefs and management, health professionals, and members of community organizations. You, the *Healthy Dining* reader and restaurant diner, play an essential role as well.

Why? Because restaurants are responsive to their customers. They need to hear from you that health-conscious menu items and nutrition information are important to you.

Here's how you can help *Healthy Dining* grow in your community:

1. Dine at the restaurants listed in the book, and tell the restaurant staff and owners that you appreciate and value their participation in *Healthy Dining*. Also, request the *Healthy Dining* menus at participating restaurants and use the discount coupons.

2. Tell friends, family and business associates about *Healthy Dining*.

3. Tell other restaurants about *Healthy Dining* and recommend that they participate next year.

4. Give *Healthy Dining* books as gifts for birthdays, holidays, etc.

5. Use *Healthy Dining* as a fund-raiser (call for information).

6. Use *Healthy Dining* restaurants for your catering and party needs.

7. Invite a *Healthy Dining* representative to give a presentation to your organization.

8. Please call us with your suggestions and feedback: (858) 541-2049.

Thanks! Together we can make Southern California a healthier place to live and dine.

Part I

Healthy Dining Tips

Realistic Guidelines and Practical Information

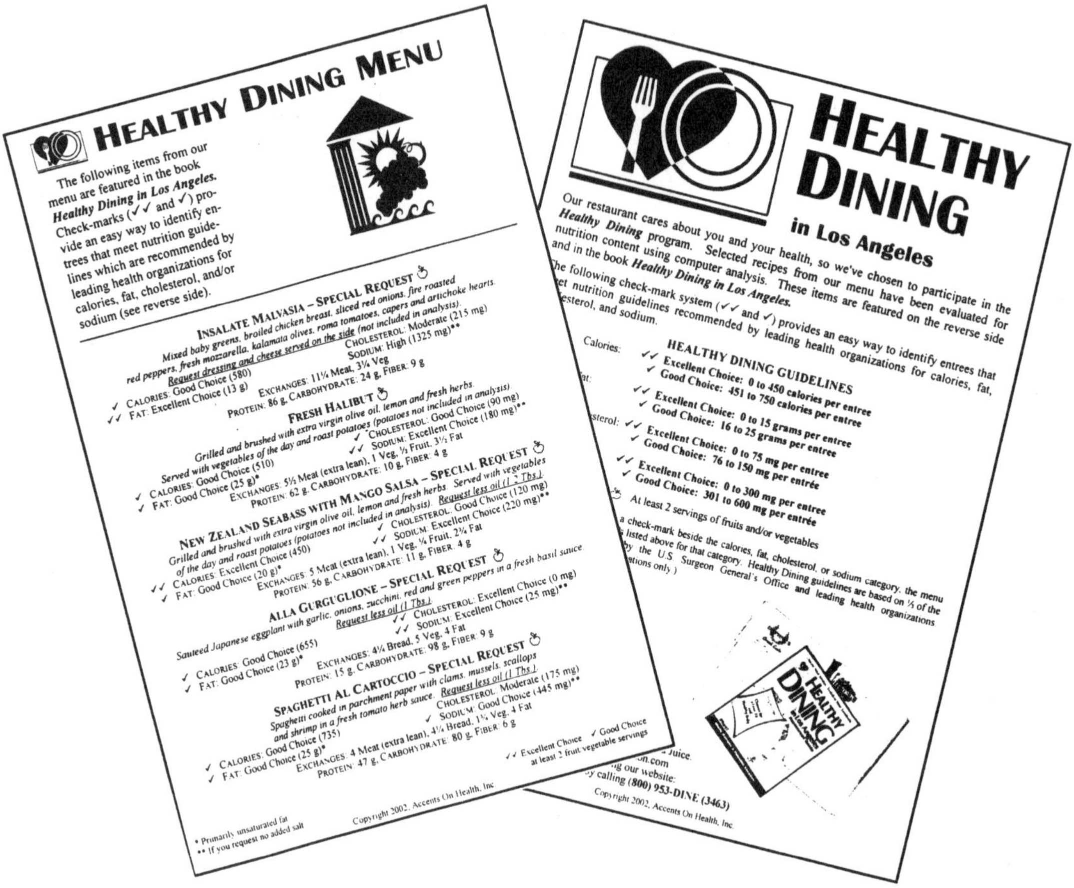

HEALTHY DINING MENU

The following items from our menu are featured in the book *Healthy Dining in Los Angeles.* Check-marks (✓✓ and ✓) provide an easy way to identify entrees that meet nutrition guidelines which are recommended by leading health organizations for calories, fat, cholesterol, and/or sodium (see reverse side).

INSALATE MALVASIA – SPECIAL REQUEST
Mixed baby greens, broiled chicken breast, sliced red onions, fire roasted red peppers, fresh mozzarella, kalamata olives, roma tomatoes, capers and artichoke hearts. *Request dressing and cheese served on the side* (not included in analysis)
- ✓ CALORIES: Good Choice (580)   CHOLESTEROL: Moderate (215 mg)
- ✓✓ FAT: Excellent Choice (13 g)   SODIUM: High (1325 mg)**
  - EXCHANGES: 11¼ Meat, 3¼ Veg
  - PROTEIN: 86 g, CARBOHYDRATE: 24 g, FIBER: 9 g

FRESH HALIBUT
Grilled and brushed with extra virgin olive oil, lemon and fresh herbs. Served with vegetables of the day and roast potatoes (potatoes not included in analysis)
- ✓ CALORIES: Good Choice (510)   ✓✓ CHOLESTEROL: Good Choice (180 mg)**
- ✓✓ FAT: Good Choice (25 g)*   ✓✓ SODIUM: Excellent Choice (90 mg)
  - EXCHANGES: 5½ Meat (extra lean), 1 Veg, ½ Fruit, 3½ Fat
  - PROTEIN: 62 g, CARBOHYDRATE: 10 g, FIBER: 4 g

NEW ZEALAND SEABASS WITH MANGO SALSA – SPECIAL REQUEST
Grilled and brushed with extra virgin olive oil, lemon and fresh herbs. Served with vegetables of the day and roast potatoes (potatoes not included in analysis) *Request less oil (1.5 Tbs.)*
- ✓✓ CALORIES: Excellent Choice (450)   ✓✓ CHOLESTEROL: Good Choice (120 mg)
- ✓ FAT: Good Choice (20 g)*   ✓✓ SODIUM: Excellent Choice (220 mg)**
  - EXCHANGES: 5 Meat (extra lean), 1 Veg, ¼ Fruit, 2¼ Fat
  - PROTEIN: 50 g, CARBOHYDRATE: 11 g, FIBER: 4 g

ALLA GURGUGLIONE – SPECIAL REQUEST
Sauteed Japanese eggplant with garlic, onions, zucchini, red and green peppers in a fresh basil sauce *Request less oil (1 Tbs.)*
- ✓ CALORIES: Good Choice (655)   ✓✓ CHOLESTEROL: Excellent Choice (0 mg)
- ✓ FAT: Good Choice (23 g)*   ✓✓ SODIUM: Excellent Choice (25 mg)**
  - EXCHANGES: 4¼ Bread, 5 Veg, 4 Fat
  - PROTEIN: 15 g, CARBOHYDRATE: 98 g, FIBER: 9 g

SPAGHETTI AL CARTOCCIO – SPECIAL REQUEST
Spaghetti cooked in parchment paper with clams, mussels, scallops and shrimp in a fresh tomato herb sauce. *Request less oil (1 Tbs.)*
- ✓ CALORIES: Good Choice (735)   ✓ CHOLESTEROL: Moderate (175 mg)
- ✓ FAT: Good Choice (25 g)*   ✓✓ SODIUM: Good Choice (445 mg)**
  - EXCHANGES: 4 Meat (extra lean), 4¼ Bread, 1¼ Veg, 4 Fat
  - PROTEIN: 47 g, CARBOHYDRATE: 80 g, FIBER: 6 g

* Primarily unsaturated fat
** If you request no added salt

Copyright 2002, Accents On Health, Inc.

HEALTHY DINING
in Los Angeles

Our restaurant cares about you and your health, so we've chosen to participate in the *Healthy Dining* program. Selected recipes from our menu have been evaluated for nutrition content using computer analysis. These items are featured on the reverse side and in the book *Healthy Dining in Los Angeles.* The following check-mark system (✓✓ and ✓) provides an easy way to identify entrees that meet nutrition guidelines recommended by leading health organizations for calories, fat, cholesterol, and sodium.

HEALTHY DINING GUIDELINES
Calories:
- ✓✓ Excellent Choice: 0 to 450 calories per entree
- ✓ Good Choice: 451 to 750 calories per entree

Fat:
- ✓✓ Excellent Choice: 0 to 15 grams per entree
- ✓ Good Choice: 16 to 25 grams per entree

Cholesterol:
- ✓✓ Excellent Choice: 0 to 75 mg per entree
- ✓ Good Choice: 76 to 150 mg per entree

Sodium:
- ✓✓ Excellent Choice: 0 to 300 mg per entree
- ✓ Good Choice: 301 to 600 mg per entrée

✓✓ At least 2 servings of fruits and/or vegetables

With a check-mark beside the calories, fat, cholesterol, or sodium category, the menu item is listed above for that category. Healthy Dining guidelines are based on ⅓ of the RDA by the U.S. Surgeon General's Office and leading health organizations (with some exceptions only.)

✓✓ Excellent Choice   ✓ Good Choice
at least 2 fruit/vegetable servings

...com.
By calling our website:
...calling (800) 953-DINE (3463)

Copyright 2002, Accents On Health, Inc.

Healthy Dining menus are available at participating restaurants for your convenience.

The *Healthy Dining* menus illustrated above are condensed versions of the menu pages in your book. We encourage all the restaurants to pass out their *Healthy Dining* menus along with their regular menus. Some restaurants, however, don't automatically provide them -- *you must request these special menus.* And please do! The more that restaurants hear customers asking for specific nutrition information and ordering "Special Requests," the more they will recognize how important healthy dining is to many people.

If nutrition information is important to you, if you want to have the choice to "order healthy," please request *Healthy Dining* menus in the restaurants and let them know that you appreciate the healthy menu choices.

How to Use This Book

This introduction summarizes how to interpret the nutrition information for the restaurant menu items. Part I of the book provides more in-depth information to help you become better informed about health and restaurant dining. Part II features nutrition profiles for specific entrees at participating restaurants at over 300 locations in Los Angeles. Part III includes a Health Resource Guide, Part IV presents a wonderful selection of Chefs' Recipes, Part V contains a Survey, a Book Order Form, and over $200 in Coupons, and finally, Part VI lists three Restaurant Indexes for quick reference.

The Check Mark System - An easy way to find entrees to fit your goals

First, let's define "healthy entree." In this book, a healthy entree is one with high-quality, nutritious calories. In general, these are low in fat, cholesterol, calories and sodium. Because many entrees are not low in all areas, the check mark system will help you easily and quickly identify which entrees best fit your individual dietary goals.

Nutritional guidelines are difficult to set because each individual has different nutritional needs. For example, caloric needs vary according to age, gender, activity level, body weight and health goals (e.g., reducing body fat, lowering cholesterol, etc.). Nevertheless, the following are general guidelines to make the menu information easy to interpret. These guidelines are based on recommendations by the U.S. Surgeon General's Office and the American Heart Association. Details about how the values were developed are included in Chapters 3 through 6, but here's a quick summary of the check mark meanings:

ENTREE GUIDELINES

Calories	✓✓ Excellent Choice = 0 to 450 calories/entree
	✓ Good Choice = 451 to 750 calories/entree
Fat	✓✓ Excellent Choice = 0 to 15 grams (g)/entree
	✓ Good Choice = 16 to 25 grams (g)/entree
Cholesterol	✓✓ Excellent Choice = 0 to 75 milligrams (mg)/entree
	✓ Good Choice = 76 to 150 milligrams (mg)/entree
Sodium	✓✓ Excellent Choice = 0 to 300 milligrams (mg)/entree
	✓ Good Choice = 301 to 600 milligrams (mg)/entree

It's important to note...

Although some individuals prefer stricter criteria for their meal guidelines (especially people on very low-fat or low-sodium diets), the *Healthy Dining* guidelines represent fairly high standards for restaurant entrees and are realistic goals for most diners, as discussed in Chapters 3 through 6.

We occasionally include a menu item that is described as "moderate" in one of the nutrient categories. "Moderate" means that the item does not meet the guidelines, but it is less than twice the cut-off value for "Good Choice." Some items are listed as "high" in sodium (meaning above 1000 mg. sodium per entree) and are **not** recommended for those watching sodium intake.

The *Healthy Dining* guidelines are general guidelines developed for the general public. You, your physician and your dietitian are responsible for setting individual nutritional guidelines according to your particular health needs. **Please note also that the numerical values for the nutrition information are approximations only, based on recipes supplied by the restaurants.**

If you are health-conscious and looking for better ways to eat and enhance your overall health, this book will provide an easy way to choose entrees that don't have the hidden calories, fat, cholesterol and sodium you'd rather avoid.

If you want to lose weight, take special note of the calorie and fat categories and select items listed as Excellent Choice (✓✓) or Good Choice (✓) in these areas (see Chapters 3 and 4). For information on calculating percentage of calories from fat, see Chapter 3.

If you want to reduce your blood cholesterol level, choose from items that are listed as Excellent Choice (✓✓) or Good Choice (✓) for both cholesterol and fat (see Chapter 5).

To reduce dietary sodium, select those menu items that are shown as Excellent Choice (✓✓) or Good Choice (✓) in sodium, and request no added salt (see Chapter 6).

If you have diabetes, the "Exchanges" (i.e., Diabetic Exchanges used by the American Diabetes Association) are particularly useful, along with values for carbohydrate and protein. For more details, see Chapter 7.

If your physician or dietitian has given you daily limits in terms of sodium, cholesterol, etc., by all means note the numerical values as well as the check marks, and be sure they fit your restrictions. You may need to ask for additional modifications to your meal.

We've included brief entree descriptions, but they are not complete ingredient lists. Therefore, if you have food allergies or sensitivities, be sure to emphasize this to the restaurant personnel so they will understand how important it is to prepare your meal according to your specifications.

Comments about serving sizes, dressings and sauces, and side dishes

The nutrition information published in this book is based on the FULL SERVING (unless stated otherwise). Restaurant portions are frequently large, so you may not want to eat the full serving. If you eat only ⅔ of the entree, you're only consuming ⅔ of the calories, fat, cholesterol, sodium, etc.

In some cases the nutrition analysis includes dressings or sauces, and in other cases it does not. We generally recommend that you order sauces and dressings on the side and use them sparingly. Dressings and sauces usually contain 5 to 10 grams of fat (45 to 90 calories) per tablespoon. Depending on your goals, you may choose to completely avoid them, or order them on the side and limit the amount you use. You will likely be served more than one tablespoon, so don't assume you can pour it all on your meal. You can measure out the amount you want using your teaspoon, keeping in mind that 3 teaspoons (tsp.) is equivalent to one tablespoon (Tbs.) or ½ ounce (oz).

The check mark system and guidelines listed on the previous page apply to main entrees only. We also feature some side dishes, appetizers, and desserts, and have set the guidelines for calories, fat, cholesterol and sodium equal to ⅓ of the Entree Guidelines. Other items such as breads are not generally shown because the nutrition values are fairly standard.

GUIDELINES for SIDE DISHES, APPETIZERS & DESSERTS†

Calories
✓✓ Excellent Choice = 0 to 150 calories/serving
✓ Good Choice = 151 to 250 calories/serving

Fat
✓✓ Excellent Choice = 0 to 5 grams (g)/serving
✓ Good Choice = 6 to 8 grams (g)/serving

Cholesterol
✓✓ Excellent Choice = 0 to 25 milligrams (mg)/serving
✓ Good Choice = 26 to 50 milligrams (mg)/serving

Sodium
✓✓ Excellent Choice = 0 to 100 milligrams (mg)/serving
✓ Good Choice = 101 to 200 milligrams (mg)/serving

KEY to FOOTNOTES

† Side dish guidelines are ⅓ of Entree Guidelines
* Primarily unsaturated fat (see Chapter 4)
** If you request no added salt (see Chapter 6)
🍎 at least 2 fruit/vegetable servings (see Chapter 8)

PRICE RANGE SYMBOL

At the end of each restaurant's introductory paragraph, a price range symbol appears:

$ Average entree under $10
$$ Average entree $10 - $20
$$$ Average entree over $20

How are restaurants selected to be included in Healthy Dining?

Our goal is to include a wide variety of restaurants. We do not specifically look for restaurants that specialize in serving "health food," but for a selection of popular restaurants that have a sincere interest in providing healthy foods and nutrition information. If you want organic and natural foods, we include restaurants that cater to these preferences as well. Vegetarian dishes are available at many of the restaurants. A good clue for vegetarian dishes is to look for items with no cholesterol (no animal products) or very low values, which may indicate small quantities of cheese or dairy products. You may, of course, double check with the restaurant personnel before ordering.

Restaurants participating in this book have a genuine interest in offering healthy choices. They pay a fee for the nutrition analysis, and they have signed an agreement with Accents On Health to prepare the selected entrees in accordance with the recipes they submitted or clearly notify customers otherwise. We highly respect the restaurants included in this book for their interest and commitment to serving healthy entrees. We purposely include many different types of cuisine with a wide range of prices and believe this will have the greatest impact in encouraging all restaurants to offer healthy, delicious choices.

How are entrees selected?

When a restaurant participates in the *Healthy Dining* Program, our staff of qualified health professionals works with the chef to select recipes low in fat, cholesterol, calories and sodium.

Our first choice is to find items already on the menu, without making any modifications. This would be the easiest for you and for the restaurant. However, in some cases the recipe analysis doesn't meet the *Healthy Dining* guidelines. So we work with the chef to develop a "Special Request" version that is lower in calories, fat, cholesterol and/or sodium than the original dish (see Chapter 2). The analyses listed in this book for the "Special Request" items correspond to the lower calorie, fat, etc. content that you will be served <u>if and only if you make the "Special Request."</u> Otherwise you will be served a meal with considerably higher fat and higher calorie values.

We need your help!

The restaurants in this book devote time, money and effort to participate in *Healthy Dining*. In many cases the restaurants have modified recipes to meet your needs. Now they need to hear that this nutrition information is important to you and that you appreciate their participation in *Healthy Dining*.

We encourage all the restaurants to pass out *Healthy Dining* menus along with their regular menus. The *Healthy Dining* menus are condensed versions of the book pages. Some restaurants, however, do not automatically provide them -- *you must request the Healthy Dining menus*. And please do! The more that restaurants hear customers asking for specific nutrition information and ordering "Special Requests," the more they will recognize how important healthy dining is to many people.

So, if this information is important to you, if you want to have the choice to "order healthy," **PLEASE tell the *Healthy Dining* restaurants**! Please tell other restaurants that you'd like them to participate. This will enable us to include more restaurants and an even greater variety of healthy choices in the next edition of *Healthy Dining in Los Angeles.*

```
Please ask for the Healthy Dining menus
at participating restaurants.
```

We welcome your ideas

This program is growing, and we welcome your ideas on how to enhance it. Please write to us with your comments. We update this publication periodically and will continue to add more restaurants, more healthy entrees, and more nutrition information.

CHAPTER 1

Health, Lifestyle, Diet, Misconceptions & ... Dining Out

In 1988, the Surgeon General made a startling announcement to the American public:

> "If you don't smoke, what you eat may be
> the biggest factor influencing your health."

We've come a long way...

Diet has always strongly influenced health and disease. Until the early decades of this century, our country suffered from problems of _undernutrition_. Rickets, pellagra, scurvy, beriberi and goiter plagued our nation. Fortunately, in the United States, advances in medicine, fortification of foods, and successful cures virtually eliminated the vicious diseases caused by a lack of essential nutrients.

Currently, we've reached a whole new perspective on health and disease. A large body of medical research shows that lifestyle greatly influences health status. It is well recognized that daily health habits -- what we eat and drink, whether or not we smoke, how much exercise we get and how effectively we manage stress -- contribute to _how well and how long_ we live.

The 1988 Surgeon General's Report on Nutrition and Health outlines the substantial impact of dietary practices on health. Today, the four leading causes of death by disease (heart disease, cancer, stroke, and diabetes), which together account for over ⅔ of all deaths in the U.S., are directly related to diet. The main conclusion of the 1988 report is:

> "_Overconsumption_ of certain dietary components is now a major concern for Americans. While many food factors are involved, chief among them is the disproportionate consumption of foods high in fats, often at the expense of foods high in complex carbohydrates and fiber that may be more conducive to health."
>
> -- 1988 Surgeon General's Report on Nutrition and Health --

Clearly, a priority for Americans is to reduce intake of total fat, and especially saturated fat, because of the relationship between excess dietary fat and the development of many leading chronic disease conditions.

Dietary guidelines for Americans

Based on extensive scientific evidence, the following recommendations were developed by the Surgeon General's Office and the American Heart Association:

1. Reduce overall consumption of fat, especially saturated fat. The American Heart Association recommends that <u>no more than 30%</u> of total calories come from fat (the average American diet contains approximately 35% fat). Saturated fat should comprise no more than 10% of the daily diet. Choose foods low in fat such as vegetables, fruits, whole grain foods, fish, lean meats and non-fat dairy products. Use food preparation methods that add little or no fat.

2. Reduce cholesterol consumption to less than 300 mg. per day, as recommended by the American Heart Association. The average American consumes about 400 - 600 mg. daily.

3. Reduce intake of sodium by choosing foods relatively low in sodium and limiting the amount of salt in food preparation and at the table. The American Heart Association recommends less than 3,000 mg. per day. The average American consumes about 4,000 - 6,000 mg. daily.

4. Achieve and maintain a desirable body weight. To do so, choose a balanced diet in which energy (caloric) intake is consistent with energy expenditure. To reduce caloric intake, limit consumption of foods relatively high in calories, fat, and sugar, and minimize alcohol consumption. Increase energy expenditure through regular exercise.

5. Eat a variety of foods. Increase consumption of complex carbohydrates and fiber, such as whole grain foods, cereals, vegetables, fruits, dried beans, peas, and lentils.

6. Limit sugar in your diet, and if you drink alcoholic beverages, do so in moderation.

Americans are catching on!

We're watching what we eat. Learning more about what we eat. Making healthier choices. We're beginning to cherish our health for its influence on all other aspects of our lives. For top performance, we're eating more high-quality fuel -- fruits, vegetables and whole grains -- and less beef, butter, whole milk and other foods high in saturated fat.

Since the mid-1970s, consumption of saturated fats has decreased significantly. In addition, U.S. death rates from heart disease have fallen dramatically, close to 25 percent in the last decade. Leading health organizations attribute some of this decline to better medical care but give most of the credit to healthier diets and lifestyles.

Food manufacturers are catching on, but...

Marketing efforts toward our increasingly health-conscious society have intensified in the past several years. Close to 30% of food advertising includes some type of health message. Although this spiraling emphasis on healthy eating from food makers is encouraging, it can be very misleading. For example, lunchmeats frequently flaunt a "96% FAT FREE" label, yet this means that only 4% of the meat's <u>weight</u> is fat, not 4% of the calories (a high percentage of the weight is water, thus decreasing the percentage weight from fat). Cookies, crackers and chips leap out from shelves with bright "NO CHOLESTEROL" or "FAT FREE" labels, yet the nutritional value seems to be of little concern (at least to the manufacturer).

Reading between the lines

Until recently, deciphering food labels was a difficult task. Nutrition information on labels was often misleading, confusing and incomplete. Terms such as "low-fat," "light," "natural," and "healthy" had virtually no standardized meaning and could be added to any package, regardless of contents.

In 1994, the Food and Drug Administration (FDA) implemented guidelines requiring almost all food packages to display a universal nutrition information label. The revised labels help you more easily identify important nutrition information. The FDA has also developed strict guidelines for several nutritional claims commonly used by food manufacturers. For example, any food package stating the product is "low-fat" must have 3 grams of fat or less per serving. A "low-calorie" food must contain 40 calories or less per serving. A food package promoting the product as "light" (e.g., light mayonnaise) must contain 50% less fat or one-third fewer calories than the food with which it is being compared (e.g., regular mayonnaise). If the original product contains more than 50% calories from fat, the fat must be reduced by at least 50% in the "light" product.

The guidelines set by the FDA for food packages are different from the *Healthy Dining* guidelines because the *Healthy Dining* guidelines represent a full meal, whereas the FDA guidelines are designed for a single product or serving.

A crusader for healthier fast foods

In April 1990, Phil Sokolof and his non-profit organization, The National Heart Savers Association, attacked American fast food restaurants with full-page ads in large newspapers accusing them of "poisoning" Americans with foods high in saturated fat. A Gallup poll showed that almost 40% of those who saw the ads immediately decreased their visits to fast food restaurants. Just three weeks later, McDonald's responded by removing beef tallow from their French fries. Other fast food chains quickly followed. Sokolof points out that his major goal was to stop fast food from being a *"fast track to a heart attack."*

With Sokolof paving the way, consumers began demanding to know -- just what are we getting in fast food meals? In response, most fast food restaurants now provide nutrition information for menu items. At last, the fast American favorites have exposed their "fat facts."

Some fat facts

A McDonald's Big Mac has 590 calories, 34 grams of fat and 1090 milligrams of sodium. If you add medium fries and a small shake, the meal adds up to 1400 calories, 65 grams of fat and 1630 mg of sodium. Even the Filet-O-Fish has 470 calories, 26 grams of fat and 890 milligrams of sodium. Add fries and a shake and you're drowning in calories, fat and sodium.

Three pieces of Original Recipe Kentucky Fried Chicken contain a whopping 790 calories, 51 grams of fat and 2285 milligrams of sodium. Add coleslaw, mashed potatoes with gravy and a biscuit, and you get a total of 1322 calories, 81 grams of fat and 3570 milligrams of sodium. That's over a full day's recommended allowance for both fat and sodium in just one meal, and 54% of the total calories come from fat!

Salads are usually considered a healthy choice. However, many salads can have over 1000 calories, over 50 grams of fat, and over 1000 milligrams of sodium. Sometimes salads are higher in calories and fat than many other items on the menu.

Better alternatives

In response to their new "fat visibility," many fast food restaurants added items that look much better on the nutritional charts. Jack in the Box now serves a Chicken Fajita Pita with under 300 calories and 9 grams of fat. Their Chicken Teriyaki Bowl, with lots of rice, is filling and very low in fat (but watch the sodium). They also provide a low calorie Italian salad dressing.

In place of traditional fast food, many people are finding healthier meals at the growing number of convenient "quick-service" restaurants. For example:

Subway offers sandwiches and salads with fresh, high quality ingredients. They bake bread fresh throughout the day and use only garden fresh veggies. Each sandwich and salad is made to your exact specifications. Light mayonnaise, low-fat potato crisps and fat-free pretzels are available.

Baja Fresh offers several delicious tacos and burritos using only fresh, quality ingredients and flavorful recipes. They're healthy and delicious!

Koo Koo Roo California Kitchen features a diverse menu, including their Original Skinless Flamebroiled Chicken Breast with only 160 calories and 4 gram of fat, chicken and turkey sandwiches, and a variety of side dishes such as Butternut Squash and Vegetable Soup that can add extra variety and nutrition to your meal.

Consumer power

As a result of health-conscious consumers speaking out, we now have the choice to "order healthy" at fast food restaurants. "The public does not realize the dramatic power it wields," Sokolof emphasizes. "The consumer's wish is big business' command."

But what about dining out in restaurants?

What's healthy and what's not?

If dining out were only for special occasions, the rich and creamy dishes could be wonderful treats. An occasional splurge might not be so bad. But because restaurant dining for business, pleasure and convenience has become so common, it is important to find healthier choices.

That's what *Healthy Dining in Los Angeles* is all about. It's the first book of its kind. Never before has so much information been available for restaurant menu items. Each restaurant has its own unique recipes, prepared in its own special way. So nutrition information must be compiled restaurant by restaurant, recipe by recipe. And that's a lot of work.

There are books that give general information for dining out. They list common entrees to avoid and those that are probably best to order. However, as restaurants become more specialized and creative, "common" entrees are not so common, and so general guidelines are not always accurate or useful.

As you read on about what we've discovered in our research, you'll find that often you can't tell what you're getting by the menu description. It may portray a healthy item, but many times there are hidden ingredients, and the method of preparation is not specified. Without complete nutrition information, you don't know what you're getting, and that can be dangerous! *Healthy Dining* makes the process of ordering healthy food much easier.

Goals of *Healthy Dining in Los Angeles:*

1. To guide you in what and how to order healthier entrees served at popular Los Angeles restaurants.

2. To provide you with easy-to-read nutrition profiles for selected entrees.

3. To give you useful, practical guidelines and advice for healthier restaurant dining.

4. To encourage restaurants to prepare and serve a wide variety of healthy choices.

CHAPTER **2**

Is Restaurant Food Fattening and Unhealthy?

It can be if you're not careful! But it doesn't have to be.

Many restaurants smother meals with excess fat, sodium, cholesterol and calories. Butter, oil, cream, cheese and salt are frequently added to achieve the taste and texture that the average American expects.   To make matters worse, many restaurant diners have the habit of adding "extras" such as salad dressing, sour cream, and butter (which push up the calorie and fat count even more). Let's take a shocking look at a favorite restaurant dinner:

Chicken Breast
Topped with a Creamy Parmesan Sauce
Served with Dinner Salad, Baked Potato and Sautéed Vegetables

	Calories	Fat (g)	Cholest. (mg)	Sodium (mg)
Dinner Salad	32	0	0	53
Blue Cheese Dressing (4 Tbs.)	308	32	36	668
Chicken Breast with Sauce	1312	91	481	1517
Baked Potato	220	0	0	16
Butter (2 Tbs.)	200	23	61	232
Sour Cream (2 Tbs.)	62	6	13	15
Sautéed Vegetables	117	11	0	207
Meal Total	2251	163	591	2708

Now let's evaluate these numbers relative to daily recommendations:

Calories: Close to a FULL day's recommended calories <u>in one meal</u>.
Fat: <u>Almost three times</u> the recommended fat intake for a FULL Day.
Cholesterol: <u>Almost twice</u> the recommended cholesterol intake for a FULL Day.
Sodium: <u>Almost the entire</u> recommended sodium intake for a FULL Day.

Other fat-filled favorites:

	Calories	Fat (g)	Cholest. (mg)	Sodium (mg)
Italian manicotti with garlic bread	1393	79	411	2330
Beef & cheese enchiladas, rice & refried beans	1510	88	210	3516
Chicken fried steak with fries	1119	77	205	1895
Ultimate cheeseburger with fries & shake	1625	96	165	1708
Chicken sandwich with onion rings & shake	1282	68	82	2290
Seafood platter - fried - with tarter sauce	1195	70	97	1780
Salmon - smothered in a cream sauce	1024	76	283	1017
Fried chicken - with potato salad & cole slaw	1124	71	239	2552
Stir fry chicken with rice & egg rolls	1213	62	99	2907
Lasagna with garlic bread & salad	1538	77	194	2805
Omelet with hashbrowns	850	53	892	852
Pizza - sausage & mushroom	1290	48	84	1656
Chimichanga with sour cream & cheese	922	68	205	2125
Salad bar - with potato & tuna salad, dressing, and muffins with butter	1715	89	310	2954

Does dining out have to be so destructive to our health?

Some say, "Order grilled fish, salads or vegetarian dishes. By avoiding red meat, fried foods and creamy sauces, you can dine out and stay on your diet."

Be careful! We've analyzed hundreds of apparently "healthy" entrees and found that many were diet disasters. Frequently, "healthy" dishes are laced with unhealthy, hidden ingredients. The menu descriptions portray healthy items, but when we looked into the preparation methods, we found the items contained too much of certain unhealthy ingredients.

Surprising nutrition information about apparently "healthy" meals:

Grilled Swordfish - *Marinated in herbs and olive oil.*

884	Calories	
71	Fat (g)	Over a full day's recommended fat intake.
115	Cholesterol (mg)	Too much olive oil used in the preparation!
846	Sodium (mg)	

Vegetarian Pasta Primavera - *Fresh vegetables and garlic sautéed in a vegetable broth. Served over fettucini noodles and tossed with Parmesan cheese.*

816	Calories	The menu description didn't mention that the pasta was
45	Fat (g)	heavily tossed with oil, and the vegetables were sautéed
139	Cholesterol (mg)	in both broth *and butter.* This brings the fat total to 75%
892	Sodium (mg)	of a FULL day's recommended fat intake.

The "Healthy" Sandwich - *Avocado, tomato & cheese on whole wheat bread.*

746	Calories	
50	Fat (g)	This is a healthy sandwich?
66	Cholesterol (mg)	Avocado, cheese, and mayonnaise add
958	Sodium (mg)	up to too much fat and sodium.

Cobb Salad - *Crispy greens topped with chicken, avocado, bacon, tomato, hard-boiled egg and blue cheese crumbles. Served with a generous portion of your favorite dressing.*

1296	Calories	
102	Fat (g)	Very unhealthy. Much too high in fat,
647	Cholesterol (mg)	cholesterol, sodium and calories.
2553	Sodium (mg)	

Shrimp Stirfry - *Shrimp and assorted vegetables with chow mein noodles.*

866	Calories	Too much fat, calories, cholesterol and sodium.
64	Fat (g)	1 oz. oil to sauté (27 g fat), butter/cream
392	Cholesterol (mg)	sauce (25 g fat), and the chow mein noodles
668	Sodium (mg)	(9 g fat) quickly add up.

Tostada - *Mexican beans, guacamole, lettuce, tomato and cheese.*

1416	Calories	
77	Fat (g)	The cheese alone contributes 519 calories,
288	Cholesterol (mg)	43 grams of fat, 137 mg cholesterol and
2010	Sodium (mg)	802 mg sodium.

We also found other items labeled "Light" or "Light-Fare" that included potato skins (deep fried), vegetables with cheese sauce, a hamburger patty and cottage cheese (too much saturated fat), cheese quesadillas (there's that saturated fat in the cheese again) and deep fried fish tacos.

Accents On Health has even analyzed entrees with a ♥ next to them, and we discovered that many were too high in fat. Here are a few examples:

??? Heart Healthy Entrees ???

♥	Eggplant Salad	34 grams fat - 86% of calories from fat
♥	Pasta with Tomatoes & Garlic	42 grams fat - 50% of calories from fat
♥	Greens Topped with Grilled Ahi	26 grams fat - 73% of calories from fat
♥	Grilled Halibut	64 grams fat - 75% of calories from fat

How can these items be designated as "healthy" or "light" when in fact they aren't? A bit of history is in order. As we noted in Chapter 1 when discussing packaged foods, health sells; and so food manufacturers were quick to tout the health benefits of their products. Restaurants soon followed, with menus and banners promoting the healthfulness of certain dishes.

As demonstrated in the previous pages, however, many dishes described as "healthy" actually are not. A restaurant may designate a meal as healthy simply because it is vegetarian or contains no butter, but in most cases, dishes with health claims have never been analyzed for nutrition content. And until recently, there were no standards for what really constituted a healthy or low-fat restaurant meal.

New restaurant regulations

In an attempt to protect consumers from vague, incorrect, or misleading information, the Food and Drug Administration (FDA) implemented regulations for restaurants that make health and nutrition claims about their food. The regulations require that dishes with descriptions such as "low fat" or "low calorie" meet specified criteria; and that restaurants provide nutrition information to substantiate any health claims made.

Unfortunately, however, the large majority of restaurants choose <u>not</u> to provide healthful menu items with credible nutrition information. This leaves diners, in most cases, at a loss for determining the nutritional content of restaurant meals.

The restaurants featured in this book lead the nation in providing meals with an eye on nutrition <u>and</u> taste, substantiated by credible nutrition data. Instead of smothering foods with excessive amounts of unhealthy ingredients, these talented chefs creatively use herbs, spices, small amounts of unsaturated oils and healthy preparation methods. They have your health <u>and</u> your tastebuds in mind.

Some scrumptious and healthy examples:

Anastasia's Asylum (Santa Monica)
ANASTASIA'S FAMOUS VEGETARIAN LASAGNA
✓✓ CALORIES: Excellent Choice (150)   ✓✓ CHOLESTEROL: Excellent Choice (10 mg)
✓✓ FAT: Excellent Choice (4 g)   ✓✓ SODIUM: Excellent Choice (195 mg)

Hotel Bel Air (Bel Air)
MAINE SCALLOP SALAD
with fennel, frisee and orange segments.
✓✓ CALORIES: Excellent Choice (215)   ✓✓ CHOLESTEROL: Excellent Choice (30 mg)
✓✓ FAT: Excellent Choice (8 g)   ✓✓ SODIUM: Excellent Choice (195 mg)

Baja Fresh (over 30 locations in Southern California)
BAJA STYLE CHICKEN TACO
✓✓ CALORIES: Excellent Choice (90)   ✓✓ CHOLESTEROL: Excellent Choice (25 mg)
✓✓ FAT: Excellent Choice (2 g)   SODIUM: not available

Café Luna (Torrance)
GRILLED SALMON
Grilled salmon served with grilled vegetables and garlic mashed potatoes.
✓ CALORIES: Good Choice (495)   ✓ CHOLESTEROL: Good Choice (100 mg)
✓ FAT: Good Choice (16 g)   ✓✓ SODIUM: Excellent Choice (100 mg)

Skew's (Los Angeles)
CALIFORNIA CHICKEN SKEWER
Fresh grilled chicken breast with no sugar added. Served with choice of two sides.
✓✓ CALORIES: Excellent Choice (235)   ✓ CHOLESTEROL: Good Choice (120 mg)
✓✓ FAT: Excellent Choice (5 g)   ✓✓ SODIUM: Excellent Choice (105 mg)

Some scrumptious and healthy examples (continued):

Changs (Brentwood)
EAST MEETS WEST CHICKEN
The juiciness of pears and crunch of apples are a snappy combo in this Chang's specialty. Refreshingly tasty.
✓✓ CALORIES: Excellent Choice (435)   CHOLESTEROL: Moderate (170 mg)
✓✓ FAT: Excellent Choice (10 g)   ✓✓ SODIUM: Excellent Choice (165 mg)

Chili My Soul (Encino)
POBLANO TURKEY CHILI
The creative blending of mild poblano and pasilla peppers enriches the character of this healthy, substantive chili reminiscent of Mexican mole. Analysis for 8oz. (cup) serving.
✓✓ CALORIES: Excellent Choice (215)   ✓ CHOLESTEROL: Good Choice (95 mg)
✓✓ FAT: Excellent Choice (4 g)   SODIUM: Moderate (635 mg)

Pane e Vino (Melrose)
CAPELLINI AL POMODORO NATURALE - SPECIAL REQUEST
Angel hair pasta, fresh tomatoes, basil, garlic, and extra virgin olive oil. <u>*Request less oil (1 Tbs.).*</u>
✓✓ CALORIES: Excellent Choice (445)   ✓✓ CHOLESTEROL: Excellent Choice (0 mg)
✓✓ FAT: Excellent Choice (15 g)   ✓✓ SODIUM: Excellent Choice (205 mg)

Chin Chin (Brentwood, Beverly Hills, Encino, W. Hollywood, Marina Del Rey, Studio City)
LITE CHICKEN WITH GARLIC AND SNOW PEAS
Velveted pieces of chicken breast stir fried with snow peas, fresh mushrooms, carrots and sliced garlic.
✓ CALORIES: Good Choice (520)   ✓ CHOLESTEROL: Good Choice (150 mg)
✓✓ FAT: Excellent Choice (12 g)   SODIUM: High (2075 mg)

Pradeep's (Santa Monica)
BAIGAN KA BHURTA
Roughly chopped roasted eggplant cooked with red onions, tomatoes, ginger, garlic, curry spices and cilantro.
✓✓ CALORIES: Excellent Choice (130)   ✓✓ CHOLESTEROL: Excellent Choice (0 mg)
✓✓ FAT: Excellent Choice (5 g)   ✓✓ SODIUM: Excellent Choice (280 mg)

Santa Monica Seafood (Santa Monica, Orange, Costa Mesa)
SUSHI ROLL COMBINATION
Includes tuna roll, cucumber roll, salmon roll and California roll.
✓✓ CALORIES: Excellent Choice (405)   ✓✓ CHOLESTEROL: Excellent Choice (55 mg)
✓✓ FAT: Excellent Choice (5 g)*   ✓✓ SODIUM: Excellent Choice (125 mg)

BeauRivage Mediterranean Restaurant (Malibu)
NEPTUNE GAZPACHO
chilled and topped with bay shrimp.
✓✓ CALORIES: Excellent Choice (160)   ✓✓ CHOLESTEROL: Excellent Choice (35 mg)
✓✓ FAT: Excellent Choice (12 g)   ✓ SODIUM: Good Choice (560 mg)

> The menu items on the previous pages and in the following chapters are just a taste of the wonderful entrees served at the restaurants participating in ***Healthy Dining in Los Angeles***. We invite you to visit the restaurants featured in this book. You'll discover a whole new world of menu items that are marvelously delicious and so good for you!

"Special Requests"

In some cases, after we analyzed the restaurant recipes, we found dishes that contained too many calories and/or too much fat, cholesterol or sodium. So we recommended that the chef modify the dishes to meet the *Healthy Dining* guidelines. We note these dishes as "Special Requests." "Special Requests" may be prepared with less oil or butter, salad dressing or sauce served on the side, less cheese, etc. When you order, you must ask for the "Special Request" for it to correspond to the published nutrition information. See the examples below to find out how many calories and grams of fat you save by ordering some of these "Special Requests."

Examples of "Special Requests:"

Crocodile Café (Burbank, Old Pasadena, Santa Monica & San Diego)
HERB CRUSTED SALMON AND TIGER SHRIMP – SPECIAL REQUEST ☙
Grilled salmon and sautéed shrimp with asparagus, red onions and tomatoes on baby field greens. Request shrimp poached and balsamic vinaigrette dressing on the side. Dressing not included in analysis.
✓✓ CALORIES: Excellent Choice (310)
✓✓ FAT: Excellent Choice (11 g)
This "**Special Request**" saves 300 calories and 32 grams of fat.

Mi Piace (Burbank, Pasadena, Calabasas)
PENNE ALL'ARRABBIATA – SPECIAL REQUEST
Pasta with crushed red pepper, fresh garlic and housemade marinara sauce. Request less oil (1/4 oz.) and no butter.
✓ CALORIES: Good Choice (565)
✓ FAT: Good Choice (22 g)
This "**Special Request**" saves 620 calories and 70 grams of fat.

Malvasia (Long Beach)
INSALATE MALVASIA – SPECIAL REQUEST
Mixed baby greens, broiled chicken breast, sliced red onions, fire roasted red peppers, fresh mozzarella, kalamata olives, roma tomatoes, capers and artichoke hearts. Request dressing and cheese served on the side (not included in analysis).
✓ CALORIES: Good Choice (560)
✓✓ FAT: Excellent Choice (13 g)
This "**Special Request**" saves 760 calories and 75 grams of fat.

Ruby's (10 locations throughout the Los Angeles area)
CHICKEN RUBYBURGER – SPECIAL REQUEST
with a tender boneless, skinless chicken breast. Request no margarine or mayonnaise.
✓ CALORIES: Good Choice (485)
✓✓ FAT: Excellent Choice (10 g)
This "**Special Request**" saves 300 calories and 32 grams of fat.

Baja Fresh (over 30 locations in the greater Los Angeles area)
GRILLED VEGETARIAN BURRITO – SPECIAL REQUEST
Request no cheese and sour cream.
✓ CALORIES: Good Choice (490)
✓✓ FAT: Excellent Choice (12 g)
This "**Special Request**" saves 340 calories and 25 grams of fat.

Remember: Any dish marked "**Special Request**" means you must specifically order the "Special Request" for it to correspond to the published nutrition information.

CHAPTER **3**

Do Your Calories Have a Purpose?

Calories have a bad reputation in our society. We're counting calories and cutting calories, as though we've forgotten that calories are what keep us alive. Food and water fuel our bodies to do the miraculous tasks we perform each day. Instead of focusing on just cutting calories, we need to look at the *quality* of the calories we consume.

Just what are you getting from your calories?

Calories add up from the amounts of protein, carbohydrate and fat in foods. Each type of calorie has a very different function in the body. The following chapters explain the functions in more detail, but briefly:

Protein calories help the body to build and restore.

Carbohydrate calories are the body's main energy source.

Fat calories turn to fat -- *easily*.

In general, protein and carbohydrate calories supply our bodies with nutrients necessary to function optimally. We need a very small amount of fat each day, but because fat is very easy to get, most Americans suffer from an excess of dietary fat, not a deficiency.

We should strive to eat foods with high-quality, nutritious calories. Recommendations vary according to individual needs, but generally 50% to 65% of total daily calories should come from carbohydrates, 10% to 20% from protein, and 15% to 30% from fat. Because most Americans get enough protein and too much fat, the best way to determine the quality of your calories is to determine the percentage of calories from fat, and keep it under 30%.

Percentage of calories from fat

The 30% fat recommendation is the suggested average for the whole day. Some foods will add little, if any, fat to your diet, while other foods may supply a big chunk of the fat for the day. Of course, it's best to avoid (or use sparingly) foods which have a high percentage of fat (e.g., butter, margarine, oils, sour cream, cheese, cream cheese, etc.).

A fattening example:

Salmon - *Smothered in a cream sauce*
Total Calories: 1024
Protein: 77 grams
Carbohydrate: 8 grams
Fat: 76 grams

How to calculate the percentage of calories from fat:

Each gram of fat has nine calories. Using this information, you can calculate the percentage of calories from fat as shown in the following example. For the **Salmon with Cream Sauce**:

1. Multiply the number of grams of fat by 9 (number of calories per gram of fat):
   76 grams x 9 cals/gram = 684 calories from fat

2. Divide by total calories to get the fraction of calories from fat:
   684 calories ÷ 1024 calories = 0.67

3. Multiply by 100 to get the percentage:
   0.67 x 100 = 67%

67% of calories in this dish come from fat!

Carbohydrate and protein percentages can be calculated in a similar way, except that the number of grams of each is multiplied by 4 rather than 9, because carbohydrates and proteins provide 4 calories per gram. The division step is the same. For this example, these calculations show that 3% of calories come from carbohydrate and 30% from protein. Cholesterol and sodium do not contribute to calories.

The small percentage of carbohydrate is common for meat, poultry, and fish entrees, but a nutritious entree should contain less fat. In this example, most of the fat comes from the cream and butter used in the sauce; however, it's not necessary to add excess fat to get a delicious tasting entree.

Let's look at a healthier salmon dish:

Grilled Salmon (Kincaid's)
*Grilled 7 oz. filet of fresh salmon, served with sweet
Sushi rice, steamed seasonal vegetables.*

Analysis for salmon alone:

Total Calories: 275
Protein: 38 grams
Carbohydrates: 0 grams
Fat: 12 grams

To calculate the percentage of calories from fat:

1. Multiply grams of fat by 9 calories per gram:
   12 grams x 9 cals/gram = 108 calories from fat

2. Divide by total calories and multiply by 100 to get a percentage:
   108 calories ÷ 275 calories x 100 = 39%

39% of calories from this dish come from fat --- much less than the example above, but still above the recommended guideline of 30% of calories from fat.

Remember, the guideline of 30% or fewer calories from fat applies to the overall diet --- an entire day or week, not just one entree. Restaurants differ greatly in the ways meals and side dishes are presented. If you order a lean meat or fish entree, it consists mainly of protein and fat, and the percentage of fat will generally appear to be high. By themselves, many lean meats and fish contain 30% to 50% fat. Even soybeans contain about 40% of their calories from fat. But generally these high-protein entrees are not eaten by themselves. If you choose quality carbohydrate side dishes such as vegetables, grains, breads, and fruits, the percentage of fat for the overall meal will be significantly less. Entrees that are made up largely of carbohydrates (such as pasta or rice dishes) will generally have a lower percentage of calories from fat.

As an example of how the side dishes change the overall percentage fat, let's include the side dishes that are served with this entree:

	Calories	Fat (g)
Salmon	275	12
Steamed Seasonal Vegetables	80	4½
Sweet Sushi Rice	225	2½
Totals	580	19

To calculate percentage of calories from fat:

19 grams of fat x 9 cals/gram = 171 calories from fat
171 calories from fat ÷ 580 total calories x 100 = 29%

Only 29% of total calories from this meal come from fat, which is within the recommended guidelines and significantly less than the percentage of fat calculated for the salmon alone.

This example demonstrates how a meal can be a good choice even when the protein-rich part of the meal by itself (the salmon in this case) exceeds 30% of calories from fat. Also, remember that a meal like this one will probably be the largest of your day, and your choices for the remainder of the day can also bring the overall percentage of fat down.

Grams of fat vs. percentage of calories from fat

We list grams of fat for each of the dishes on the menu pages rather than percentage of calories from fat. The previous example illustrates how calculating the percentage of calories from fat for a single menu item does not adequately reflect values for the entire meal or the entire day. Chapter 4 discusses in more detail how to choose guidelines for fat intake that are appropriate for you.

How the check mark guidelines for calories are set

The *Healthy Dining* guidelines assume an average intake of 2,000 calories per day. Next, we assume that the restaurant meal accounts for the largest of the day's meals, up to 40% of the daily calories allotment, or 800 calories. So 750 calories for the main entree would fit into the calorie budget. Thus, an upper limit of 750 calories is labeled as a "Good Choice" for calories. The "Excellent Choice" value of 450 calories represents a proportionately lower level, corresponding to about 1200-1500 calories per day:

✓✓ Excellent Choice = 0 to 450 calories/entree
  ✓ Good Choice = 451 to 750 calories/entree

> Glance through the restaurant pages and use the quick, easy check mark system to see the wide variety of entrees which contain high-quality, nutritious calories and are "Excellent Choice" (✓✓) or "Good Choice" (✓) for calories.

CHAPTER 4

Fat - How Much and What Type?

Fat -- it clogs our arteries and builds up around the stomach, thighs and buttocks. Too much body fat, almost always caused by <u>too much fat in our diet, too many calories</u> and/or <u>too little exercise</u> in our day, increases the risks of high blood pressure, elevated blood fats (triglycerides and cholesterol), heart disease, stroke, diabetes, cancer and other health problems.

How much is too much?

The guidelines recommended by the American Heart Association and the Surgeon General's Office (see Chapter 1) suggest that fat should contribute no more than 30% of total calories. Chapter 3 shows examples of calculating percentage of calories from fat. This section deals with counting grams of fat. If we assume a daily intake of 2000 calories, then no more than 600 calories per day (30%) should come from fat. Since each gram of fat contributes 9 calories, then about 66 grams of fat (600 ÷ 9) is the suggested upper limit of fat intake per day. If you're not careful, it's very easy to exceed that with just one meal!

How the check mark guidelines for fat are set

What is a reasonable limit per meal or per entree? If we assume the restaurant meal is the largest meal of the day, and allow up to 40% of the daily fat allotment (66 grams) for that meal, that sets a limit of 26 grams of fat. Main entrees usually contribute the largest amount of fat to the meal (assuming you're careful about side dishes), so we set guidelines of:

✓✓ Excellent Choice = 0 to 15 grams of fat/entree
✓ Good Choice = 16 to 25 grams of fat/entree

If you're very active and take in more calories, then a higher limit would be appropriate. If you're on a <u>weight loss diet</u> or <u>very low fat diet</u>, then the <u>"Excellent Choice" guideline of up to 15 grams</u> of fat per entree is probably more appropriate.

Notice that these recommended guidelines represent an average intake for an average meal. Don't be overly concerned about the cutoff between our designations of "Good Choice" and "Excellent Choice." Unless you're on a very restricted diet, the difference between an entree with 16 grams of fat (which would receive one check mark) and one with 15 grams of fat (two check marks) is probably not worth worrying about. An occasional meal with somewhat more fat (but don't overdo it!) can be fairly easily compensated for by reducing fat intake during other meals.

Portion sizes

Be aware of portion sizes. Restaurant portions tend to be very large. The entrees listed in this book often represent 6 to 10 ounces of a very filling, protein-rich meal. In some cases, for a large serving, we may note that the nutrition information is based on only a part (e.g., ½ or ⅔) of a full serving. This means that only the recommended portion of the meal corresponds to the nutrition information. So, because it is a large serving, eat ½ or ⅔ and save the rest for the next day – or share with a friend.

Types of fat

Together with protein, fats form the structures in our bodies, including muscles, nerves, membranes and blood vessels. However, we need very little fat to perform these functions, and only *unsaturated* sources of fat aid in these processes. "Saturated" and "unsaturated" refer to the chemical structure of the fat molecules.

Unsaturated Fats - Monounsaturated, Polyunsaturated. These are the *"good"* types of fat. A low total fat intake, with the majority of fat from unsaturated sources, appears to lower blood cholesterol levels. The best sources for these "good" fats are natural grains, seeds and nuts, and fish. Many oils are primarily unsaturated, such as olive, canola, peanut, corn, safflower, sesame, cottonseed and soybean. Once again, these fats are "good" only in very small amounts! Look for menu items with the * alongside the fat content for dishes that contain primarily unsaturated fat.

Omega-3 Fats. Some types of fish contain unique polyunsaturated fats called Omega-3 fatty acids. These fatty acids seem to make blood platelets less likely to clot, thus decreasing risk of artery blockage and heart attack. Fish with high amounts of Omega-3 include salmon, albacore tuna, mackerel, herring and rainbow trout.

Saturated Fats. Saturated fats are the *very unhealthy* fats that raise blood cholesterol levels. Excess saturated fat is related to an increased risk of cardiovascular disease. Foods that contain saturated fats are usually hard at room temperature. Saturated fat is found mostly in animal products (beef, chicken, butter, ice cream, and cheese), processed and fast foods and some vegetable oils (palm oil, coconut oil, and partially hydrogenated oils).

Hydrogenated Oils and Trans-Fatty Acids. The vegetable oils found in most margarines and in packaged and processed foods (such as cookies, pastries, crackers, chips, etc.) are "hydrogenated." During the hydrogenation process, hydrogen is added to liquid oil, thereby changing its chemical structure. The result is a harder, more saturated fat product, which many people find appealing for spreads and in cooking. Manufacturers use the hydrogenation process because it increases product stability and shelf life, saving them money. Unfortunately, consumption of hydrogenated products contributes to elevated blood cholesterol levels and an increase in heart disease risk.

In addition to making the fat more saturated, hydrogenation also produces unnatural compounds called trans-fatty acids that have a more rigid molecular structure than natural fats do. Many scientists now believe that these trans-fatty acids are harmful because they block the important functions of the "good" types of fat. It is probably wise to opt for unprocessed foods rather than foods that contain "hydrogenated" or "partially hydrogenated" oils.

A summary of fat

When assessing the fat content of food, it is important to look at:
1. The <u>number of grams</u> of fat
2. The <u>percentage of calories</u> from fat
3. The <u>type</u> of fat - minimize or avoid saturated and hydrogenated fats

<u>One Last Word on Fat:</u> Although unsaturated fats do not raise blood cholesterol levels, too much fat -- saturated <u>or</u> unsaturated -- may make you fat, and excess body fat is a risk factor for many chronic diseases.

> On the restaurant menu pages, the asterisk (*) next to the grams of fat indicates that the fat is primarily unsaturated (the "good" type). Look for it!

Some delicious examples of "Excellent" and "Good" choices for fat:
Notice that many contain primarily unsaturated fat (designated with the *).

Coco's (38 Los Angeles locations)
EGG WHITE OMELETTE
Garden-fresh spinach, red-ripe tomato, sautéed onion, fresh basil and crumbled Feta cheese folded into a fluffy omelette. Served with fresh, seasonal fruit instead of breakfast potatoes.
✓✓ FAT: Excellent Choice (13 g)

Empress Harbor Seafood (Monterey Park)
STIR-FRIED SHRIMP, SCALLOPS & CHICKEN
in garlic chili sauce.
✓✓ FAT: Excellent Choice (11 g)

Junior's (Westwood)
GARDEN BURGER
A vegetarian burger served with fresh fruit.
✓✓ FAT: Excellent Choice (15 g)*

Il Moro (West Los Angeles)
TRANCIO DI TONNO
Tartare of ahi tune (raw), mixed with anchovies, onions and garlic, in a lemon and olive oil dressing on a bed of baby lettuces and julienne of leeks.
✓✓ FAT: Excellent Choice (9 g)*

Havana Mania (Redondo Beach)
FILETE DE POLLO
Chicken breast (boneless) grilled in our own garlic sauce and sautéed onions, served with black beans and rice.
✓✓ FAT: Excellent Choice (13 g)

Some delicious examples of "Excellent" and "Good" choices for fat (continued):

Ruby's (10 Los Angeles locations)
TURKEY RUBYBURGER
with a full ⅓ lb. of lean ground turkey.
✓ FAT: Good Choice (19 g)

Shenandoah Café (Long Beach)
SAN FRANCISCO SWORDFISH - SPECIAL REQUEST
Marinated in soy, dijon, lemon and garlic and charbroiled. Request vegetables steamed.
✓✓ FAT: Excellent Choice (13 g)*

Wahoo's Fish Taco's (6 Los Angeles locations)
CHARBROILED FISH BURRITO
✓✓ FAT: Excellent Choice (12 g)

Wasabi Japanese Restaurant (Long Beach)
CHICKEN TERIYAKI
Chicken breast grilled with teriyaki sauce. Served with white rice and veggies.
✓✓ FAT: Excellent Choice (6 g)

McCormick & Schmick's (Pasadena, Los Angeles, Beverly Hills, El Segundo)
GRILLED HALIBUT WITH FRESH SALSA - SPECIAL REQUEST
served with Chefs special salsa of the day. Request steamed vegetables.
✓✓ FAT: Excellent Choice (9 g)*

Now - how well are YOU doing?

Now that Los Angeles restaurants are watching how much fat they're adding to your diet, just *how well are you watching?* Here are some easy ways to add too much fat to your diet - quickly!

High-fat culprits:

	Calories	Fat (g)	Cholest.(mg)	Sodium (mg)
Salad Dressings: (3 Tbs.)				
Blue Cheese	231	24	27	501
Thousand Island	176	17	15	327
French	201	19	6	642
Italian	206	21	0	348
Oil & Vinegar	215	24	0	0
Ranch	162	17	12	291
Toppings: (2 Tbs.)				
Butter	200	23	61	232
Margarine	202	23	0	264
Sour Cream	67	6	13	15
Cream Cheese	100	10	31	85
Tarter Sauce	150	16	18	196
Mayonnaise	198	22	16	157
Cheese (1 oz. cheddar)	114	9	30	176

High-fat culprits (continued):

Desserts:

Cheesecake	386	24	82	284
Apple Pie	323	14	28	207
Chocolate Cake	407	17	5	300
Ice Cream (1 cup)	349	24	88	108

Instead try:

- Fat-free or low-fat salad dressings
- Salsa, low-fat cottage cheese, or plain yogurt as salad dressing or topping for potatoes
- Only very small amounts of regular or high-fat salad dressings
- Frozen yogurt, sorbet, sherbet or fruit for dessert

CHAPTER 5

Cholesterol - A Hot Topic

Cholesterol continues to be a hot topic enmeshed in controversy. Medical research is progressing on this subject, and we hope to clear up some misconceptions concerning cholesterol.

Where does cholesterol come from?

Most of the cholesterol in your blood is manufactured by your liver. The body produces about 1,000 milligrams (mg) of cholesterol each day. In addition, the average American consumes 400 to 600 mg daily from food. Cholesterol from our food is found only in animal products. The cholesterol we derive from our diets is essentially the same as the cholesterol our bodies manufacture. Our bodies use cholesterol to form hormones and cell membranes.

However, the average high-fat/high-cholesterol diet tends to add too much cholesterol to the bloodstream. The excess cholesterol and other substances accumulate in the walls of the blood vessels. Over time the arteries become narrowed, and eventually the flow of blood is cut off, leading to a heart attack or stroke.

How should blood cholesterol be measured?

For an accurate and complete cholesterol measure, a tube of blood should be drawn from the arm by a qualified health professional. You should not eat or drink anything (except water) for 12 hours before the blood draw. The laboratory which analyzes the blood sample should follow the reference methods set by the U. S. Centers for Disease Control. The fingertip method found in shopping malls and health fairs may not provide results that are as accurate.

What determines blood cholesterol levels?

1. **Genetics**. Some individuals, no matter how prudent their diet or how regularly they exercise, can't achieve a low cholesterol level without the help of a physician and cholesterol-lowering medications.

2. **Lipoproteins**. Cholesterol is carried through the blood in protein packages called lipoproteins. The amounts and types of lipoproteins are an important indicator of your heart disease risk.

LDLs (low-density lipoproteins) are commonly termed "bad" cholesterol. LDLs increase heart disease risk because they keep cholesterol in blood circulation and carry it to the arteries to be deposited. Excess body fat and a diet high in saturated fat tend to increase LDL levels.

HDLs (high-density lipoproteins) are the "good" cholesterol that protect against heart disease. They actually carry cholesterol AWAY from the arteries to the liver to be excreted from the body. Individuals with high HDL levels have a lower risk of heart disease. Regular exercise, maintaining appropriate body weight, and not smoking help to increase HDL levels.

3. **Diet**. Foods high in saturated fat increase cholesterol levels. These include butter, whole milk products, palm and coconut oils, cheese, beef, pork, and eggs. In addition, many packaged and processed foods are high in saturated fat or (partially) hydrogenated oils, which also have a cholesterol-raising effect.

A diet *low in total fat*, with fat intake primarily from unsaturated fat sources, reduces cholesterol levels. Unsaturated fats include olive, corn, safflower, sesame, canola, soybean, and sunflower oils. *High fiber foods*, especially oat bran, apples, carrots, oranges, and legumes (beans, peas and lentils) decrease cholesterol levels by inhibiting the absorption of cholesterol into the bloodstream. *Fish and fish oils*, which contain omega-3 fatty acids, also decrease cholesterol levels.

4. **Smoking, stress and some medications** also raise cholesterol levels.

Important facts on dietary cholesterol and fat

Too much of any fat (even unsaturated oils!) can increase body fat, and excess body fat may increase blood cholesterol levels. Oils, margarine, and butter all have approximately the same number of calories and fat grams per ounce, and so all have the same potential to make you fat. Therefore it's important to limit your total intake of all types of fat.

Even though oils, margarine, and butter have about the same calorie and fat counts, there is a big difference in the chemical make-up of these fats. Butter is high in saturated fat, and saturated fats increase blood cholesterol levels. Saturated fats stimulate the production of LDLs ("bad cholesterol"), resulting in increased blood cholesterol levels. Therefore, if you avoid only dietary cholesterol in the food you eat, without reducing the amount of saturated fat, you may not decrease your blood cholesterol level at all.

Avoid hydrogenated fats too, because they are also saturated. Margarine, although cholesterol-free, is partially hydrogenated and contains trans-fatty acids, which have been shown to have a cholesterol-raising effect.

Vegetable oils are generally unsaturated fats. Liquid oils (such as olive, corn, canola, etc.) in small amounts may help to decrease cholesterol levels. Remember though, that all oils are 100% fat, so use only small amounts.

The amount of cholesterol found in foods is not as important as the amount of saturated fat. But you should minimize intake of very concentrated sources of cholesterol such as egg yolks and liver. Shellfish is very low in saturated fat, but moderately high in cholesterol. Most medical experts agree that shellfish, in small quantities, is a healthy choice.

Cholesterol is found only in animal products. Don't be misled, though --- just because foods don't contain cholesterol doesn't mean they are also low in fat! In fact, many "no-cholesterol" foods are loaded with fat. Be sure to check the number of fat grams on nutrition labels.

How the check mark guidelines for cholesterol are set

The Surgeon General's Office and the American Heart Association recommend that cholesterol consumption be limited to 300 mg per day. If the day's total were evenly divided in thirds, this would suggest a limit of 100 mg per meal. We set our guidelines for cholesterol as follows:

✓✓　Excellent Choice = 0 to 75 mg cholesterol/entree
✓　Good Choice = 76 to 150 mg cholesterol/entree

If every meal in your day were at the "Good Choice" limit of 150 mg, you would exceed the recommended amount. But since a restaurant meal usually contains a larger portion of meat or other cholesterol-containing foods than side dishes or other meals of the day, we assumed that this cholesterol intake can easily be compensated for by choosing foods with little or no cholesterol for the remaining selections.

If you are watching your blood cholesterol level, select items that are:

1.　"Excellent Choice" or "Good Choice" for fat
2.　Primarily unsaturated (designated with the *)
3.　"Excellent Choice" or "Good Choice" for cholesterol

Some flavorful examples of "Excellent" and "Good" choices for cholesterol:

Charo Chicken (11 Los Angeles locations)
CHICKEN BOWL
Generous portions of our critically acclaimed rice, pinto or black beans, mild pico de gallo salsa and shredded chicken.
✓ FAT: Good Choice (23 g)　　✓✓ CHOLESTEROL: Excellent Choice (70 mg)

El Torito (24 Los Angeles locations)
SPINACH ENCHILADAS
Two corn tortillas filled with sautéed spinach, mushrooms, mild chiles and melted cheese – then topped with our zesty fire-roasted tomatillo sauce. Served with fresh fruit relish, Mexican-style rice and frijoles de la olla.
✓ FAT: Good Choice (25 g)　　✓✓ CHOLESTEROL: Excellent Choice (45 mg)

Mi Piace (Pasadena, Burbank, & Calabasas)
CAPPELLINI PRIMAVERA
Pasta with fresh seasonal julienned vegetables.
✓ FAT: Good Choice (22 g)*　　✓✓ CHOLESTEROL: Excellent Choice (10 mg)

PJ's Thai Restaurant (Long Beach)
CHICKEN - SPICY MINT WITH GREEN CHILE PEPPER & ONION
✓✓ FAT: Excellent Choice (13 g)　　✓✓ CHOLESTEROL: Excellent Choice (60 mg)

Examples of "Good" and "Excellent" choices for cholesterol (continued):

CHAYA Venice (Venice Beach)
JAVA CHICKEN SALAD
with spicy peanut sauce.
✓ FAT: Good Choice (16 g)   ✓✓ CHOLESTEROL: Excellent Choice (65 mg)

China Grill (Manhattan Beach)
WOK-SEARED YELLOW FIN TUNA
Served with steamed vegetables, seaweed salad and pickled ginger.
✓✓ FAT: Excellent Choice (7 g)*   ✓✓ CHOLESTEROL: Excellent Choice (70 mg)

Susan's Healthy Gourmet (Conveniently located pick-up throughout LA County)
TROPICAL SALMON
Citrus–marinated baked Atlantic Salmon, topped with pineapple jalapeño salsa, and served over organic brown rice.
✓✓ FAT: Excellent Choice (10 g)*   ✓✓ CHOLESTEROL: Excellent Choice (50 mg)

Riviera Mexican Grill (Redondo Beach)
VEGGIE BURRITO
Grilled red and yellow bell peppers, avocado, red onion, roasted chilies, black beans and rice with two salsas and guacamole. Served with Zuni chopped salad and black beans.
✓ FAT: Good Choice (19 g)*   ✓✓ CHOLESTEROL: Excellent Choice (5 mg)

Palomino (Westwood Village)
BRICK OVEN-ROASTED VEGETABLES
Balsamic-shallot marinade, almond wood-charred vegetables, romaine greens. Also available with garlic prawns or wood-grilled chicken.
✓ FAT: Good Choice (24 g)   ✓✓ CHOLESTEROL: Excellent Choice (25 mg)

CHAPTER 6

Sodium - To Salt or Not to Salt?

That is the question. Sodium is an essential nutrient. It helps to maintain blood volume, regulate the balance of water in the cells, and transmit nerve impulses. The kidneys control sodium balance by increasing or decreasing sodium in the urine.

In general, Americans consume more sodium than the body needs. Many foods contain sodium naturally, and it is commonly added to foods during preparation or processing. Sodium is also found in drinking water, prescription drugs and over-the-counter medications.

One teaspoon of salt contains about 2,000 milligrams of sodium, approximately ⅔ of the American Heart Association's recommended daily amount. Other condiments contain significant amounts of sodium, such as seasoning salts (1620 - 1850 mg per teaspoon), monosodium glutamate (MSG, 492 mg per teaspoon), soy sauce (343 mg per teaspoon), and meat tenderizer (1750 mg per teaspoon). Packaged and processed foods also tend to be very high in sodium.

In the United States, about one in four adults has elevated blood pressure. Sodium intake is only one of the factors known to affect blood pressure, and not everyone is equally susceptible. The sensitivity to sodium seems to be very individualized. At present, there is not a good method to predict who is salt-sensitive or who will develop high blood pressure. Low-sodium diets may help some people avoid high blood pressure. Low-sodium diets may help some people with high blood pressure to control their blood pressure. And in some individuals, a low-sodium diet will not affect blood pressure at all.

Since most Americans consume more sodium than needed, consider reducing your sodium intake. Use less table salt, read labels carefully, and eat sparingly those foods which have large amounts of sodium. Remember that a substantial amount of the sodium you eat may be "hidden" - either occurring naturally in foods or as part of a preservative or flavoring agent that has been added.

To avoid too much sodium:

- Learn to enjoy the flavors of unsalted foods.
- Cook without salt or with only small amounts of added salt.
- Flavor foods with herbs, spices, and lemon juice.
- Add little or no salt to food at the table.
- Limit your intake of salty foods such as potato chips, pretzels, salted nuts and popcorn, condiments (soy sauce, steak sauce, garlic salt), pickled foods, cured meats, cheeses, and canned foods.
- Read food labels carefully to determine the amounts of sodium.
- Use lower sodium products, when available, to replace those with higher sodium content.

To avoid too much sodium when dining out:

1. Order entrees listed as "Excellent Choice" or "Good Choice" for sodium levels, <u>and</u>
2. Request no added salt whenever possible.

The analyses shown in this book reflect the sodium content that occurs naturally in food, as well as salt that is included in a prepared sauce or recipe where the sodium cannot be reduced for an individual portion. In addition, many chefs cook with salt "to taste" that was not included in the recipes they provided for analysis. Therefore it's important to <u>specify very clearly</u> that you want "no added salt."

The double asterisk (**) next to the sodium values reminds you to specify "no added salt" to get the values as published.

Note: Many items included in this book are listed as "moderate" (meaning 600 to 1000 mg sodium per entree) or "high" in sodium (meaning above 1000 mg sodium per entree) and are <u>not</u> recommended for those watching sodium intake.

How the check mark guidelines for sodium are set

Of the 3000 mg of sodium recommended per day, we consider a value of 1000 mg per meal (⅓ of 3000) to be a reasonable level. We assume 600 mg can reasonably come from the main entree as a "Good Choice" value, and the remainder from side dishes. An "Excellent Choice" level is ½ of the "Good" value, or 300 mg:

✓✓ Excellent Choice = 0 to 300 mg sodium/entree
✓ Good Choice = 301 to 600 mg sodium/entree

Examples of "Excellent" and "Good" choices for sodium:

CHAYA Brasserie (Los Angeles)
KING SALMON WITH SUNDRIED TOMATOES
with sundried tomato basil pesto.
✓✓ SODIUM: Excellent Choice (165 mg)**

Riviera Mexican Grill (Redondo Beach)
PAPAYA & GRILLED CHICKEN SALAD
Field greens, sliced avocado and ripe papaya with charbroiled chicken breast and mango vinaigrette.
✓✓ SODIUM: Excellent Choice (170 mg)**

il forno (Santa Monica)
SCAMPI MEDITERRANEA
Scampi baked in the oven with a touch of brandy, fresh grapefruit juice,
green peppercorn and Dijon mustard. Served with seasonal vegetables.
✓ SODIUM: Good Choice (385 mg)**

Examples of "Good" and "Excellent" choices for sodium (continued):

Allegria (Malibu)
INSALATA DI MARE
Seafood salad of calamari, shrimp, clams & homemade marinated vegetables in a garlic & lemon vinaigrette.
✓✓ SODIUM· Excellent Choice (250 mg)**

Gaetano's (Torrance)
SWORDFISH - CATCH OF THE DAY
Fresh swordfish grilled with garlic, olive oil and lemon juice and served with assorted vegetables and pasta.
✓ SODIUM: Good Choice (350 mg)**

Pinot Restaurants (Studio City, Los Angeles, Hollywood, Pasadena)
JAPANESE SOBA NOODLES WITH GINGERED CHICKEN AND SHIITAKE BROTH
✓✓ SODIUM: Excellent Choice (165 mg)**

Café Santorini (Pasadena)
RISOTTO CON VERDURE ALLA GRIGLIA
Italian arborio rice with grilled vegetables, balsamic vinegar, garlic and chicken broth.
✓✓ SODIUM: Excellent Choice (80 mg)**

Zax (Brentwood)
GRILLED ALASKAN HALIBUT
with roasted fingerling potatoes, baby turnips, and haricots verts..
✓✓ SODIUM: Excellent Choice (235 mg)**

Malvasia (Long Beach)
NEW ZEALAND SEABASS WITH MANGO SALSA
Grilled and brushed with extra virgin olive oil, lemon and fresh herbs. Served with vegetables of the day and roast potatoes (potatoes not included in analysis).
✓✓ SODIUM: Excellent Choice (220 mg)**

CHAPTER 7

Protein, Carbohydrates & Diabetic Exchanges

Protein: the building blocks

Protein is very important for a healthy body. Protein provides materials for growth, helps to maintain and repair tissues, manufactures the lipoproteins to carry fat, and assists in the maintenance of proper fluid levels.

Generally it's easy to get protein in your diet, and most Americans consume 2 - 3 times more than necessary. Excess protein does not create muscle, as many hope, but is stored as fat. Excess protein puts a strain on the liver and kidneys. In addition, some protein sources are also high in fat, cholesterol and calories, such as: beef, whole milk products, eggs, poultry with skin, cheese and nuts.

The best sources of protein are low-fat foods, including fish, poultry without skin, skim or low-fat milk products and tofu. Whole grains, vegetables and especially legumes (dried beans, peas and lentils) also contain some protein. Unless you are a very strict vegetarian, you probably get adequate protein with a balanced diet. If you are a strict vegetarian, a dietitian can analyze your present diet to make sure you're getting adequate amounts of protein.

Carbohydrates: energy

Total carbohydrates are made up of simple sugars, complex carbohydrates, and fiber.

Simple carbohydrates. Sources of simple carbohydrates include table sugar, candies and other sweets, sodas and bakery goods. These foods contain little or no vitamins and minerals. They provide empty calories, i.e., calories that supply no nutrients and should therefore be minimized.

Fruits and some vegetables contain sugar naturally, and they also provide other nutrients, so they are valuable to a healthy diet. The sugar in simple carbohydrates is in a form that is absorbed quickly by the body, as opposed to the slower-digesting complex carbohydrates.

Complex carbohydrates. These carbohydrates contain many essential nutrients and are the body's most effective source of energy. They are very low in fat and should be the primary source of calories. It is recommended that 50% to 65% of total daily calories come from nutrient-dense carbohydrates. Foods high in complex carbohydrates include:

- breads and cereals
- dried beans, peas, and lentils
- rice and other grain products
- vegetables
- pasta

Dietary Fiber. The typical American diet is much too low in fiber. The American Cancer Society recommends 20 - 30 grams of fiber daily. The average American consumes only 7 - 8 grams of fiber daily. Dietary fiber is a term used to describe parts of plant foods that are generally not digestible by humans. By increasing your intake of foods containing complex carbohydrates, you will add dietary fiber to your diet.

There are two main types of fiber: soluble and insoluble. Soluble fiber may help lower blood cholesterol and control blood sugar and is found in oats, beans, carrots, apples and oranges. Insoluble fiber helps to move food through the body quickly and protect against colorectal cancer. Insoluble fiber is found in wheat bran and whole grains. Because both types of fiber have different functions for improving health, a variety of foods with fiber should be included in your diet. Fruits and vegetables are a significant source of nutrients and fiber. Thus, a diet rich in whole grains, breads, cereals, fruits and vegetables will provide optimal amounts of nutrients, fiber and energy.

Diabetic food exchanges

A well-balanced and carefully controlled diet is essential for those with diabetes. Recently carbohydrate counting is becoming more common as a way of choosing foods and serving sizes. The grams of carbohydrate are listed on most menu items in this *Healthy Dining* book. However "Diabetic Exchanges" was the system traditionally recommended by the American Diabetes Association and it is still used extensively. Foods are grouped into the various exchange lists according to their similarities in calories, carbohydrate, protein and fat content, which influence how they are utilized by the body. Although carbohydrates have the largest influence on blood sugar levels, protein and fat also contribute calories and influence the rates of digestion, so they are important to the overall plan.

Even for those without diabetes, exchanges can give useful information about portion size and the overall balance between protein and simple and complex carbohydrates, as explained below.

One meat exchange is equivalent to approximately 7 grams of protein and 3 grams of fat. One bread (starch) exchange contains approximately 15 grams of carbohydrate and 3 grams of protein. Starchy vegetables (potatoes, corn, beans, etc.) are counted as bread (starch) exchanges rather than vegetable exchanges. Vegetable exchanges have less starch (5 grams of carbohydrate and 2 grams of protein) and lots of fiber. A fruit exchange contains approximately 15 grams of more easily digested (simple) carbohydrate. A milk exchange contains 12 grams of carbohydrate, 8 grams of protein, and only a trace of fat, assuming skim milk is used. A fat exchange represents 5 grams of fat.

Some diabetic exchange lists use separate categories for lean, medium-fat, and high-fat meats. The computerized system used for the *Healthy Dining* analysis uses the lean meat category, which assumes approximately 7 grams of protein and 3 grams of fat per meat exchange. In most entrees included in the book, the meat is very lean and the total fat from the meat is lower than the 3 grams of fat per meat exchange normally assumed. In these cases we have designated the meat exchanges as "(extra lean)," which indicates that the meat exchange contains less fat than the assumed standard of 3 grams of fat per meat exchange. Any added fat from additional ingredients (e.g., butter or oil used in preparation, sauces, spreads, etc.) is counted as separate fat exchanges. This means that the fat exchanges reflect additional fat added to the meat.

In many entrees shown in this book, extra fat (often unsaturated) is added, but with the very lean meat, the total grams of fat still come out very low. So you don't necessarily need to shy away from a selection that shows fat exchanges. Looking at the grams of fat probably gives better information about the overall fat content.

The food exchange system used by some weight loss programs is similar to the diabetic food exchange system. A dietitian can help you interpret these numbers to meet your own dietary needs.

CHAPTER 8

Fruits & Vegetables – Nutrition Heavyweights

Science is finding that the saying "An apple a day keeps the doctor away" may be closer to the truth than most of us realize. And your mother was right — you should eat your vegetables! An abundance of research is in progress, and it is becoming increasingly clear that natural, whole foods such as fruits and vegetables contain more valuable substances than previously imagined, and certainly a more diverse range than available in nutrition supplements.

Fruits and vegetables deserve a special chapter in this book because of their importance in a healthy diet, and because their contributions overlap those of the other chapters so much. In addition to providing carbohydrates and high quality calories, they are packed full of other essentials — vitamins, minerals, fiber, antioxidants, and the more-recently discovered classes of compounds called phytochemicals (discussed in more detail below). Although numerical values are generally not available for these other substances, they are important and deserve special consideration as you make your food selections.

The World Health Organization, the National Cancer Institute, the American Cancer Society and other organizations emphasize a clear relationship between the amounts of fruits and vegetables consumed and several diseases, especially cancer and cardiovascular diseases. These organizations encourage Americans to eat at least 5 servings of fruits and vegetables each day. Eating "5 a day" is important to ensure that your body gets a variety of health-promoting nutrients. Research has shown that people who eat at least 5 servings of fruits and vegetables a day have only half the cancer risk of those who eat only one or two servings a day.

Fruits and vegetables are nutritional powerhouses which:

- are excellent sources of vitamins and minerals
- contain fiber (most Americans don't eat enough fiber)
- are virtually fat-free (exceptions: coconut, olives and avocado) and cholesterol-free
- are particularly helpful in weight management, due to their high-fiber and low-fat content
- contain antioxidants and phytochemicals (discussed below)

Vitamins and minerals

Vitamins and minerals are essential for many bodily functions. They play a prominent role in maintaining the health of the brain, heart, bones, teeth and nerves, in making and repairing red blood cells, in regulating the body's balance of fluids, and in other vital functions. The absence of any one vitamin or mineral may result in a unique deficiency that can only be corrected by supplying that specific nutrient. In some cases, people who have a certain disease or condition may need to adjust their intake of a particular vitamin or mineral. However, consuming mega (large) doses of certain fat-soluble vitamins (particularly vitamins A and D) can be toxic. It's best to get most of your vitamins and minerals from natural, healthy foods.

It is important to consume a wide variety of fruits and vegetables in order to benefit fully from the antioxidants, vitamins and minerals they contain. For example, the following tables show fruits and vegetables that contain significant amounts of Vitamins A and C (the other major vitamins B, D and E come primarily from other food sources such as grains, seeds, nuts, dairy or meat):

<u>Fruits and Vegetables High in Vitamin A</u>:

Apricots (fresh or dried)	Broccoli	Carrots	Chinese cabbage
Cantaloupe & melons	Collards & other greens	Green onions	Mangoes
Papayas	Peaches & Nectarines	Persimmons	Spinach
Tomatoes	Sweet potatoes	Winter squash & pumpkins	

<u>Fruits and Vegetables High in Vitamin C</u>:

Bell peppers	Broccoli	Brussels sprouts	Cantaloupe & melons
Cauliflower	Grapefruit	Guavas	Kiwifruit
Lemons & other citrus	Mangoes	Oranges	Papayas
Raspberries	Strawberries		

Notice that there is little overlap among the fruits and vegetables that are high in vitamins A and C. Some fruits and vegetables that don't appear on either list may be high in other important nutrients. For example, bananas are high in potassium. Some fruits and vegetables, especially leafy green vegetables, citrus, berries, melons, and beans are high in folate (from "foliage"), a B vitamin important in preventing heart disease, some types of anemia, and neural tube birth defects. There is no one food that "has it all." So be careful not to depend on a limited selection of fruits and vegetables to supply your nutrients. A glass of orange juice at breakfast and carrots at dinner, for example, move you toward your "5 a day" goal, but a wider variety of fruits and vegetables throughout the day is optimal.

Antioxidants

Antioxidants are disease-fighting compounds found in many foods. They neutralize free radicals, compounds that damage cells and lead to cardiovascular disease, cancer, cataracts, premature aging, and impaired immunity. Antioxidants include some vitamins (A, C, and E), beta carotene, some minerals (for example, selenium, copper, zinc, and manganese) and some of the phytochemicals discussed below. Fruits and vegetables are excellent sources of many of these antioxidants.

Phytochemicals

Phytochemicals are substances found in plant foods that are now recognized as powerful disease-fighting compounds. They have been shown to protect against cancer, cardiovascular disease, diabetes, and other medical conditions. "Phyto" means plant, and chemicals — well not all chemicals are bad for you. Our bodies are made of chemicals, and some kinds are essential for our health. Fruits and vegetables contain thousands, perhaps tens or hundreds of thousands of different phytochemical compounds.

Scientists have grouped phytochemicals into at least 14 different classes, but still little is known about their functions and their interactions. Many appear to stimulate or block the effects of enzymes in the body, some of which can fight diseases such as cancer or cardiovascular disease. Some phytochemicals have received a great deal of media attention, such as resveratrol, a substance found in grapes that appears to lower blood cholesterol. The resveratrol in grapes may explain the initial studies showing a beneficial effect of wine in reducing the risk of cardiovascular disease. Soybeans contain genistein, which nutritionists now link to lowering hormone-related cancer risk and stimulating the immune system. Other examples include the vegetables from the cabbage family (cabbage, brussel sprouts and broccoli), which contain phytochemicals that interact with estrogens and prostaglandins in fighting cancer.

A phytochemical-rich diet includes lots of fruits, vegetables, legumes (beans, peas and lentils), herbs and spices, whole grains, soy products, and also tea and nuts. With literally thousands of different phytochemicals already identified, this area of nutrition continues to be a rich field for scientific study. The table below lists beneficial effects of some of the fruits and vegetables studied so far.

Food:	Beneficial effects:
Berries, melons, cucumbers, squash & pumpkins	Aids immune system and helps lower blood cholesterol
Broccoli & cabbage family and leafy green vegetables	Lowers risk of hormone-related cancers, boosts ability to fight cancer and protects DNA in cells
Carrots, apricots, other orange & deep yellow fruits & vegetables	Helps protect against cancer, plaque in arteries, blood clotting and loss of eyesight
Citrus (orange, grapefruit, lemon, lime)	Helps body resist carcinogens, avoid blindness, and prevents blood clotting
Grapes (red)	Prevents blood clotting, protects DNA in cells and helps body resist carcinogens
Onions, garlic, leeks & chives	Controls cancer cells, blocks carcinogens, eliminates toxins & lowers blood cholesterol
Soybeans and soy foods	Helps block hormone-related cancers, slow tumor growth, and stimulate the immune system
Tomatoes & eggplant	Shields against carcinogens, reduces cancer and heart attack risk

The most effective approach is to eat as wide a variety of foods as possible to gain benefits from many sources. Studies have demonstrated that not all the foods listed above have the same cancer or blood cholesterol-fighting substances, and the phytochemicals may appear in different concentrations or be absorbed differently. Even different varieties of foods within the same category (such as various varieties of apples or lettuce) may have widely varying concentrations and kinds of phytochemicals. Unfortunately, there is no "magic" pill or supplement which can supply as much as whole foods can, or we would have long ago found an easier way to combat diet-related diseases such as cancer, heart disease, diabetes, and obesity.

What is considered one serving?

Fruits
1 medium whole fruit (apple, banana)
½ cup of canned or fresh fruit
6 oz. (or ¾ cup) 100% fruit juice
¼ cup of dried fruit

Vegetables
½ cup of raw or cooked vegetables
1 cup raw, leafy vegetables
6 oz. (or ¾ cup) vegetable juice

How can I get more fruits and vegetables in my diet?

For a snack or on the go, select nectarines, plums, berries, apple wedges, baby carrots, broccoli spears, or cherry tomatoes. Also, dried fruit is a healthy option over candy. You can easily pack it in a bag and take it with you on the road or eat it at your office.

At home, top your hot or cold cereal with fresh fruit, and drink a glass of 100% juice for breakfast. Smoothies made with fresh or frozen fruits and juices make a great breakfast or lunch choice. Fruit and vegetable juices are also delicious, sweet alternatives to soft drinks. At dinner, include a salad or raw vegetables with low-fat/non-fat dressing to reduce fat and calories. Steamed vegetables are always a good side dish, but you can also add vegetables to your favorite entrees, like tacos, lasagna, casseroles, and pasta dishes. Add pureed vegetables to sauces to fortify them and help get your "5 a day." Try more vegetarian meals, like tofu, rice or pasta with vegetables, or Oriental stir-fries. For dessert, bake apples, peaches, pears, or bananas, or make fruit cobblers.

Experiment with new recipes that emphasize fruits and vegetables, such as those starting on page 133 of this *Healthy Dining* book. Many cookbooks specialize in fruits, vegetables and other natural foods so you can try great-tasting dishes that will help you toward your 5 a Day goal. The California 5 a Day — for Better Health! Campaign offers a recipe booklet "Discover the Secret" which has 37 wonderful recipes incorporating fruits and vegetables. You can obtain a free copy of this recipe booklet and other information by contacting 1-888-EAT-FIVE or www.ca5aday.com.

When dining out, order meals that include vegetables or fruits as a major component. For example, Chicken with Vegetables at **Pick Up Stix**, will provide better nutritional balance than a dish with chicken alone. **Roundtable's** Gourmet Veggie Pizza, which includes artichoke hearts, zucchini, spinach, mushrooms and tomatoes, is a better choice than plain cheese pizza. For a quick meal and a great contribution to your "5 a day," try a blended fruit smoothie at **Jamba Juice**. You can also request substitutions for side dishes. For example, if French fries normally come as part of a meal, request steamed vegetables or seasonal fresh fruit instead. Most restaurants are happy to make substitutions if you ask.

In choosing a restaurant meal from this book, you can determine if the meal contributes significantly to your "5 a day" goal. Look for the ☙ symbol next to the entrée's name. The ☙ indicates the dish provides at least 2 servings of fruits or vegetables (one serving for side dishes).

Examples of Restaurant Meals with two or more servings of fruits or vegetables

Acapulco (25 Los Angeles locations)
HALIBUT TACOS ☙
Unique...delicious! Grilled filet of Alaskan halibut, our fresh cabbage slaw, and
a touch of Mexican spices rolled in two flour tortillas. Served with fresh vegetables and rice.
✓ CALORIES: Good Choice (660)   ✓✓ CHOLESTEROL: Excellent Choice (35 mg)
✓ FAT: Good Choice (25 g)*   SODIUM: High (1485 mg)
EXCHANGES: 2¼ Meat (extra lean), 4 Bread, 2¾ Veg, 4½ Fat
PROTEIN: 36 g, CARBOHYDRATE: 77 g, FIBER: 4 g

China Grill (Manhattan Beach)
GRILLED SEA SCALLOPS WITH JULIENNED SQUASH ☙
in black bean chili sauce.
✓✓ CALORIES: Excellent Choice (430)   ✓ CHOLESTEROL: Good Choice (105 mg)
✓ FAT: Good Choice (17 g)*   SODIUM: High (1124 mg)**
EXCHANGES: 3¾ Meat (extra lean), ¼ Bread, 1¼ Veg, ½ Fruit, 2¾ Fat
PROTEIN: 48 g, CARBOHYDRATE: 25 g, FIBER: 2 g

Examples of Restaurant Meals with fruits or vegetables (continued):

Chang's of Brentwood (Brentwood)
WESTLAKE HOT FISH ☃

White fish filets sautéed & served spicy hot in sweet & sour sauce with bell peppers, mushrooms & chili.

✓ CALORIES: Good Choice (550) CHOLESTEROL: Moderate (230 mg)
✓✓ FAT: Excellent Choice (7 g)* ✓ SODIUM: Good Choice (365 mg)**
EXCHANGES: 11½ Meat (extra lean), 1 Bread, 2¼ Veg, ¼ Fat
PROTEIN: 85 g, CARBOHYDRATE: 33 g, FIBER: 5 g

Il Forno (Santa Monica)
SPAGHETTI VECCHIO STYLE ☃

Spaghetti with eggplant, mushrooms, parsley, basil and radicchio in homemade tomato sauce.

✓ CALORIES: Good Choice (495) ✓✓ CHOLESTEROL: Excellent Choice (0 mg)
✓✓ FAT: Excellent Choice (3 g)* ✓✓ SODIUM: Excellent Choice (30 mg)**
EXCHANGES: 5½ Bread, 2¾ Veg
PROTEIN: 18 g, CARBOHYDRATE: 100 g, FIBER: 9 g

Chin Chin (7 Los Angeles locations)
LITE SHRIMP WITH BLACK BEANS ☃

Plump shrimp with green bell pepper, carrots and onions in a garlic and black bean sauce.

✓✓ CALORIES: Excellent Choice (405) CHOLESTEROL: Moderate (275 mg)
✓✓ FAT: Excellent Choice (2 g)* SODIUM: High (3560 mg)
EXCHANGES: 4¼ Meat (extra lean), ½ Bread, 5¼ Veg
PROTEIN: 35 g, CARBOHYDRATE: 57 g, FIBER: 6 g

Junior's (West Los Angeles)
VEGETABLE OMELETTE WITH EGG WHITES – SPECIAL REQUEST ☃

Served with fresh fruit and toasted rye bread. Request egg whites.

✓✓ CALORIES: Excellent Choice (295) ✓✓ CHOLESTEROL: Excellent Choice (0 mg)
✓✓ FAT: Excellent Choice (2 g)* SODIUM: Moderate (655 mg)**
EXCHANGES: 3¾ Meat (extra lean), 1 Bread, 1¼ Veg, 1 Fruit, ¼ Fat
PROTEIN: 33 g, CARBOHYDRATE: 37 g, FIBER: 5 g

Jamba Juice (50 locations in Los Angeles)
CARIBBEAN PASSION™ SMOOTHIE *(24 oz.)* ☃

Passionfruit mango juice, peaches, strawberries, orange sherbet and ice.

✓✓ CALORIES: Excellent Choice (415) ✓✓ CHOLESTEROL: Excellent Choice (10 mg)
✓✓ FAT: Excellent Choice (2 g) ✓✓ SODIUM: Excellent Choice (70 mg)
PROTEIN: 4 g, CARBOHYDRATE: 105 g

Rosti (Beverly Hills, Brentwood, Encino, Santa Monica, and Westlake)
PENNE PUTTANESCA – SPECIAL REQUEST ☃

Penne with capers, olives, white wine and garlic in a pomodoro sauce with herbs. Request less oil (½ oz.).

✓ CALORIES: Good Choice (540) ✓✓ CHOLESTEROL: Excellent Choice (0 mg)
✓ FAT: Good Choice (19 g)* SODIUM: High (1345 mg)**
EXCHANGES: 4¼ Bread, 2¼ Veg, 2¾ Fat
PROTEIN: 14 g, CARBOHYDRATE: 78 g, FIBER: 6 g

* Primarily unsaturated fat
** If you request no added salt

CHAPTER 9

Additional Tips for Healthy Dining

Here are some additional dining tips, adapted from "Eating Better When Eating Out," from the USDA Human Nutrition Information Service:

Appetizers: Enjoy raw vegetables dipped in salsa or low-calorie dressing, fruit or steamed seafood. Limit rich sauces, dips and batter-fried foods.

Soups: Choose broth or tomato-based soups rather than creamed soups. Lentil, bean and split pea soups are high in fiber. Most soups are high in sodium.

Breads: Bread supplies complex carbohydrates, vitamins, and minerals. Whole grain breads provide fiber. Watch out for breads with added fat or sugar such as croissants, biscuits, cornbread, muffins (e.g., bran, corn, blueberry) and sweet rolls. Use toppings (butter, cream cheese and margarine) very sparingly.

Vegetables and Salads: Plain vegetables are high in fiber and nutrients and very low in calories, fat and sodium. However, butter, margarine and sauces increase calories, fat, cholesterol and sodium considerably. Look for vegetables seasoned with lemon, herbs or spices rather than fat and salt. Remember -- salad dressings and toppings can add a lot of calories, fat and sodium.

Watch out for prepared salads that contain mayonnaise, salad dressing or oil, such as macaroni salad, potato salad, creamy coleslaw, tuna and chicken salad, and marinated vegetables. Some pasta salads are made with large amounts of oily dressing.

Main Entrees: Ask how meals are prepared and what ingredients are used. Is the fish or chicken broiled with butter or other fat? Is it served with a sauce? How large is the portion? Are vegetables fresh or canned, buttered or creamed?

Fish or poultry that is broiled, grilled, baked, steamed or poached is a good choice. However, entrees are often basted with large amounts of fat. Ask to have your entree prepared without added fat, and that chicken be prepared without skin (or remove the skin before eating). Request that lemon juice, wine or only a small amount of fat be used and that no salt be added.

Watch out for menu selections termed "light fare" or "light." "Light" may or may not mean lower in fat and calories. We have found restaurants in which "On the Light Side" means anything from smaller portions to lower prices!

Choose dishes flavored with herbs and spices rather than rich sauces, gravies, or dressings. If that's not an option, ask for gravies, sour cream, sauces, and other toppings to be served on the side and use sparingly. Limit your use of soy sauce, steak sauce, catsup, mustard, pickles and other condiments to help control sodium.

Portions are often very large. Ask for a take-home bag and eat the remaining portion the next day. Or share an entree with a friend and get an extra appetizer.

Many stir-fried entrees are prepared with very little oil, while some are prepared with too much. Request that yours be prepared with very little.

Pizza can be a low-fat, nutritious choice if you order yours with half the cheese and only vegetable toppings.

Sandwiches can be an excellent choice if you choose lean deli meats such as turkey or ham (but watch portion size!) instead of higher fat cold cuts, such as bologna or salami. Choose whole grain breads and go easy on or avoid oil, butter, avocado, and mayonnaise.

Desserts: Fruits are great! Sherbet, sorbet and frozen yogurt are much lower in fat than ice cream. If temptation gets to you, share the dessert with a dinner partner.

Words that signal _high fat_ include:

buttered or buttery	creamed or creamy	rich
scalloped	fried	breaded
fritters	tempura	croquettes
crispy	with gravy	in cheese sauce
Hollandaise	au gratin	à la king
Béarnaise	Alfredo	Newburg

Words that signal _high sodium_ include:

smoked	barbecued	pickled
broth	soy sauce	teriyaki
Creole sauce	marinated	cocktail sauce
tomato base	Parmesan	mustard sauce

Appendix:
Analysis Methods and Accuracy

How is the nutrition analysis done?

Using recipes supplied by the restaurant, a computerized nutritional analysis is performed with the Nutritionist IV computer program. Research shows the Nutritionist IV Program to be one of the most current and reliable nutrition analysis programs available. It uses the US Department of Agriculture (USDA) database. We regularly update our program with new data values published by the USDA. When values for recipe ingredients are not available from the USDA database, we contact the manufacturer for nutritional information. If the manufacturer does not have nutritional information, we match ingredients as closely as possible to another product, which does have nutritional information.

The numbers coming from the USDA database and the computer analysis imply a high degree of accuracy. In reality, the USDA found that nutritional values of foods can vary between similar food samples by as much as 20%, and the numbers coming from their measurements represent their average data. As recommended by the FDA, we rounded the data as follows: for calories, cholesterol and sodium, to the nearest 5 (mg). For fat, protein and carbohydrates, to the nearest whole number, and for diabetic exchanges to the nearest ¼ exchange. Therefore it is important to note that the numerical values for the selected menu items published in this book are approximations only.

Notes about accuracy

The most accurate method to obtain nutritional information is a chemical analysis performed in a professional laboratory. That is, in fact, how the USDA obtained the information for their database. It is very expensive (over $1,000 per item) and time-consuming, and therefore not feasible for this project. Every effort was made to ensure accurate information from the computerized analysis and the USDA database.

Two main obstacles were encountered with the computerized analysis. First, how much marinade do meats actually absorb? Second, how much oil is absorbed in flash-frying (a method commonly used in Chinese foods)? After numerous conversations with experts throughout the U.S., we found that there has been very little research in these areas. As recommended by nutritionists at the USDA and the Human Nutrition Information Service, we calculate that one gram per one ounce of marinade is absorbed, and that one teaspoon per six ounces of meat is absorbed with flash-frying.

Part II
Healthy Dining Menus

Arranged alphabetically
Also see indexes at back, arranged by cuisine, location, and alphabetically.

Summary of check mark system:

ENTREE GUIDELINES†

Calories	✓✓ Excellent Choice = 0 to 450 calories/entree
	✓ Good Choice = 451 to 750 calories/entree
Fat	✓✓ Excellent Choice = 0 to 15 grams (g)/entree
	✓ Good Choice = 16 to 25 grams (g)/entree
Cholesterol	✓✓ Excellent Choice = 0 to 75 milligrams (mg)/entree
	✓ Good Choice = 76 to 150 milligrams (mg)/entree
Sodium	✓✓ Excellent Choice = 0 to 300 milligrams (mg)/entree
	✓ Good Choice = 301 to 600 milligrams (mg)/entree

Footnotes
*   Primarily unsaturated fat
**   If you request no added salt
†   Side dish guidelines are ⅓ of entree guidelines
🍎   at least 2 fruit/vegetable servings

Price Range Symbols
$ Average entree under $10
$$ Average entree $10 - $20
$$$ Average entree over $20

Special Request - modification of the usual restaurant recipe or preparation method. You must ask for the "Special Request" for the dish to correspond to the published nutrition information.

ACAPULCO

MEXICAN RESTAURANT Y CANTINA

Voted #1 Mexican Restaurant for two years in a row by the Readers of La Opinion Newspaper. Acapulco Restaurant offers a festive atmosphere to enjoy deliciously prepared Mexican dishes. Acapulco's executive chef has worked with time-tested recipes to refine their food for the more health conscious guest. Please stop in and enjoy a delicious, health-consciously prepared meal at Acapulco Mexican Restaurant. $

Acapulco participating locations: Atwater, Azusa, Burbank, Cerritos, Del Amo, Downey, Glendale, Hollywood, La Cienega, Los Angeles, Manhattan Beach, Montclair, Monrovia, Moreno Valley, Northridge, Pasadena, Puente Hills, San Pedro, Santa Fe Springs, Santa Monica, Simi Valley, Sun Valley, Ventura, Westwood & Woodland Hills. For more participating locations, call (800) 735-3501 or visit www.acapulcorestaurants.com.

HALIBUT FILET WITH TOMATILLO SAUCE – SPECIAL REQUEST ☙
Filet of halibut grilled with distinctly delicious
tomatillo sauce. Served with rice and fresh vegetables.
<u>*Request Healthy Dining preparation.*</u>
- ✓ CALORIES: Good Choice (545)
- ✓ FAT: Good Choice (17 g)*
- ✓ CHOLESTEROL: Good Choice (80 mg)
- SODIUM: High (1330 mg)

EXCHANGES: 4½ Meat (extra lean), 2 Bread, 1¾ Veg, 2 Fat
PROTEIN: 55 g, CARBOHYDRATE: 43 g, FIBER: 4 g

ENCHILADAS RANCHERAS – SPECIAL REQUEST ☙
Two corn tortillas filled with grilled chicken and topped
with salsa ranchera. Served with black beans and fresh vegetables.
<u>*Request Healthy Dining preparation.*</u>
- ✓ CALORIES: Good Choice (560)
- ✓ FAT: Good Choice (17 g)
- ✓ CHOLESTEROL: Good Choice (80 mg)
- SODIUM: High (1000 mg)

EXCHANGES: 4 Meat (extra lean), 3 Bread, 1¾ Veg, 2½ Fat
PROTEIN: 42 g, CARBOHYDRATE: 59 g, FIBER: 10 g

HALIBUT TACOS – SPECIAL REQUEST ☙
Unique...delicious! Grilled filet of Alaskan halibut, our fresh cabbage slaw, and
a touch of Mexican spices rolled in two flour tortillas. Served with fresh vegetables and rice.
<u>*Request Healthy Dining preparation.*</u>
- ✓ CALORIES: Good Choice (660)
- ✓ FAT: Good Choice (25 g)*
- ✓✓ CHOLESTEROL: Excellent Choice (35 mg)
- SODIUM: High (1485 mg)

EXCHANGES: 2¼ Meat (extra lean), 4 Bread, 2¾ Veg, 4½ Fat
PROTEIN: 36 g, CARBOHYDRATE: 77 g, FIBER: 4 g

☙ at least 2 fruit/vegetable servings
✓ Good Choice   ✓✓ Excellent Choice

Allegria

The dictionary defines "allegria" as "joy" and "gaiety" --- food reviewers have called it "the best Italian restaurant to open this year" (Merrill Shindler), and "another hit," serving "real country cooking" with "exemplary" service (Los Angeles Times). Allegria is a restaurant that you can take your family to for an early dinner, or enjoy later in the evening for a relaxed and intimate meal with friends. If you can't make it for a meal in the original watery city, Allegria might just be the next best thing! $ - $$

Allegria 22821 Pacific Coast Hwy., Malibu, CA 90265 (310) 456-3132

CALAMARI AFFOGATI - SPECIAL REQUEST ☺
Sautéed calamari with green peas in a spicy tomato sauce. Request less oil (½ oz.).

✓✓ CALORIES: Excellent Choice (335)   CHOLESTEROL: Moderate (265 mg)
✓ FAT: Good Choice (18 g)   ✓ SODIUM: Good Choice (445 mg)**
EXCHANGES: 2½ Meat (extra lean), ½ Bread, 1¾ Veg, 3¼ Fat
PROTEIN: 23 g, CARBOHYDRATE: 22 g, FIBER: 5 g

INSALATA DI MARE ☺
Seafood salad of calamari, shrimp, clams & homemade marinated vegetables in a garlic & lemon vinaigrette.

✓✓ CALORIES: Excellent Choice (320)   CHOLESTEROL: Moderate (250 mg)
✓ FAT: Good Choice (16 g)*   ✓✓ SODIUM: Excellent Choice (250 mg)**
EXCHANGES: 3¼ Meat (extra lean), 2¼ Veg, ¼ Fruit, 2¾ Fat
PROTEIN: 28 g, CARBOHYDRATE: 21 g, FIBER: 6 g

SPAGHETTI ALLEGRIA - SPECIAL REQUEST
Sautéed clams, arugula, chopped tomatoes with roasted garlic and wine sauce. Request less oil (½ oz.).

✓ CALORIES: Good Choice (635)   ✓✓ CHOLESTEROL: Excellent Choice (40 mg)
✓ FAT: Good Choice (17 g)*   ✓ SODIUM: Good Choice (360 mg)**
EXCHANGES: 2 Meat (extra lean), 5¼ Bread, 1 Veg, 2¾ Fat
PROTEIN: 30 g, CARBOHYDRATE: 88 g, FIBER: 5 g

PIZZA ORTOLANA (½ PIZZA)
Focaccina topped with fresh chopped tomatoes, garlic, basil and olive oil. Analysis is for ½ pizza.

✓✓ CALORIES: Excellent Choice (375)   ✓✓ CHOLESTEROL: Excellent Choice (0 mg)
✓ FAT: Good Choice (16 g)*   SODIUM: Moderate (630 mg)**
EXCHANGES: 2¾ Bread, 1¼ Veg, 3 Fat
PROTEIN: 7 g, CARBOHYDRATE: 52 g, FIBER: 3 g

CAPPELINI ALLA CHECCA - SPECIAL REQUEST ☺
Angel hair pasta with fresh organic tomatoes, roasted garlic, fresh basil & olive oil Request less oil (1 Tbs.).

✓ CALORIES: Good Choice (620)   ✓✓ CHOLESTEROL: Excellent Choice (5 mg)
✓ FAT: Good Choice (19 g)*   ✓ SODIUM: Good Choice (600 mg)**
EXCHANGES: 5¼ Bread, 3¼ Veg, 3¼ Fat
PROTEIN: 17 g, CARBOHYDRATE: 98 g, FIBER: 8 g

MINESTRONE SOUP†
Old fashioned farmer style fresh vegetable soup.

✓✓ CALORIES: Excellent Choice (65)   ✓ CHOLESTEROL: Good Choice (30 mg)
✓✓ FAT: Excellent Choice (3 g)*   SODIUM: Moderate (220 mg)**
EXCHANGES: ¼ Bread, ¾ Veg
PROTEIN: 9 g, CARBOHYDRATE: 8 g, FIBER: 1 g

---

* Primarily unsaturated fat
** If you request no added salt

† Side dish guidelines are 1/3 of entree guidelines

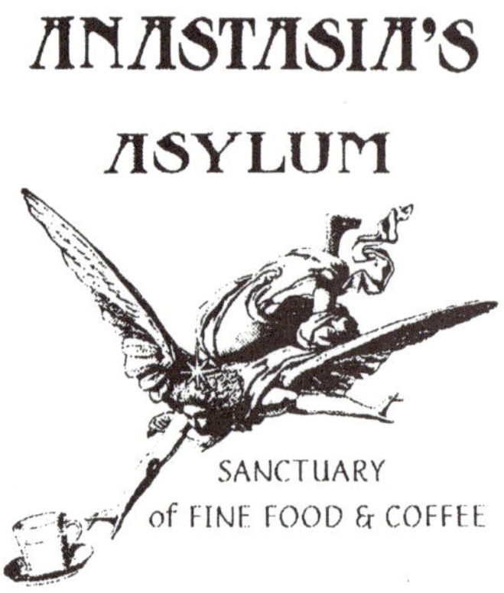

ANASTASIA'S ASYLUM
SANCTUARY of FINE FOOD & COFFEE

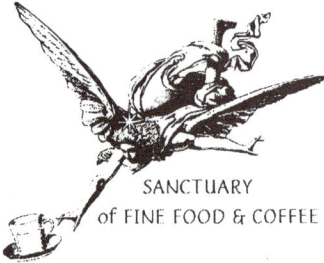

This unique, 10 year old, award winning café combines a beautiful interior design with rotating art exhibits and nightly music performances, and sets a high standard for its moderately priced, and surprisingly varied menu. Anastasia's Asylum features a wide range of delicious and healthy menu options, many of them vegetarian, including quesadillas, panini sandwiches, salads, burritos and soups, as well as a number of chicken and tuna entrees. It has excellent coffee, espresso and specialty drinks as well as a large assortment of outstanding desserts. Anastasia's Asylum is an extremely popular café delivering high quality breakfast, lunch and dinner, available 6:30am until midnight, 7 days a week. $

Anastasia's Asylum
SANCTUARY OF FINE FOOD AND COFFEE
1028 Wilshire Boulevard, Santa Monica 90401 (310) 394-7113

ANASTASIA'S FAMOUS VEGETARIAN LASAGNA
[handwritten: ← 3 Pts ☺]
Anastasia's secret recipe.

✓✓ CALORIES: Excellent Choice (150)   ✓✓ CHOLESTEROL: Excellent Choice (10 mg)
✓✓ FAT: Excellent Choice (4 g)   ✓✓ SODIUM: Excellent Choice (195 mg)**
EXCHANGES: ¾ Meat, 1 Bread, 1 Veg, ¼ Fat   *[handwritten: dairy?]*
PROTEIN: 11 g, CARBOHYDRATE: 20 g, FIBER: 5 g

ANASTASIA'S NICOISE ☙
Albacore tuna, tomatoes, red onions, artichoke hearts and kalamata olives.

✓✓ CALORIES: Excellent Choice (285)   ✓✓ CHOLESTEROL: Excellent Choice (45 mg)
✓✓ FAT: Excellent Choice (11 g)*   SODIUM: Moderate (630 mg)**
EXCHANGES: 4¼ Meat (extra lean), 2 Veg, 1¼ Fat
PROTEIN: 34 g, CARBOHYDRATE: 13 g, FIBER: 5 g

QUESADILLA ISABELLA
Artichoke hearts, avocado, mild Ortega chiles and mozzarella.

✓✓ CALORIES: Excellent Choice (390)   ✓✓ CHOLESTEROL: Excellent Choice (30 mg)
✓ FAT: Good Choice (16 g)   SODIUM: Moderate (730 mg)**
EXCHANGES: 1¾ Meat, 2 Bread, 1½ Veg, 2½ Fat
PROTEIN: 22 g, CARBOHYDRATE: 43 g, FIBER: 8 g

OPEN FACE TOFU VEGGIE MELT ☙
[handwritten: ← 4 Pts ☺]
Grilled tofu, artichoke hearts, sundried tomatoes, red peppers and melted mozzarella. *[handwritten: Sub soy cheese?]*

✓✓ CALORIES: Excellent Choice (235)   ✓✓ CHOLESTEROL: Excellent Choice (15 mg)
✓✓ FAT: Excellent Choice (6 g)   ✓ SODIUM: Good Choice (520 mg)**
EXCHANGES: 2 Meat, 2¼ Veg, ¼ Fat
PROTEIN: 20 g, CARBOHYDRATE: 29 g, FIBER: 4 g

VEGGIE POT PIE ☙
[handwritten: 9 Pts!]
Baked flaky pie crust filled with fresh vegetables and baked tofu.

✓✓ CALORIES: Excellent Choice (440)   ✓✓ CHOLESTEROL: Excellent Choice (0 mg)
✓✓ FAT: Excellent Choice (6 g)*   ✓✓ SODIUM: Excellent Choice (170 mg)**
EXCHANGES: ¾ Meat, 4¾ Bread, 1½ Veg, ¾ Fat
PROTEIN: 16 g, CARBOHYDRATE: 81 g, FIBER: 5 g

GRILLED TOFU & PEAR SALAD
Tofu, cucumbers, pears & sunseeds tossed with pear vinaigrette.

✓✓ CALORIES: Excellent Choice (275)   ✓✓ CHOLESTEROL: Excellent Choice (0 mg)
✓ FAT: Good Choice (16 g)*   ✓✓ SODIUM: Excellent Choice (110 mg)**
EXCHANGES: 1¼ Meat, 1 Fruit, 2¾ Fat
PROTEIN: 15 g, CARBOHYDRATE: 24 g, FIBER: 5 g

☙ at least 2 fruit/vegetable servings
✓ Good Choice   ✓✓ Excellent Choice

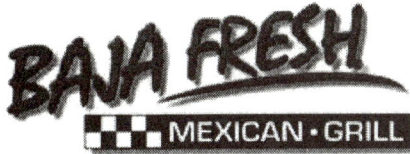

Baja Fresh is not your ordinary Mexican restaurant. All of our food is prepared fresh at each location. This ensures the FRESH, quality difference that you taste in our food. We believe we have developed recipes that provide you with the fullest and most pleasing FLAVORS for each of our offerings. While we have worked to develop products that reflect the best FLAVORS and quality for each of our items, many of our customers modify their orders to satisfy their individual taste or dietary needs (i.e., no onions, no sour cream, etc.). $

Baja Fresh Locations

Locations in: Alhambra, Bakersfield, Belmont Shores, Beverly Hills, Burbank, Beverly Connection, Brentwood, Encino, Canyon Country, Chatsworth, Culver City, Glendale, La Crescenta, Lakewood, Long Beach, Manhattan Beach, Marina Del Rey, Miracle Mile, Monrovia, Northridge, Palmdale, East Pasadena, South Pasadena, Porter Ranch, Rowland Heights, Santa Monica, Sherman Oaks, Studio City, Toluca Lake, Torrance, Valencia, West Hills, West Hollywood, West L.A., Westwood, Whittier, Woodland Hills. For a complete list of all locations visit www.bajafresh.com.

ENCHILADAS VERANO
Charbroiled chicken, grilled peppers, chilis & onions, topped with salsa verde & shaved cheese, served with rice, beans, and pico de gallo.

✓ CALORIES: Good Choice (580)   ✓✓ CHOLESTEROL: Excellent Choice (60 mg)
✓✓ FAT: Excellent Choice (9 g)   SODIUM: High (2140 mg)
PROTEIN: 38 g, CARBOHYDRATE: 87 g, Fiber 21 g

BARE BURRITO (SERVED IN A BOWL, NO TORTILLA)
Charbroiled chicken, grilled peppers, chilis & onions, rice, beans, pico de gallo and salsa verde.

✓ CALORIES: Good Choice (650)   ✓✓ CHOLESTEROL: Excellent Choice (75 mg)
✓✓ FAT: Excellent Choice (7 g)   SODIUM: High (2410 mg)
PROTEIN: 45 g, CARBOHYDRATE: 99 g, Fiber 22 g

VEGETARIAN BARE BURRITO (SERVED IN A BOWL, NO TORTILLA)
Grilled peppers, chilis & onions, rice, beans, lettuce, jack cheese, pico de gallo and "Salsa Baja."

✓ CALORIES: Good Choice (560)   ✓✓ CHOLESTEROL: Excellent Choice (10 mg)
✓✓ FAT: Excellent Choice (8 g)   SODIUM: High (2040 mg)
PROTEIN: 20 g, CARBOHYDRATE: 102 g, Fiber 22 g → wow

GRILLED VEGGIE TACOS
Two soft tacos on corn tortillas, shaved cheese, guacamole, beans, grilled peppers, chilis & onions, lettuce, pico de gallo and salsa verde.

✓✓ CALORIES: Excellent Choice (420)   ✓✓ CHOLESTEROL: Excellent Choice (10 mg)
✓✓ FAT: Excellent Choice (10 g)   ✓✓ SODIUM: Excellent Choice (110 mg)
PROTEIN: 16 g, CARBOHYDRATE: 72 g, Fiber 14 g

BAJA MAHI MAHI TACO
Fresh mahi mahi, sliced avocado, cabbage, fresh pico de gallo salsa, and zesty avocado salsa.

✓✓ CALORIES: Excellent Choice (260)   ✓✓ CHOLESTEROL: Excellent Choice (20 mg)
✓✓ FAT: Excellent Choice (10 g)   ✓ SODIUM: Good Choice (460 mg)
PROTEIN: 13 g, CARBOHYDRATE: 32 g, Fiber 6 g

FRESH MAHI MAHI ENSALADA
Charbroiled mahi mahi, romaine lettuce, pico de gallo & salsa verde, topped with avocado, tomato slices and shaved cheese.

✓✓ CALORIES: Excellent Choice (280)   ✓✓ CHOLESTEROL: Excellent Choice (70 mg)
✓✓ FAT: Excellent Choice (9 g)   SODIUM: High (1010 mg)
PROTEIN: 34 g, CARBOHYDRATE: 20 g, Fiber 7 g

Nutrition information provided by Baja Fresh.

* Primarily unsaturated fat
** If you request no added salt

Established in 1982, BeauRivage is the premier Mediterranean restaurant to offer innovative as well as authentic and creative specialties from the countries bordering this captivating sea. Our award-winning chef will delight in preparing the freshest food with delicate sauces or simply treated, grilled, or steamed with locally grown fresh herbs. Located on the shore of the Pacific, BeauRivage offers a breathtaking view from every one of its seven dining areas, including the spectacular patio or the romantic atmosphere with candlelight and fireplace featuring soft piano or guitar dinner music. $$$

BeauRivage   26025 W. Pacific Coast Highway, Malibu, CA 90265 (310) 456-5733
(2 miles north of Pepperdine at Corral Canyon)

BEAURIVAGE SALADE EXOTIQUE ☾
Hearts of palm, Belgian endive, watercress and tomatoes with Chutney Vinaigrette.

✓✓ CALORIES: Excellent Choice (185)   ✓✓ CHOLESTEROL: Excellent Choice (0 mg)
✓✓ FAT: Excellent Choice (14 g)*   ✓✓ SODIUM: Excellent Choice (155 mg)**
EXCHANGES: ¾ Veg, ¾ Fruit, 2¾ Fat
PROTEIN: 1 g, CARBOHYDRATE: 15 g, FIBER: 2 g

NEPTUNE GAZPACHO ☾
chilled and topped with bay shrimp.

✓✓ CALORIES: Excellent Choice (160)   ✓✓ CHOLESTEROL: Excellent Choice (35 mg)
✓✓ FAT: Excellent Choice (12 g)   ✓ SODIUM: Good Choice (560 mg)**
EXCHANGES: ½ Meat, ¼ Bread, ½ Veg, 2¼ Fat
PROTEIN: 5 g, CARBOHYDRATE: 7 g, FIBER: 1 g

BRANZINO ALLA GRIGLIA - SPECIAL REQUEST ☾
Grilled striped Italian bass with Mediterranean herbs and virgin olive oil. Request vegetables steamed.

✓✓ CALORIES: Excellent Choice (440)   ✓ CHOLESTEROL: Good Choice (115 mg)
✓ FAT: Good Choice (20 g)*   ✓✓ SODIUM: Excellent Choice (240 mg)**
EXCHANGES: 7 Meat (extra lean), 1¾ Veg, 2¾ Fat
PROTEIN: 57 g, CARBOHYDRATE: 9 g, FIBER: 6 g

PENNE ALL'ARRABBIATA - SPECIAL REQUEST
Spicy fresh tomato sauce, garlic and olive oil. Request less oil (½ oz.).

✓ CALORIES: Good Choice (580)   ✓✓ CHOLESTEROL: Excellent Choice (0 mg)
✓ FAT: Good Choice (19 g)*   SODIUM: Moderate (890 mg)**
EXCHANGES: 5¼ Bread, 1½ Veg, 3¼ Fat
PROTEIN: 15 g, CARBOHYDRATE: 88 g, FIBER: 6g

PENNE AL POMODORO AND BASILICO - SPECIAL REQUEST ☾
with fresh tomatoes and basil. Request less oil (½ oz.).

✓ CALORIES: Good Choice (570)   ✓✓ CHOLESTEROL: Excellent Choice (0 mg)
✓ FAT: Good Choice (16 g)*   ✓✓ SODIUM: Excellent Choice (300 mg)**
EXCHANGES: 5¼ Bread, 1¾ Veg, 2¾ Fat
PROTEIN: 16 g, CARBOHYDRATE: 91 g, FIBER: 7 g

☾ at least 2 fruit/vegetable servings

✓ Good Choice   ✓✓ Excellent Choice

BLUEWATER GRILL

SEAFOOD RESTAURANT
& OYSTER BAR

At the Bluewater Grill, the fish is so fresh the menu is printed daily! We feature over fifteen varieties of fresh fish which are prepared over a mesquite wood fired barbecue. In addition, we have numerous salads, pastas and an oyster bar with oysters, shrimp, crab, clams, mussels, sushi, sashimi, and much more. Our menu philosophy is to purchase the freshest fish possible and to serve it simply, without sauces filled with lots of calories. $$

Bluewater Grill 665 N. Harbor Dr., Redondo Beach, CA 90277 (310) 318-3474

FRESH FISH

Analyses for 8 oz. portions (except lobster) are listed in the table below.
Each is served with 2 side dishes – fresh broccoli and sliced tomatoes recommended (see analysis below).

	Calories	Fat (g)	Cholesterol (mg)	Sodium (mg)	Protein (g)
Orange Roughy	150	2	45	140	32
Lingcod	190	2	115	130	39
Mahi Mahi	195	2	165	200	42
Ahi Tuna	220	2	90	75	48
Lobster Tail *(without butter)*	265	2	195	1025	56
Lobster *(without butter)*	445	3	325	1725	93
Monkfish	165	3	55	40	32
Red Snapper	225	3	85	100	47
Walleye Pike	270	4	250	150	56
Halibut	245	5	75	125	47
Seabass	280	6	120	200	54
Rainbow Trout	270	8	130	60	47
Shark	265	9	105	160	43
Swordfish	275	9	90	205	45
Bluefin Tuna	295	10	80	80	48
Yellowtail	300	11	115	80	47
Atlantic Salmon	315	14	120	95	44
Mississippi Catfish	345	18	145	180	42
King Salmon	365	21	135	95	41

SLICED TOMATOES AND FRESH BROCCOLI

CALORIES: 35, FAT: ½ g, CHOLESTEROL: 0 mg, SODIUM: 30 mg, Fiber: 3 g
EXCHANGES: 1¼ Veg; PROTEIN: 3 g, CARBOHYDRATE: 7 g

* Primarily unsaturated fat

** If you request no added salt

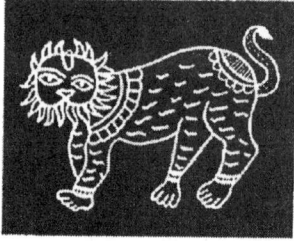

BOMBAY CAFE

Unique among Los Angeles' Indian restaurants, Bombay Cafe offers a mix of savory "street" foods, tandoor-cooked fish, chicken, lamb, breads, and light traditional Indian home cooking. See for yourself why "Gourmet" magazine raved "I've never tasted better spicing." Sample one of our 15 house-made chutneys and see why Ruth Reichl put them in her list of LA restaurants' top 40 dishes. Try our California Tandoori Salad and see why Zagat Survey consistently rates us LA's best Indian restaurant. Open Tues. to Fri. 11:30 am to 10:00 pm; Sat. & Sun. 4:00 pm to 10:00 pm. $$

Bombay Cafe 12021 West Pico Boulevard, West Los Angeles (310) 473-3388

CALIFORNIA TANDOORI SALAD - SPECIAL REQUEST ☙

Warm tandori chicken, mushrooms, paneer, romaine, scallions and cilantro.
Request dressing on the side (60 calories, 7 g fat, 240 mg sodium per Tbs., not included in analysis).

✓✓ CALORIES: Excellent Choice (325)   ✓ CHOLESTEROL: Good Choice (105 mg)
✓✓ FAT: Excellent Choice (13 g)   ✓✓ SODIUM: Excellent Choice (220 mg)**
EXCHANGES: 4¾ Meat, 1½ Veg, ¼ Milk, ¾ Fat
PROTEIN: 39 g, CARBOHYDRATE: 14 g, FIBER: 4 g

TANDOORI CHICKEN

Boneless pieces of chicken marinated with ginger, cilantro, garlic and green chilies,
mesquite fired in the tandoor oven, and served with mint yogurt chutney.

✓✓ CALORIES: Excellent Choice (420)   CHOLESTEROL: Moderate (185 mg)
✓ FAT: Good Choice (16 g)   ✓ SODIUM: Good Choice (445 mg)**
EXCHANGES: 8½ Meat, ¼ Veg, ¼ Fat
PROTEIN: 60 g, CARBOHYDRATE: 4 g, FIBER: 0 g

UTTAPAM

A semolina griddle cake topped with tomato, onion, green chili and cilantro and served with coconut chutney.

✓✓ CALORIES: Excellent Choice (410)   ✓✓ CHOLESTEROL: Excellent Choice (10 mg)
✓ FAT: Good Choice (19 g)   SODIUM: Moderate (635 mg)**
EXCHANGES: 2¾ Bread, ½ Veg, ¼ Milk, 2¼ Fat
PROTEIN: 10 g, CARBOHYDRATE: 50 g, FIBER: 2 g

JALPARI TIKKA

Marinated fish of the day, mesquite fired in the tandoor oven.

✓✓ CALORIES: Excellent Choice (390)   ✓ CHOLESTEROL: Good Choice (110 mg)
✓✓ FAT: Excellent Choice (8 g)*   ✓✓ SODIUM: Excellent Choice (235 mg)**
EXCHANGES: 6¾ Meat (extra lean), ¼ Veg
PROTEIN: 71 g, CARBOHYDRATE: 3 g, FIBER: 0 g

GOBI SABZI ☙

Cauliflower sautéed with green chilies, ginger, coriander, tumeric and cumin seeds.

✓✓ CALORIES: Excellent Choice (210)   ✓✓ CHOLESTEROL: Excellent Choice (0 mg)
✓✓ FAT: Excellent Choice (14 g)*   SODIUM: Moderate (650 mg)**
EXCHANGES: 3½ Veg, 2¾ Fat
PROTEIN: 7 g, CARBOHYDRATE: 20 g, FIBER: 1 g

☙ at least 2 fruit/vegetable servings
✓ Good Choice   ✓✓ Excellent Choice

Mary Sue Milliken and Susan Feniger, the celebrated chefs/owners of Border Grill, have developed a menu which pays homage to the bold flavors from the border, coastal Mexico and beyond. With a colorful, festive ambiance and a surprisingly light cuisine that is more authentic than the fat-laden food served in the majority of Mexican restaurants, Border Grill is undoubtedly an original, and one of the city's 40 best restaurants according to the LA Times. $$

Border Grill   1445 Fourth St., Santa Monica, CA 90401 (310) 451-1655

CHICKEN GRIDDLED TACOS
Our homemade corn tortillas with chicken, avocado and red salsa. Analysis is for 3 tacos.
✓✓ CALORIES: Excellent Choice (370)   ✓✓ CHOLESTEROL: Excellent Choice (40 mg)
✓ FAT: Good Choice (16 g)   ✓ SODIUM: Good Choice (465 mg)**
EXCHANGES: 1½ Meat, 2½ Bread, ½ Veg, 2¼ Fat
PROTEIN: 17 g, CARBOHYDRATE: 41 g, FIBER: 3 g

GRIDDLED FISH TACOS
Our homemade corn tortillas with grilled fish, avocado and cucumber relish. Analysis is for 2 tacos.
✓✓ CALORIES: Excellent Choice (210)   ✓✓ CHOLESTEROL: Excellent Choice (30 mg)
✓✓ FAT: Excellent Choice (4 g)*   ✓✓ SODIUM: Excellent Choice (170 mg)**
EXCHANGES: 2 Meat (extra lean), 1½ Bread, ¼ Veg, ¼ Fruit, ½ Fat
PROTEIN: 17 g, CARBOHYDRATE: 27 g, FIBER: 1 g

BORDER VEGETARIAN 🍎
Plateful of assorted steamed, grilled and roasted vegetables with rice and beans.
✓ CALORIES: Good Choice (550)   ✓✓ CHOLESTEROL: Excellent Choice (5 mg)
✓ FAT: Good Choice (21 g)*   SODIUM: Moderate (605 mg)**
EXCHANGES: 3¾ Bread, 3¼ Veg, 4 Fat
PROTEIN: 14 g, CARBOHYDRATE: 77 g, FIBER: 7 g

PESCADO VERACRUZANA
Pan seared and baked fish with tomatoes, jalapenos, olives and oregano, served with rice.
✓✓ CALORIES: Excellent Choice (445)   ✓✓ CHOLESTEROL: Excellent Choice (70 mg)
✓ FAT: Good Choice (20 g)*   ✓ SODIUM: Good Choice (545 mg)**
EXCHANGES: 3 Meat (extra lean), 1½ Bread, ½ Veg, 3¼ Fat
PROTEIN: 38 g, CARBOHYDRATE: 27 g, FIBER: 1 g

CHICKEN AL CARBON - SPECIAL REQUEST
Marinated with citrus and morita chile and topped with orange salsa. Served with rice (included in analysis)
& black beans (130 cal, 6 g fat, 0 cholesterol, 315 mg sodium, not included in analysis). Request no skin.
✓ CALORIES: Good Choice (525)   CHOLESTEROL: Moderate (175 mg)
✓ FAT: Good Choice (19 g)   SODIUM: Moderate (855 mg)**
EXCHANGES: 9 Meat (extra lean), ¾ Bread, ½ Veg, ¼ Fruit, 2¼ Fat
PROTEIN: 66 g, CARBOHYDRATE: 20 g, FIBER: 1 g

* Primarily unsaturated fat
** If you request no added salt

Bristol's Café

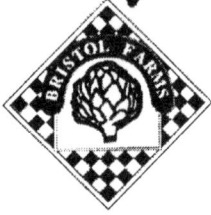

Located inside Bristol Farms markets, Bristol's Café offers breakfast, lunch and dinner menus. We feature a variety of farm fresh breakfasts, a selection of classic sandwiches, crisp salads, and homemade soups for lunch, and an array of wonderful dinners and fresh baked desserts. Bristol's Café also offers beer and wine tastings, special winery dinners, patio dining and free cooking classes. Hours: 8 am to 9 pm daily. $

Bristol's Café & Bristol Farms' Deli

Hollywood: 7880 Sunset Blvd.	(323) 874-6301
Long Beach: 2080 Bellflower Blvd.	(562) 430-4134
Los Angeles: 1515 Westwood Blvd.	(310) 481-0100
Manhattan Beach: 1570 Rosecrans Ave.	(310) 643-5229
Redondo Beach: 1700 S Pacific Coast Hwy. #A	(310) 303-3922
Rolling Hills Estates: 837 Silver Spur Rd.	(310) 541-9157
South Pasadena: 606 Fair Oaks Ave.	(626) 441-5450
West Hollywood: 9039 Beverly Blvd.	(310) 248-2804

GRILLED VEGGIE MOZZARELLA - SPECIAL REQUEST ❀
Fresh mozzarella, grilled eggplant, zucchini, summer squash, onions, mushrooms, tomatoes and fresh herbs on a French baguette. Served in Café. Request no butter.
- ✓ CALORIES: Good Choice (520)
- ✓ FAT: Good Choice (17 g)
- ✓✓ CHOLESTEROL: Excellent Choice (30 mg)
- SODIUM: Moderate (880 mg)**

EXCHANGES: 1¾ Meat, 3¾ Bread, 1¾ Veg, 1¾ Fat
PROTEIN: 26 g, CARBOHYDRATE: 66 g, FIBER: 3 g

TURKEY ASPARAGUS MELT
Fresh asparagus wrapped with sliced turkey, topped with alfalfa sprouts, tomato, onions, reduced-fat Swiss cheese and non-fat thousand island dressing on pumpernickel. Served in Café.
- ✓ CALORIES: Good Choice (550)
- ✓✓ FAT: Excellent Choice (14 g)
- ✓ CHOLESTEROL: Good Choice (95 mg)
- SODIUM: High (1690 mg)

EXCHANGES: 4¼ Meat (extra lean), 4 Bread, 1¼ Veg, 5 Fat
PROTEIN: 38 g, CARBOHYDRATE: 71 g, FIBER: 5 g

BIKINI BURGER
A veggie patty topped with onion, lettuce, tomato and low-cal mayo on a onion roll. Served in Café.
- ✓ CALORIES: Good Choice (575)
- ✓ FAT: Good Choice (17 g)
- ✓✓ CHOLESTEROL: Excellent Choice (30 mg)
- SODIUM: High (1445 mg)

EXCHANGES: 3¼ Meat, 3¾ Bread, 1¼ Veg, 2¾ Fat
PROTEIN: 35 g, CARBOHYDRATE: 71 g, FIBER: 8 g

JADE SALAD (DELI ITEM, ½ POUND) ❀
- ✓✓ CALORIES: Excellent Choice (100)
- ✓✓ FAT: Excellent Choice (4 g)*
- ✓✓ CHOLESTEROL: Excellent Choice (10 mg)
- ✓ SODIUM: Good Choice (460 mg)

EXCHANGES: 1¼ Veg, ½ Fat
PROTEIN: 7 g, CARBOHYDRATE: 14 g, FIBER: 5 g

POACHED SALMON FILLETS (DELI ITEM, 6 OZ.)
- ✓✓ CALORIES: Excellent Choice (340)
- ✓✓ FAT: Excellent Choice (14 g)*
- ✓ CHOLESTEROL: Good Choice (120 mg)
- ✓✓ SODIUM: Excellent Choice (100 mg)

EXCHANGES: 5¾ Meat, ¼ Veg, ¼ Fruit
PROTEIN: 44 g, CARBOHYDRATE: 5 g, FIBER: 1 g

BROWN RICE SALAD (DELI ITEM, ½ POUND)
with kidney beans, grilled corn, pumpkin seeds, feta cheese, turkey and seasonings.
- ✓✓ CALORIES: Excellent Choice (275)
- ✓✓ FAT: Excellent Choice (10 g)
- ✓✓ CHOLESTEROL: Excellent Choice (35 mg)
- SODIUM: Moderate (880 mg)

EXCHANGES: 1¾ Meat, 1¼ Bread, ½ Veg, 3½ Fat
PROTEIN: 14 g, CARBOHYDRATE: 34 g, FIBER: 4 g

❀ at least 2 fruit/vegetable servings
✓ Good Choice ✓✓ Excellent Choice

Enjoy award-winning authentic Italian cuisine in a pleasant and relaxing atmosphere. We offer a unique and imaginative menu that features fresh homemade pasta dishes, delicious chicken, veal, seafood specialties and gourmet pizza. Join us for an unforgettable indoor or outdoor dining experience. Banquet and party facilities available. $$

Buon Gusto

5755 East Pacific Coast Highway
Long Beach 90803 (562) 498-1135

CHICKEN LEMON

Boneless breast sautéed with fresh garlic, lemon and a splash of white wine, served with rigatoni.
Served with soup or salad and fresh Italian bread, not included in analysis.

✓ CALORIES: Good Choice (720)
✓ FAT: Good Choice (25 g)
CHOLESTEROL: Moderate (185 mg)
✓ SODIUM: Good Choice (385 mg)**
EXCHANGES: 9¾ Meat (extra lean), 2 Bread, ¼ Veg, ½ Fruit, 3 Fat
PROTEIN: 75 g, CARBOHYDRATE: 40 g, FIBER: 2 g

PASTA WITH MARINARA SAUCE

Your choice of pasta with marinara sauce. Served with fresh Italian bread, not included in analysis.

✓ CALORIES: Good Choice (495)
✓✓ FAT: Excellent Choice (13 g)
✓✓ CHOLESTEROL: Excellent Choice (10 mg)
✓✓ SODIUM: Excellent Choice (250 mg)**
EXCHANGES: ¾ Meat, 4¼ Bread, 1¾ Veg, 1¾ Fat
PROTEIN: 18 g, CARBOHYDRATE: 77 g, FIBER: 6 g

ALLA BUON GUSTO ♻

Pasta with zucchini, mushrooms, fresh tomato sauce and garlic.
Includes fresh Italian bread, not included in analysis.

✓ CALORIES: Good Choice (505)
✓✓ FAT: Excellent Choice (15 g)*
✓✓ CHOLESTEROL: Excellent Choice (0 mg)
✓✓ SODIUM: Excellent Choice (15 mg)**
EXCHANGES: 4¼ Bread, 1½ Veg, 2¾ Fat
PROTEIN: 13 g, CARBOHYDRATE: 74 g, FIBER: 6 g

SEAFOOD LINGUINI BUON GUSTO

Fresh steamed clams, calamari and scampi with herbs, mushrooms and diced tomato.
Served with soup or salad and fresh Italian bread, not included in analysis.

✓ CALORIES: Good Choice (625)
✓ FAT: Good Choice (17 g)*
CHOLESTEROL: Moderate (250 mg)
✓✓ SODIUM: Excellent Choice (245 mg)**
EXCHANGES: 4¼ Meat (extra lean), 4¼ Bread, ¾ Veg, 2¾ Fat
PROTEIN: 41 g, CARBOHYDRATE: 70 g, FIBER: 4 g

* Primarily unsaturated fat
** If you request no added salt

Buona Vita has been described as a trattoria that you can only find it in Italy, or perhaps in New York City. Says the LA Times, "Simplicity sells"... and that is what we are. Buona Vita serves uncomplicated food, using the best ingredients. We are health conscious and none of our staff are "aspiring actors or actresses"—just nice people that want to make you feel at home. Buona Vita and Mezzaluna, our sister restaurant in Puerto Vallarta, Mexico as well as Buona Vita on Main and Buona Vita Provo in Utah are owned and operated by the Galeano and Nastari families. We are open every day at 5:00 pm. We take reservations for parties of 15 or more. $$

Buona Vita

Buona Vita Pizzeria 425 Pier Avenue, Hermosa Beach 90254 (310) 372-2233
Buona Vita Trattoria 439 Pier Avenue, Hermosa Beach 90254 (310) 379-7626
Buona Vita On Main 427 Main Street, Park City Utah 84060 (435) 658-0999

CHICKEN PAILLARD – SPECIAL REQUEST ☼

Chicken sautéed in extra virgin olive oil, fresh vegetables, calamata olives & garlic. <u>Request less oil (1 Tbs.).</u>
✓ CALORIES: Good Choice (545)   ✓ CHOLESTEROL: Good Choice (110 mg)
✓ FAT: Good Choice (20 g)   ✓✓ SODIUM: Excellent Choice (235 mg)**
EXCHANGES: 5¾ Meat (extra lean), 6 Veg, 2¾ Fat
PROTEIN: 52 g, CARBOHYDRATE: 45 g, FIBER: 11 g

PASTA POMODORO ☼

Spaghetti, marinara sauce, garlic and fresh basil.
✓ CALORIES: Good Choice (670)   ✓✓ CHOLESTEROL: Excellent Choice (0 mg)
✓ FAT: Good Choice (18 g)*   SODIUM: High (1040 mg)**
EXCHANGES: 6¼ Bread, 2½ Veg, 3 Fat
PROTEIN: 19 g, CARBOHYDRATE: 110 g, FIBER: 8 g

SCAMPI BELLO – SPECIAL REQUEST ☼

Jumbo shrimp, fresh basil, carrots, tomato, sundried tomato, mushrooms, calamata olives, sautéed in extra-virgin olive oil and garlic, served with spaghetti. <u>Request less oil (1 Tbs.).</u>
CALORIES: Moderate (815)   CHOLESTEROL: Moderate (275 mg)
✓ FAT: Good Choice (20 g)*   ✓ SODIUM: Good Choice (545 mg)**
EXCHANGES: 4¼ Meat (extra lean), 4¾ Bread, 4¾ Veg, 2¾ Fat
PROTEIN: 50 g, CARBOHYDRATE: 112 g, FIBER: 11 g

ALLA CHECCA – SPECIAL REQUEST ☼

Spahgettini, fresh tomato, basil, sundried tomato and extra virgin olive oil. <u>Request less oil (1 Tbs.).</u>
CALORIES: Moderate (785)   ✓✓ CHOLESTEROL: Excellent Choice (0 mg)
✓ FAT: Good Choice (16 g)*   ✓✓ SODIUM: Excellent Choice (120 mg)**
EXCHANGES: 4¾ Bread, 5¾ Veg, 2¾ Fat
PROTEIN: 24 g, CARBOHYDRATE: 145 g, FIBER: 12 g

POLLO PRIMAVERA ☼

Chicken sautéed with vegetables and served with spaghetti in a marinara sauce.
CALORIES: Moderate (990)   ✓ CHOLESTEROL: Good Choice (110 mg)
✓ FAT: Good Choice (23 g)   SODIUM: High (1195 mg)**
EXCHANGES: 5¾ Meat (extra lean), 6¼ Bread, 6½ Veg, 3 Fat
PROTEIN: 64 g, CARBOHYDRATE: 134 g, FIBER: 15 g

LOW-FAT PEACH CHEESECAKE†

✓ CALORIES: Good Choice (175)   ✓✓ CHOLESTEROL: Excellent Choice (6 mg)
✓ FAT: Good Choice (4 g)   SODIUM: Moderate (230 mg)
EXCHANGES: 1 Bread, 1½ Milk, ¾ Fat
PROTEIN: 10 g, CARBOHYDRATE: 26 g, FIBER: 0 g

† Side dish guidelines are 1/3 of entree guidelines
✓ Good Choice   ✓✓ Excellent Choice

Ca'Brea serves the finest in Northern Italian cuisine in a comfortable setting of casual country elegance. Local and national publications continue to pick Ca'Brea as one of Los Angeles' best restaurants. Daily specials augment the regular menu, allowing for plenty of variety for even the most frequent patrons. Private rooms available for parties up to 60. Excellent food quality and reasonable prices along with attentive service keep Ca'Brea full and reservations advisable. $$

Ca'Brea
(323) 938-2863
346 South La Brea Avenue, Los Angeles, CA 90036

INSALATA TIEPIDA DI FRUTTI DI MARE CON ORTAGGI
Fresh seafood salad with marinated vegetables in a lemon and garlic dressing.

✓✓ CALORIES: Excellent Choice (285)   CHOLESTEROL: Moderate (155 mg)
✓ FAT: Good Choice (16 g)*   ✓ SODIUM: Good Choice (490 mg)**
EXCHANGES: 3 Meat (extra lean), 1 Veg, 2¾ Fat
PROTEIN: 24 g, CARBOHYDRATE: 11 g

LINGUINETTE ALLE VONGOLE ALL'AGLIO DI FRANTOIO
Linguine pasta with fresh clams in a garlic and white wine sauce.

✓ CALORIES: Good Choice (650)   ✓✓ CHOLESTEROL: Excellent Choice (50 mg)
✓ FAT: Good Choice (17 g)*   ✓✓ SODIUM: Excellent Choice (85 mg)**
EXCHANGES: 2½ Meat (extra lean), 5¼ Bread, ½ Veg, 2¾ Fat
PROTEIN: 32 g, CARBOHYDRATE: 85 g

PENNETTE RUSTICHE AL POMODORO ED ERBETTE AROMATICHE
Short tube pasta with aromatic herbs in a garlic tomato sauce (spicy).

✓ CALORIES: Good Choice (515)   ✓✓ CHOLESTEROL: Excellent Choice (<1 mg)
✓✓ FAT: Excellent Choice (9 g)*   ✓ SODIUM: Good Choice (410 mg)**
EXCHANGES: 5¼ Bread, 1½ Veg, 1½ Fat
PROTEIN: 16 g, CARBOHYDRATE: 90 g

RISOTTO AL RAGU' DI BOLETI CON ERBETTE DI BOSCO - SPECIAL REQUEST
Risotto with a ragout of mixed porcini mushrooms and wild herbs. Request less butter (¼ oz).

✓ CALORIES: Good Choice (460)   ✓✓ CHOLESTEROL: Excellent Choice (60 mg)
✓ FAT: Good Choice (20 g)   ✓ SODIUM: Good Choice (365 mg)**
EXCHANGES: ½ Meat, 3½ Bread, 1½ Veg, 2¾ Fat
PROTEIN: 20 g, CARBOHYDRATE: 59 g

PESCE DEL GIORNO ☍
Red snapper grilled with rosemary and served with steamed spinach and roasted potatoes.

✓✓ CALORIES: Excellent Choice (450)   ✓ CHOLESTEROL: Good Choice (85 mg)
✓ FAT: Good Choice (16 g)*   SODIUM: Moderate (630 mg)**
EXCHANGES: 4¼ Meat (extra lean), 1¼ Bread, 1¼ Veg, 2½ Fat
PROTEIN: 51 g, CARBOHYDRATE: 26 g

* Primarily unsaturated fat
** If you request no added salt

☍ at least 2 fruit/vegetable servings

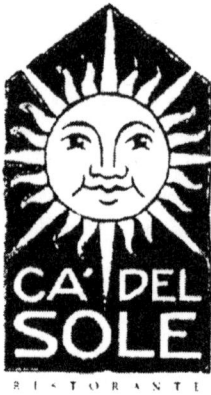

Ca' del Sole offers Northern Italian fare in a friendly, comfortable, airy and sunny setting. We have the rustic country style feel of a Venetian Trattoria --- simple yet classic, elegant but not pretentious. We have a full bar and extensive wine list. Ca' del Sole has three unique dining rooms, a private banquet room and an exquisite outside patio. $$

Ca' del Sole

(818) 985-4669

4100 Cahuenga Blvd., North Hollywood, CA 91602

MISTICANZA DI VERDURE GRIGLIATE ☼

Zucchini, yellow squash, mushrooms, eggplant, carrots, red onions, bell peppers, vine-ripened tomatoes, and asparagus grilled to perfection. Dressing served on the side is not included in analysis.

- ✓✓ CALORIES: Excellent Choice (205)
- ✓✓ FAT: Excellent Choice (14 g)*
- ✓✓ CHOLESTEROL: Excellent Choice (0 mg)
- ✓✓ SODIUM: Excellent Choice (10 mg)**

EXCHANGES: ¾ Bread, 2 Veg, 2¾ Fat
PROTEIN: 4 g, CARBOHYDRATE: 21 g, FIBER: 3g

CAPELLINI ALLA CHECCA ☼

Angel hair pasta with fresh tomato, garlic, olive oil, and basil pesto.

- ✓ CALORIES: Good Choice (570)
- ✓ FAT: Good Choice (17 g)*
- ✓✓ CHOLESTEROL: Excellent Choice (0 mg)
- ✓✓ SODIUM: Excellent Choice (20 mg)**

EXCHANGES: 5¼ Bread, 1¼ Veg, 2¾ Fat
PROTEIN: 16 g, CARBOHYDRATE: 90 g, FIBER: 8 g

STUFATINO DI GAMBERI E POMODORO CON PATATINE AL VAPORE ☼

Tiger shrimp sautéed with steamed potatoes in a spicy tomato and garlic sauce.

- ✓ CALORIES: Good Choice (500)
- ✓ FAT: Good Choice (16 g)*
- CHOLESTEROL: High (350 mg)
- SODIUM: High (1200 mg)

EXCHANGES: 3¼ Meat (extra lean), 2 Bread, 2½ Veg, 2¾ Fat
PROTEIN: 43 g, CARBOHYDRATE: 44 g, FIBER: 6 g

PENNETTE AI POMODORI DI SAN MARZANO, PEPERONCINO E ROSMARINO

Penne pasta, sautéed in a spicy sauce of tomato, olive oil, rosemary and garlic.

- ✓✓ CALORIES: Excellent Choice (435)
- ✓✓ FAT: Excellent Choice (9 g)*
- ✓✓ CHOLESTEROL: Excellent Choice (0 mg)
- SODIUM: Moderate (920 mg)**

EXCHANGES: 4¼ Bread, 2 Veg, 1¼ Fat
PROTEIN: 13 g, CARBOHYDRATE: 76 g, FIBER: 4 g

PAPPARDELLE DI SPINACI - SPECIAL REQUEST

Wide ribbon spinach pasta sautéed with shiitake mushrooms, leeks, extra virgin olive oil and garlic. Request chicken breast instead of sausage.

- ✓ CALORIES: Good Choice (615)
- ✓ FAT: Good Choice (17 g)
- CHOLESTEROL: Moderate (220 mg)
- ✓✓ SODIUM: Excellent Choice (255 mg)**

EXCHANGES: 5 Meat, 4 Bread, ¾ Veg, 2¼ Fat, FIBER: 4 g
PROTEIN: 49 g, CARBOHYDRATE: 65 g

☼ at least 2 fruit/vegetable servings
✓ Good Choice   ✓✓ Excellent Choice

Café Luna is a long time favorite place for great Italian cuisine in Torrance. We offer an warm and inviting atmosphere that is perfect for family-style dining and social occasions. Come and enjoy our wonderful Italian cuisine. The Café Luna family looks forward to seeing you soon. $-$$

Café Luna

1870 W. Carson St., Torrance 90501   (310) 787-1223
2933 Rolling Hills Road, Torrance 90505   (310) 891-0111

MARINATED GRILLED CHICKEN ☺

Chicken breast deeply marinated. Served with grilled vegetables and garlic mashed potatoes.

✓ CALORIES: Good Choice (630)   ✓ CHOLESTEROL: Good Choice (130 mg)
   FAT: Moderate (26 g)   ✓✓ SODIUM: Excellent Choice (260 mg)**

EXCHANGES: 5½ Meat (extra lean), 2¾ Bread, 1 Veg, 4 Fat
PROTEIN: 45 g, CARBOHYDRATE: 55 g, FIBER: 5 g

GRILLED SALMON ☺

Grilled salmon served with grilled vegetables and garlic mashed potatoes.

✓ CALORIES: Good Choice (495)   ✓ CHOLESTEROL: Good Choice (100 mg)
✓ FAT: Good Choice (16 g)   ✓✓ SODIUM: Excellent Choice (100 mg)**

EXCHANGES: 3½ Meat, 2¾ Bread, 1 Veg, 1½ Fat
PROTEIN: 33 g, CARBOHYDRATE: 54 g, FIBER: 5 g

VERDURE GRIGLIATE ☺

Grilled eggplant, zucchini, tomatoes, red onions, mushrooms brushed with extra virgin olive oil.

✓✓ CALORIES: Excellent Choice (295)   ✓✓ CHOLESTEROL: Excellent Choice (0 mg)
✓ FAT: Good Choice (21 g)*   ✓✓ SODIUM: Excellent Choice (20 mg)**

EXCHANGES: ¼ Bread, 2 Veg, 4 Fat
PROTEIN: 3 g, CARBOHYDRATE: 17 g, FIBER: 4 g

SHRIMP DIABLO

Sautéed shrimp over a bed of linguini topped with a red spicy garlic sauce.

✓ CALORIES: Good Choice (550)   CHOLESTEROL: Moderate (170 mg)
✓ FAT: Good Choice (18 g)*   SODIUM: Moderate (860 mg)**

EXCHANGES: 2½ Meat (extra lean), 3¼ Bread, 1¼ Veg, 3¼ Fat
PROTEIN: 29 g, CARBOHYDRATE: 63 g, FIBER: 5 g

CAPELLINI POMODORO

Fresh roma tomatoes, basil, garlic and olive oil over capellini.
Also available with chicken or shrimp (not included in analysis. Analysis for lunch portion.

✓✓ CALORIES: Excellent Choice (415)   ✓✓ CHOLESTEROL: Excellent Choice (0 mg)
✓✓ FAT: Excellent Choice (15 g)*   ✓✓ SODIUM: Excellent Choice (10 mg)**

EXCHANGES: 3¼ Bread, 1¼ Veg, 2¾ Fat
PROTEIN: 9 g, CARBOHYDRATE: 60 g, FIBER: 5 g

SPICY CHICKEN SICILLIANO ☺

Sautéed chicken breast topped with a red spicy garlic sauce, capers, black olives and mushrooms.
Served with pasta (not included in analysis).

✓ CALORIES: Good Choice (475)   ✓ CHOLESTEROL: Good Choice (110 mg)
✓ FAT: Good Choice (23 g)   SODIUM: Moderate (915 mg)**

EXCHANGES: 5¾ Meat (extra lean), 2 Veg, 3¼ Fat
PROTEIN: 45 g, CARBOHYDRATE: 18 g, FIBER: 4 g

SPAGHETTI WITH MARINARA SAUCE

✓✓ CALORIES: Excellent Choice (330)   ✓✓ CHOLESTEROL: Excellent Choice (5 mg)
✓✓ FAT: Excellent Choice (4 g)*   ✓ SODIUM: Good Choice (475 mg)**

EXCHANGES: 3¼ Bread, 1¼ Veg, ½ Fat
PROTEIN: 11 g, CARBOHYDRATE: 61 g, FIBER: 5 g

* Primarily unsaturated fat
** If you request no added salt

CAFÉ SANTORINI
The Mediterranean Cuisine

If you like Mediterranean food and atmosphere, don't miss a chance to dine at Café Santorini in Old Pasadena. You'll find dishes from Italy, Greece, the Middle East and France, "the best Mediterranean food in LA," claims one restaurant critic. This "hidden treasure" features "fantastic alfresco dining" on the second floor of a historic mall; with a "lovely balcony" for people watching and "dishes that are worth going back for." $$

Cafe Santorini 64 W. Union Street, Pasadena, CA 91103 (626) 564-4200
www.cafesantorini.com

FRICASSE OF PACIFIC SEAFOOD ☙
High temperature sautéed shrimp, salmon, calamari with mushrooms, onions, basil and marinara sauce.
✓✓ CALORIES: Excellent Choice (345)   CHOLESTEROL: Moderate (290 mg)
✓✓ FAT: Excellent Choice (12 g)*   ✓ SODIUM: Good Choice (405 mg)**
EXCHANGES: 5 Meat (extra lean), 2 Veg, 1¼ Fat
PROTEIN: 40 g, CARBOHYDRATE: 14 g

BAKED BUTTERNUT SQUASH ☙
Roasted Mediterranean vegetables with buttered rice and wilted greens in a baked butternut squash.
✓✓ CALORIES: Excellent Choice (420)   ✓✓ CHOLESTEROL: Excellent Choice (10 mg)
✓✓ FAT: Excellent Choice (9 g)   SODIUM: Moderate (785 mg)**
EXCHANGES: 4¾ Bread, 1¾ Veg, 1¾ Fat
PROTEIN: 10 g, CARBOHYDRATE: 80 g

RISOTTO CON VERDURE ALLA GRIGLIA
Italian arborio rice with grilled vegetables, balsamic vinegar, garlic and chicken broth.
✓✓ CALORIES: Excellent Choice (400)   ✓✓ CHOLESTEROL: Excellent Choice (30 mg)
✓✓ FAT: Excellent Choice (8 g)   ✓✓ SODIUM: Excellent Choice (80 mg)**
EXCHANGES: 1 Meat, 4¼ Bread, ¾ Veg, 1 Fat
PROTEIN: 15 g, CARBOHYDRATE: 72 g

VEGETARIAN MEZZE TASTING ☙
Our vegetarian sampling platter of baked eggplant, hummus, grape leaves and lentil pilaf.
✓ CALORIES: Good Choice (570)   ✓✓ CHOLESTEROL: Excellent Choice (<5 mg)
✓ FAT: Good Choice (20 g)*   SODIUM: High (1045 mg)
EXCHANGES: ¾ Meat, 4½ Bread, 3 Veg, 3¾ Fat
PROTEIN: 21 g, CARBOHYDRATE: 84 g

PENNE ALL'ARRABBIATA ☙
Tender penne pasta in our house-made marinara sauce with crushed chili flakes.
✓✓ CALORIES: Excellent Choice (390)   ✓✓ CHOLESTEROL: Excellent Choice (0 mg)
✓✓ FAT: Excellent Choice (8 g)*   ✓ SODIUM: Good Choice (380 mg)**
EXCHANGES: 3¾ Bread, 2¼ Veg, 1 Fat
PROTEIN: 12 g, CARBOHYDRATE: 71 g

☙ at least 2 fruit/vegetable servings
✓ Good Choice   ✓✓ Excellent Choice

California Wok

Whoever said you can't have healthy food that tastes great at a reasonable price? In our restaurants, we serve the finest and freshest ingredients in all of our dishes. Each dish is prepared to your liking with any modifications necessary to meet your dietary preferences. We cook without MSG and use low-sodium soy sauce in our cooking preparations. With more than three decades of restaurant experience, it's no wonder California Wok has become one of the most popular places to dine. CALIFORNIA WOK..."you've never imagined that healthy food can be this tasty." $

California Wok locations:

16656 Ventura Blvd., Encino   (818) 386-0561
12004 Wilshire Blvd., West Los Angeles   (310) 479-0552

Analyses below assume the entree is shared between two people.

CHICKEN WITH MUSHROOMS AND PEA PODS (½ SERVING)
Sliced white meat chicken, mushrooms and pea pods in our special light sauce.
- ✓ CALORIES: Good Choice (500)
- ✓ FAT: Good Choice (16 g)
- ✓ CHOLESTEROL: Good Choice (85 mg)
- ✓ SODIUM: Good Choice (440 mg)

PROTEIN: 67 g, CARBOHYDRATE: 17 g, FIBER: 2 g

CHA CHA CHICKEN (½ SERVING)
White meat chicken and spinach sautéed in our special mandarin B.B.Q. sauce.
- ✓✓ CALORIES: Excellent Choice (390)
- ✓✓ FAT: Excellent Choice (12 g)
- ✓✓ CHOLESTEROL: Excellent Choice (70 mg)
- SODIUM: Moderate (615 mg)

PROTEIN: 53 g, CARBOHYDRATE: 12 g, FIBER: 3 g

SHRIMP WITH GARLIC SAUCE (½ SERVING)
Tender shrimp, celery, and water chestnuts in a hot garlic sauce.
- ✓✓ CALORIES: Excellent Choice (280)
- ✓✓ FAT: Excellent Choice (6 g)*
- ✓ CHOLESTEROL: Good Choice (140 mg)
- SODIUM: High (1520 mg)

PROTEIN: 34 g, CARBOHYDRATE: 38 g, FIBER: 6 g

SHRIMP WITH ASPARAGUS (OR BROCCOLI OR MIXED VEGETABLES) (½ SERVING)
Tender shrimp and fresh asparagus sautéed in our special delicious light sauce.
Nutrition values for the Shrimp with Broccoli and Shrimp with Mixed Vegetables are similar.
- ✓✓ CALORIES: Excellent Choice (165)
- ✓✓ FAT: Excellent Choice (6 g)*
- ✓ CHOLESTEROL: Good Choice (135 mg)
- ✓ SODIUM: Good Choice (495 mg)

PROTEIN: 26 g, CARBOHYDRATE: 14 g, FIBER: 3 g

HOUSE SPECIAL BEEF STEAK (½ SERVING)
Juicy fillet mignon stir-fried with chopped onions and green peppers with a touch of black pepper.
Only a few Chinese restaurants carry this top quality steak, and we are one of the best.
- ✓✓ CALORIES: Excellent Choice (380)
- ✓✓ FAT: Excellent Choice (14 g)
- ✓ CHOLESTEROL: Good Choice (115 mg)
- ✓ SODIUM: Good Choice (420 mg)

PROTEIN: 42 g, CARBOHYDRATE: 19 g, FIBER: 3 g

BEAN CURD WITH SPINACH (½ SERVING)
Bean curd and spinach sautéed in our special brown sauce.
- ✓✓ CALORIES: Excellent Choice (190)
- ✓✓ FAT: Excellent Choice (7 g)*
- ✓✓ CHOLESTEROL: Excellent Choice (0 mg)
- SODIUM: Moderate (890 mg)

PROTEIN: 19 g, CARBOHYDRATE: 18 g, FIBER: 7 g

Analysis provided by California Wok from results of laboratory analysis.

* Primarily unsaturated fat
** If you request no added salt

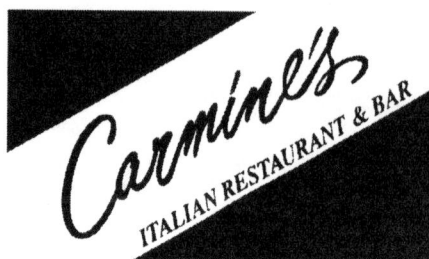

The Sabatella Family prides itself on serving great tasting traditional Italian meals, including fresh veal and chicken dishes, lasagna, specialties such as eggplant parmigiana, a variety of pastas, pizza and salads. The owner, Carmine Sabatella, says that "if you try us once you will definitely be back." At Carmine's Restaurant you can enjoy eating large portions at a fair price in a warm and friendly atmosphere. So come in and try us and we will make your "dining out" a pleasure. $-$$

Carmine's Italian Restaurant & Bar

424 Fair Oaks Ave., South Pasadena   (626) 799-2266
311 East Live Oak Ave., Arcadia   (626) 445-4726

SPINACH LASAGNA
Spinach lasagna baked with mozzarella cheese.
✓✓ CALORIES: Excellent Choice (420)   ✓✓ CHOLESTEROL: Excellent Choice (50 mg)
✓✓ FAT: Excellent Choice (10 g)   ✓ SODIUM: Good Choice (450 mg)
EXCHANGES: 1¾ Meat, 3½ Bread, ½ Veg, 1 Fat
PROTEIN: 18 g, CARBOHYDRATE: 58 g

MEDITERRANEAN GRILLED CHICKEN SALAD – SPECIAL REQUEST ᕬ
Baby greens, grilled chicken breast, artichokes, olives, red onion, bell pepper, romano cheese and sun dried tomatoes. Served with dressing on the side, not included in analysis. Request less cheese (1 Tbs.).
✓ CALORIES: Good Choice (730)   CHOLESTEROL: Moderate Choice (220 mg)
✓ FAT: Good Choice (20 g)   SODIUM: High (1020 mg)
EXCHANGES: 11½ Meat (extra lean), 8 Veg, 2 Fat
PROTEIN: 95 g, CARBOHYDRATE: 44 g

MUSHROOM MARINARA PASTA ᕬ
Made with fresh tomato, mushroom, eggplant, garlic and basil in a delicate mushroom marinara sauce.
CALORIES: Moderate (780)   ✓✓ CHOLESTEROL: Excellent Choice (35 mg)
✓ FAT: Good Choice (19 g)   SODIUM: High (1160 mg)
EXCHANGES: 6½ Bread, 6¾ Veg, 2¾ Fat
PROTEIN: 26 g, CARBOHYDRATE: 134 g

WHITE PIZZA – SPECIAL REQUEST
This is a "no sauce" pizza. We top it with our own garlic spread, ricotta cheese, mozzarella and your choice of two items, not included in analysis. Analysis for 2 slices of a large pizza. Request lowfat cheese.
✓ CALORIES: Good Choice (585)   ✓✓ CHOLESTEROL: Excellent Choice (50 mg)
✓ FAT: Good Choice (22 g)   SODIUM: Moderate (725 mg)
EXCHANGES: 2½ Meat, 4 Bread, 2¾ Fat
PROTEIN: 27 g, CARBOHYDRATE: 67 g

LEMON CHICKEN – SPECIAL REQUEST ᕬ
Diced chicken breasts, sautéed in a light butter, lemon, romano and paprika sauce topped with crisp red bell pepper and accompanied by a side of spaghetti and broccoli & cauliflower florets. Request less butter (½ Tbs.).
CALORIES: Moderate (810)   CHOLESTEROL: Moderate (235 mg)
✓ FAT: Good Choice (19 g)   ✓ SODIUM: Good Choice (380 mg)**
EXCHANGES: 11¼ Meat (extra lean), 2½ Bread, 4¼ Veg, 1½ Fat
PROTEIN: 97 g, CARBOHYDRATE: 64 g

SPAGHETTI LIGHT ᕬ
Made with fresh tomato, mushrooms, eggplant, garlic and basil in a delicate, light marinara sauce.
✓ CALORIES: Good Choice (635)   ✓✓ CHOLESTEROL: Excellent Choice (0 mg)
✓✓ FAT: Excellent Choice (6 g)*   SODIUM: High (1030 mg)
EXCHANGES: 6½ Bread, 5¼ Veg, ¼ Fat
PROTEIN: 22 g, CARBOHYDRATE: 127 g

ᕬ at least 2 fruit/vegetable servings

    ✓ Good Choice   ✓✓ Excellent Choice

CHANG'S
of BRENTWOOD

Chang's is a Chinese restaurant serving Mandarin and Szechwan cuisine with your health in mind. Owners Polly and Albert Chang use fresh ingredients, no MSG, and only slight amounts of vegetable oil, preferring to cook as much as possible in the natural juices of the food. Chang's menu of more than 100 choices includes authentic Chinese dishes, a large selection of traditional, specialty dishes and a Health & Fitness Fare menu with steamed items low in calories, cholesterol and sodium. Restaurant reviewers have credited Chang's with bringing "happiness to your tummy" and creating food that is "distinctive, flavorful, very fresh and good." Portions are large, and you may wish to share. $

Chang's   11726 San Vicente Blvd., Los Angeles (Brentwood), CA 90049 (310) 207-2295

STEAMED CHICKEN FILET WITH VEGETABLES ☺
Boneless, skinless chicken breast steamed with fresh vegetables.

✓ CALORIES: Good Choice (475)   CHOLESTEROL: Moderate (170 mg)
✓✓ FAT: Excellent Choice (9 g)   ✓✓ SODIUM: Excellent Choice (205 mg)**
EXCHANGES: 9 Meat (extra lean), ¼ Bread, 4¾ Veg, ¼ Fat
PROTEIN: 70 g, CARBOHYDRATE: 27 g, FIBER: 8 g

CHICKEN STEAMED WITH FRESH FRUIT ☺
Skinless breast of chicken steamed with fresh fruit and served with a lite lemon sauce.

✓ CALORIES: Good Choice (645)   CHOLESTEROL: Moderate (170 mg)
✓✓ FAT: Excellent Choice (8 g)   ✓✓ SODIUM: Excellent Choice (165 mg)**
EXCHANGES: 9 Meat (extra lean), 1¾ Bread, 3 Fruit
PROTEIN: 65 g, CARBOHYDRATE: 81 g, FIBER: 8 g

EAST MEETS WEST CHICKEN
The juiciness of pears and crunch of apples are a snappy combo in this Chang's specialty. Refreshingly tasty.

✓✓ CALORIES: Excellent Choice (435)   CHOLESTEROL: Moderate (170 mg)
✓✓ FAT: Excellent Choice (10 g)   ✓✓ SODIUM: Excellent Choice (165 mg)**
EXCHANGES: 9 Meat (extra lean), ¼ Bread, 1 Fruit, ½ Fat
PROTEIN: 64 g, CARBOHYDRATE: 19 g, FIBER: 2 g

ASIAN PEAR SCALLOPS ☺
Juicy and crunchy 20th century Asian pears combined with sliced jumbo steamed scallops.

✓✓ CALORIES: Excellent Choice (375)   ✓ CHOLESTEROL: Good Choice (120 mg)
✓✓ FAT: Excellent Choice (4 g)*   SODIUM: Moderate (610 mg)**
EXCHANGES: 4¾ Meat (extra lean), ½ Bread, 1¼ Veg, 1 Fruit
PROTEIN: 55 g, CARBOHYDRATE: 32 g, FIBER: 8 g

WESTLAKE HOT FISH ☺
White fish filets sautéed & served spicy hot in sweet & sour sauce with bell peppers, mushrooms & chili.

✓ CALORIES: Good Choice (550)   CHOLESTEROL: Moderate (230 mg)
✓✓ FAT: Excellent Choice (7 g)*   ✓ SODIUM: Good Choice (365 mg)**
EXCHANGES: 11½ Meat (extra lean), 1 Bread, 2¼ Veg, ¼ Fat
PROTEIN: 85 g, CARBOHYDRATE: 33 g, FIBER: 5 g

SEAFOOD MEDLEY ☺
Our Oriental version of the taco salad. Shrimp and scallops tossed with shredded lettuce, vegetables and a light fresh lemon sauce. Egg roll pastry shell not included in analysis.

✓✓ CALORIES: Excellent Choice (375)   CHOLESTEROL: Moderate (200 mg)
✓✓ FAT: Excellent Choice (4 g)*   ✓ SODIUM: Good Choice (410 mg)**
EXCHANGES: 4 Meat (extra lean), 2 Veg, ¼ Fruit
PROTEIN: 38 g, CARBOHYDRATE: 52 g, FIBER: 4 g

---

* Primarily unsaturated fat

** If you request no added salt

Our mission is to provide the best tasting fast food anywhere. We do this by selecting the finest ingredients and preparing our delicious food hourly at each location. Our expert cooks combine the most expensive herbs and spices with the freshest produce available to give you an unforgettable dining experience. $

Charo Chicken   www.charochicken.com

Costa Mesa: 1170 Baker St., G1	(714) 540-9700	Long Beach: 4752 E. PCH	(562) 498-5600
Dana Point: 24831 Del Prado Pkwy.	(949) 496-0044	Los Alamitos:	
Foothill Ranch: 26696 Portola Pkwy	(949) 837-7800	11105 Los Alamitos Blvd.	(562) 598-7979
Huntington Beach: 6531 Edinger Av.	(714) 892-2900	Redondo Bch: 1617 S. PCH, #101	(310) 792-0388
Irvine: 18040-A Culver Dr.	(949) 786-2000	Seal Beach: 333 Main St.	(562) 594-0909
Lake Forest: 22611 Lake Forest Dr.	(949) 581-3770	Tustin: 17612 E. 17th St.	(714) 832-1300

WE DELIVER!

2 PIECES WHITE MEAT CHICKEN - SKINLESS
✓✓ CALORIES: Excellent Choice (185)   ✓ CHOLESTEROL: Good Choice (90 mg)
✓✓ FAT: Excellent Choice (5 g)   ✓✓ SODIUM: Excellent Choice (80 mg)**
EXCHANGES: 4¾ Meat
PROTEIN: 33 g, CARBOHYDRATE: 0 g, FIBER: 0 g

CHARO SALAD – SPECIAL REQUEST ☺
Warm shredded chicken, pinto or black beans, guacamole and lettuce. Request cheese and sour cream on the side (not included in analysis). Served with salsa and tortillas on the side (not included in analysis).
✓ CALORIES: Good Choice (575)   ✓ CHOLESTEROL: Excellent Choice (70 mg)
✓ FAT: Good Choice (22 g)   SODIUM: High (2095 mg)
EXCHANGES: 3¼ Meat, 2¼ Bread, 1¾ Veg, ¼ Fruit, 3 Fat
PROTEIN: 43 g, CARBOHYDRATE: 54 g, FIBER: 13 g

CHICKEN BOWL
Generous portions of our critically acclaimed rice, pinto or black beans, mild pico de gallo salsa and shredded chicken.
✓ CALORIES: Good Choice (750)   ✓✓ CHOLESTEROL: Excellent Choice (70 mg)
✓ FAT: Good Choice (23 g)   SODIUM: High (3010 mg)
EXCHANGES: 3½ Meat, 5 Bread, 1½ Veg, 3¼ Fat
PROTEIN: 44 g, CARBOHYDRATE: 93 g, FIBER: 11 g

VEGGIE BOWL
Generous portions of our critically acclaimed rice, pinto or black beans, and mild pico de gallo salsa.
✓ CALORIES: Good Choice (675)   ✓✓ CHOLESTEROL: Excellent Choice (0 mg)
✓ FAT: Good Choice (20 g)*   SODIUM: High (2565 mg)
EXCHANGES: 5¾ Bread, 1¾ Veg, 3¾ Fat
PROTEIN: 21 g, CARBOHYDRATE: 105 g, FIBER: 11 g

BLACK BEANS (¾ CUP SERVING) †
CALORIES: Moderate (205)   ✓✓ CHOLESTEROL: Excellent Choice (0 mg)
✓ FAT: Good Choice (6 g)   SODIUM: High (780 mg)
PROTEIN: 10 g, CARBOHYDRATE: 28 g, FIBER: 5g; EXCHANGES: 1¾ Bread, 1¼ Fat

RICE (¾ CUP SERVING) †
✓ CALORIES: Good Choice (175)   ✓✓ CHOLESTEROL: Excellent Choice (0 mg)
✓ FAT: Good Choice (6 g)   SODIUM: Moderate (325 mg)
PROTEIN: 3 g, CARBOHYDRATE: 28 g, FIBER: 1g; EXCHANGES: 1¾ Bread, 1 Fat

CORN ON THE COB (3 INCH COB) †
✓✓ CALORIES: Excellent Choice (40)   ✓✓ CHOLESTEROL: Excellent Choice (0 mg)
✓✓ FAT: Excellent Choice (0 g)   ✓✓ SODIUM: Excellent Choice (5 mg)**
PROTEIN: 1 g, CARBOHYDRATE: 10 g, FIBER: 1g; EXCHANGES: ½ Bread

† Side dish guidelines are 1/3 of entree guidelines

64 *Healthy Dining in Los Angeles*   ✓ Good Choice   ✓✓ Excellent Choice

Executive Chef Shigefumi Tachibe has been at the helm of Chaya since its inception in the 1980's. Almost twenty years later, Chef Tachibe commands the menus and kitchens of three California restaurants including Chaya Brasserie Los Angeles, Chaya Venice and Chaya Brasserie San Francisco. Chaya's continued success in Los Angeles is testament to the passion and consistent ability of the acclaimed chef, who at a recent appearance at the James Beard House in New York received a standing ovation. Chef Tachibe, a pioneer of what is now called "Franco-Japanese" cuisine, travels the world as inspiration for the ever-evolving Chaya menus. $$-$$$

CHAYA
BRASSERIE
8741 Alden Dr., Los Angeles 90048
(310) 859-8833

CHAYA
VENICE
110 Navy St., Venice 90291
(310) 396-1179

SEAWEED SALAD – available at CHAYA Venice & CHAYA Brasserie ☙
Mixed greens with ginger, soy and rice vinaigrette.

✓✓ CALORIES: Excellent Choice (205) ✓✓ CHOLESTEROL: Excellent Choice (0 mg)
✓✓ FAT: Excellent Choice (11 g)* SODIUM: High (3180 mg)
EXCHANGES: ¼ Bread, 3¼ Veg, 2¼ Fat
PROTEIN: 7 g, CARBOHYDRATE: 19 g, FIBER: 12 g

JAVA CHICKEN SALAD – available at CHAYA Venice
with spicy peanut sauce.

✓✓ CALORIES: Excellent Choice (330) ✓✓ CHOLESTEROL: Excellent Choice (65 mg)
✓ FAT: Good Choice (16 g) SODIUM: High (1450 mg)
EXCHANGES: 3¾ Meat (extra lean), ¼ Bread, ¼ Veg, 2¼ Fat
PROTEIN: 30 g, CARBOHYDRATE: 14 g, FIBER: 3 g

LINGUINE VONGOLE – SPECIAL REQUEST – available at CHAYA Venice
Fresh linguine, Manilla clams with white wine olive oil sauce. Request less oil (1/2 oz.).

✓ CALORIES: Good Choice (540) ✓ CHOLESTEROL: Good Choice (130 mg)
✓ FAT: Good Choice (18 g)* ✓✓ SODIUM: Excellent Choice (130 mg)**
EXCHANGES: 3½ Meat (extra lean), 3 Bread, 1¼ Veg, 3¼ Fat
PROTEIN: 35 g, CARBOHYDRATE: 55 g, FIBER: 1 g

PEPPERED SALMON "TORO" SASHIMI – available at CHAYA Brasserie
with lemon-mustard ponzu.

✓✓ CALORIES: Excellent Choice (180) ✓✓ CHOLESTEROL: Excellent Choice (45 mg)
✓✓ FAT: Excellent Choice (6 g) SODIUM: High (1265 mg)
EXCHANGES: 2¼ Meat, ¼ Bread, ¼ Veg, ¼ Fruit
PROTEIN: 19 g, CARBOHYDRATE: 12 g, FIBER: 2 g

ANGEL HAIR – SPECIAL REQUEST – available at CHAYA Brasserie
with organic tomato and fresh basil. Request less oil (1/2 oz.).

✓ CALORIES: Good Choice (595) ✓ CHOLESTEROL: Good Choice (125 mg)
✓ FAT: Good Choice (19 g) ✓✓ SODIUM: Excellent Choice (70 mg)**
EXCHANGES: ¾ Meat, 5 Bread, 1¾ Veg, 3¾ Fat
PROTEIN: 22 g, CARBOHYDRATE: 85 g, FIBER: 3 g

KING SALMON WITH SUNDRIED TOMATOES – SPECIAL REQUEST – available at CHAYA Brasserie
with sundried tomato basil pesto. Request less oil (1/4 oz.).

✓ CALORIES: Good Choice (500) ✓ CHOLESTEROL: Good Choice (105 mg)
✓ FAT: Good Choice (22 g) ✓✓ SODIUM: Excellent Choice (165 mg)**
EXCHANGES: 5 Meat, ¾ Bread, 1½ Veg, 2 Fat
PROTEIN: 45 g, CARBOHYDRATE: 32 g, FIBER: 3 g

---

* Primarily unsaturated fat
** If you request no added salt

☙ at least 2 fruit/vegetable servings

CHILI MY SOUL
Gourmet Chili
www.chilimysoul.com

Delicious, hearty, and healthy, all "Chili My Soul®" gourmet chilis cook for a minimum of 40 hours to achieve an unparalleled flavor and texture. Our chili is much lower in salt and fat due to an exclusive 4-stage de-fatting process. We rotate our flavors and feature about 12 varieties daily including at least one of our five, 100% vegetarian chilis. Samples are always free and we're certain you'll appreciate the difference great care, quality and attention to every detail make in creating, "Quite simply... The finest chili anywhere! ™". **For our daily flavor list visit www.chilimysoul.com or call our "flavor Line" at (818) 386-9966. $**

Chili My Soul   4928 Balboa Blvd., Encino 91316 (818) 981-SOUL (7685)

POBLANO TURKEY CHILI
The creative blending of mild poblano and pasilla peppers enriches the character of this healthy, substantive chili reminiscent of Mexican mole. Analysis for 8oz. (cup) serving.
✓✓ CALORIES: Excellent Choice (215)   ✓ CHOLESTEROL: Good Choice (95 mg)
✓✓ FAT: Excellent Choice (4 g)   SODIUM: Moderate (635 mg)
EXCHANGES: 5 Meat, 1¼ Veg, ½ Fat
PROTEIN: 36 g, CARBOHYDRATE: 9 g, FIBER: 2 g

DURANGO CHILI
Smoked chipotle peppers enhance this intense, spicy beef chili accented with beef chorizo and tender maize. Hot and piquant with an earthy undertone. Analysis for 8oz. (cup) serving.
✓✓ CALORIES: Excellent Choice (325)   ✓✓ CHOLESTEROL: Excellent Choice (70 mg)
✓ FAT: Good Choice (17 g)   SODIUM: Moderate (715 mg)
EXCHANGES: 3 Meat, ½ Bread, 1¼ Veg, 1½ Fat
PROTEIN: 24 g, CARBOHYDRATE: 19 g, FIBER: 2 g

ESPRESSO BLACK BEAN CHILI
Spicy and zesty, this all vegetarian ultra-low fat chili is enhanced by the unmistakable aroma of premium decaf espresso and earthy-rich Jamaican black beans, garlic and lime. Analysis for 8oz. (cup) serving.
✓✓ CALORIES: Excellent Choice (240)   ✓✓ CHOLESTEROL: Excellent Choice (0 mg)
✓✓ FAT: Excellent Choice (4 g)   SODIUM: Moderate (640 mg)
EXCHANGES: 2 Bread, 1 Veg, ½ Fat
PROTEIN: 12 g, CARBOHYDRATE: 42 g, FIBER: 8 g

BLANCO Y VERDE CHILI
Fragrant tomatillos replace sweeter red tomatoes with Northern white beans, Anaheim chiles and garlic in this elegant cutting-edge all white meat chicken chili.
✓✓ CALORIES: Excellent Choice (270)   ✓ CHOLESTEROL: Good Choice (85 mg)
✓✓ FAT: Excellent Choice (4 g)   SODIUM: Moderate (860 mg)
EXCHANGES: 4¾ Meat, ½ Bread, 1½ Veg
PROTEIN: 37 g, CARBOHYDRATE: 20 g, FIBER: 6 g

CURRY CHICKEN CHILI
Crave the exotic? This mystical blend of Mid-Eastern and Indonesian curry and Western chiles gives a unique twist to this non-traditional spicy theme. Analysis for 8oz. (cup) serving.
✓✓ CALORIES: Excellent Choice (235)   ✓ CHOLESTEROL: Good Choice (85 mg)
✓✓ FAT: Excellent Choice (7 g)   ✓ SODIUM: Good Choice (490 mg)
EXCHANGES: 4¼ Meat, 1 Veg, ½ Fat
PROTEIN: 33 g, CARBOHYDRATE: 11 g, FIBER: 4 g

HICKORY TURKEY CHILI
All the warmth and sweet-smokiness of our Hickory Beef chili without the steer. If you like Southern BBQ flavor that's lean and light, this is a perfect chili for you. Analysis for 8oz. (cup) serving.
✓✓ CALORIES: Excellent Choice (230)   ✓ CHOLESTEROL: Good Choice (100 mg)
✓✓ FAT: Excellent Choice (5 g)   SODIUM: Moderate (615 mg)
EXCHANGES: 5 Meat, 1 Veg, ½ Fat
PROTEIN: 37 g, CARBOHYDRATE: 11 g, FIBER: 4 g

🍎 at least 2 fruit/vegetable servings

✓ Good Choice   ✓✓ Excellent Choice

Chin Chin locations:

West Hollywood: 8618 Sunset Blvd.   (310) 652-1818
Brentwood: 11740 San Vicente Blvd.   (310) 826-2525
Beverly Hills: 206 So. Beverly Dr.   (310) 248-5252
Studio City: 12215 Ventura Blvd.   (818) 985-9090
Marina Del Rey: 13455 Maxella Ave.   (310) 823-9999
Encino: 16101 Ventura Boulevard   (818) 783-1717

*"Chin Chin" not only means "to your health" but it is also known as a popular hotspot for Chinese food, offering generous portions served in a contemporary setting with a bustling atmosphere. Chin Chin is committed to preparing light and healthy food, and now offers its new **Chin Chin Lite Menu.** Visit www.chinchin.com. $$*

You may request any of the first 3 items LITE and they will be prepared without added oil.

SHRIMP WITH BLACK BEANS – LITE ☃

Shrimp stir-fried with green bell pepper, carrots and onions in a garlic and black bean sauce.

✓ CALORIES: Good Choice (460)   CHOLESTEROL: Moderate (255 mg)
✓✓ FAT: Excellent Choice (2 g)*   SODIUM: High (4600 mg)
EXCHANGES: 4 Meat (extra lean), 1½ Bread, 6 Veg, ¼ Fruit
PROTEIN: 34 g, CARBOHYDRATE: 75 g, FIBER: 6 g

CHICKEN WITH GARLIC & SNOW PEAS – LITE ☃

Velveted pieces of chicken breast stir-fried with snow peas, fresh mushrooms, carrots and sliced carrots.

✓ CALORIES: Good Choice (475)   ✓ CHOLESTEROL: Good Choice (135 mg)
✓✓ FAT: Excellent Choice (8 g)   SODIUM: High (3675 mg)
EXCHANGES: 7 Meat (extra lean), 1½ Bread, 3 Veg, ¼ Fruit, ½ Fat
PROTEIN: 54 g, CARBOHYDRATE: 44 g, FIBER: 6 g

CLASSIC CHICKEN SALAD – LITE – SPECIAL REQUEST ☃

Roasted chicken, shredded lettuce, scallions, shredded carrots and toasted almonds in a tart red ginger dressing. Request crunchies on the side (not included in analysis).

✓✓ CALORIES: Excellent Choice (230)   ✓✓ CHOLESTEROL: Excellent Choice (60 mg)
✓✓ FAT: Excellent Choice (7 g)   SODIUM: High (3225 mg)
EXCHANGES: 3 Meat (extra lean), 1 Veg, ¾ Fat
PROTEIN: 28 g, CARBOHYDRATE: 15 g, FIBER: 4 g

SZECHUAN DUMPLINGS (DIM SUM)†

Made with chopped chicken and tossed with a spicy cilantro sauce.
Five dumplings per order. Analysis is for one dumpling plus ⅕ of szechuan sauce.

✓✓ CALORIES: Excellent Choice (80)   ✓✓ CHOLESTEROL: Excellent Choice (20 mg)
✓✓ FAT: Excellent Choice (4 g)   SODIUM: Moderate (335 mg)**
EXCHANGES: ½ Meat, ¼ Bread, ¼ Fat
PROTEIN: 5 g, CARBOHYDRATE: 6 g, FIBER: 0 g

VEGETABLE BAO (DIM SUM)†

Fluffy steamed buns filled with vegetables. Three bao per order. Analysis is for one bao.

✓✓ CALORIES: Excellent Choice (90)   ✓✓ CHOLESTEROL: Excellent Choice (0 mg)
✓✓ FAT: Excellent Choice (1 g)*   SODIUM: Moderate (250 mg)**
EXCHANGES: 1 Bread, ¼ Veg, ¼ Fat
PROTEIN: 2 g, CARBOHYDRATE: 18 g, FIBER: 1 g

---

* Primarily unsaturated fat

** If you request no added salt

† Side dish guidelines are 1/3 of entree guidelines

CHINA GRILL

CONTEMPORARY CHINESE BISTRO

Our challenge has always been to create a cuisine, one that would make use of the familiar, prepared and presented in an altogether fresh and intriguing way. We are gratified that our efforts have met with the cheerful recognition of satisfied palates. And we promise to keep trying hard to earn further the trust and confidence with which we've been entrusted. $$

China Grill

3282 Sepulveda Blvd., Manhattan Beach 90266 (310) 546-7284

STEAMED SALMON FILLET WITH SOY-LEMON SAUCE
Served with grilled artichoke hearts, black shiitake mushrooms and asparagus.

✓✓ CALORIES: Excellent Choice (425)   ✓ CHOLESTEROL: Good Choice (125 mg)
✓ FAT: Good Choice (17 g)*   SODIUM: Moderate (720 mg)**
EXCHANGES: 5¾ Meat, ½ Bread, 1½ Veg, ½ Fat
PROTEIN: 50 g, CARBOHYDRATE: 19 g, FIBER: 7 g

GRILLED SEA SCALLOPS WITH JULIENNED SQUASH ☙
in black bean chili sauce.

✓✓ CALORIES: Excellent Choice (430)   ✓ CHOLESTEROL: Good Choice (105 mg)
✓ FAT: Good Choice (17 g)*   SODIUM: High (1124 mg)**
EXCHANGES: 3¾ Meat (extra lean), ¼ Bread, 1¼ Veg, ½ Fruit, 2¾ Fat
PROTEIN: 48 g, CARBOHYDRATE: 25 g, FIBER: 2 g

SAUTEED CHILEAN SEABASS FILLET
in a spicy tomato Asian basil sauce, served with garlic noodles.

✓ CALORIES: Good Choice (610)   ✓ CHOLESTEROL: Good Choice (110 mg)
✓ FAT: Good Choice (23 g)*   SODIUM: Moderate (785 mg)**
EXCHANGES: 7 Meat, 1 Bread, 1½ Veg, 4 Fat
PROTEIN: 54 g, CARBOHYDRATE: 31 g, FIBER: 2 g

ROASTED HALIBUT IN PARCHMENT PAPER ☙
Halibut chunks roasted in cumin and orange zest with vegetable medley.

✓ CALORIES: Good Choice (495)   ✓ CHOLESTEROL: Good Choice (85 mg)
✓ FAT: Good Choice (20 g)*   SODIUM: Moderate (825 mg)**
EXCHANGES: 7½ Meat (extra lean), ¼ Bread, 1¼ Veg, ¾ Fruit, 2¾ Fat
PROTEIN: 57 g, CARBOHYDRATE: 22 g, FIBER: 4 g

MIXED VEGETABLE STIR-FRY ☙
Fresh vegetables in season, tofu, and black mushrooms in a garlic-scallion sauce.

✓✓ CALORIES: Excellent Choice (400)   ✓✓ CHOLESTEROL: Excellent Choice (10 mg)
✓ FAT: Good Choice (21 g)*   SODIUM: High (1105 mg)**
EXCHANGES: 1½ Meat, 3 Veg, ¾ Fruit, 3¼ Fat
PROTEIN: 18 g, CARBOHYDRATE: 37 g, FIBER: 9 g

WOK-SEARED YELLOW FIN TUNA ☙
Served with steamed vegetables, seaweed salad and pickled ginger.

✓✓ CALORIES: Excellent Choice (390)   ✓✓ CHOLESTEROL: Excellent Choice (70 mg)
✓✓ FAT: Excellent Choice (7 g)*   SODIUM: High (1115 mg)**
EXCHANGES: 5 Meat (extra lean), 1½ Bread, 2¼ Veg, ¾ Fat
PROTEIN: 46 g, CARBOHYDRATE: 40 g, FIBER: 6 g

☙ at least 2 fruit/vegetable servings

✓ Good Choice   ✓✓ Excellent Choice

Coco's

Bakery Restaurant

What more could you want?

For family dining, Coco's Bakery Restaurant is in a class by itself, providing just the right setting: friendly service in a casual, comfortable atmosphere and a menu that emphasizes quality, freshness and value. Breakfast, lunch and dinner selections cover a wide range of choices, from fresh vegetable omelettes to terrific pastas and fresh fish. Freshly baked muffins, cakes, and a wide variety of freshly baked pies, including delicious no-sugar-added pies, are available all day long. Coco's Bakery Restaurants are located throughout California. Hours vary by location. $

38 Los Angeles area locations. Visit www.cocosbakery.com for a list of all locations.

EGG WHITE OMELETTE

Garden-fresh spinach, red-ripe tomato, sautéed onion, fresh basil and crumbled Feta cheese folded into a fluffy omelette. Analysis assumes fresh, seasonal fruit instead of breakfast potatoes and does not include bread.

✓✓ CALORIES: Excellent Choice (360)
✓✓ FAT: Excellent Choice (13 g)
✓✓ CHOLESTEROL: Excellent Choice (50 mg)
SODIUM: Moderate (970 mg)**

PROTEIN: 32 g, CARBOHYDRATE: 30 g, Fiber 5 g

ROASTED TURKEY

Hand-carved, oven-roasted turkey and mashed potatoes topped with traditional turkey gravy, served with seasonal vegetables and cranberry sauce. Bread and choice of salad or soup not included in analysis.

✓ CALORIES: Good Choice (725)
✓ FAT: Good Choice (18 g)
CHOLESTEROL: Moderate (180 mg)
SODIUM: High (4,065 mg)

PROTEIN: 65 g, CARBOHYDRATE: 76 g, Fiber 12 g

TERIYAKI CHICKEN

Grilled chicken breast glazed with our special, ginger teriyaki sauce, and sprinkled with toasted sesame seeds and diced green onion, on a bed of garden-fresh, steamed spinach and served with rice pilaf and seasonal vegetables. Basket of freshly baked bread, hot from our ovens, not included in analysis.

✓ CALORIES: Good Choice (505)
✓✓ FAT: Excellent Choice (7 g)
✓ CHOLESTEROL: Good Choice (85 mg)
SODIUM: High (3,390 mg)

PROTEIN: 38 g, CARBOHYDRATE: 61 g, Fiber 3 g

SPAGHETTI

with marinara sauce. Bread and choice of salad or soup not included in analysis.

✓ CALORIES: Good Choice (680)
✓✓ FAT: Excellent Choice (13 g)
✓✓ CHOLESTEROL: Excellent Choice (2 mg)
SODIUM: High (1,065 mg)

PROTEIN: 20 g, CARBOHYDRATE: 100 g, Fiber 15 g

COCO'S FRESH CATCH OF THE DAY- SPECIAL REQUEST

Always the freshest fish available. Served with baked potato and seasoned vegetables.
Analysis for charbroiled mahi mahi; most other fish similar, salmon higher.
Bread and choice of soup or salad not included in analysis. Request no butter.

✓ CALORIES: Good Choice (560)
✓✓ FAT: Excellent Choice (6 g)
✓ CHOLESTEROL: Good Choice (90 mg)
SODIUM: High (1,830 mg)

PROTEIN: 49 g, CARBOHYDRATE: 78 g, Fiber: 2 g

Nutrition information supplied by Coco's.

* Primarily unsaturated fat
** If you request no added salt

Healthy Dining in Los Angeles **69**

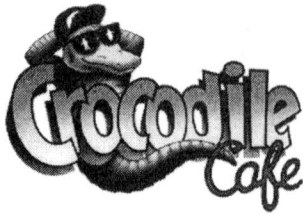

Crocodile Café is an upscale experience at a moderate price. The design of the restaurants emphasizes a lively, bright, airy environment with a high energy level. The focal point is the exhibition-style kitchen featuring a wood burning pizza oven and Oakwood grill where diners can watch their food being prepared. The restaurant's eclectic menu includes innovative twists on such items as gourmet pizzas, pastas, salads, and sandwiches, all made from scratch using the freshest ingredients. $-$$

Crocodile Cafe

Burbank: 201 N. San Fernando Blvd. (818) 843-7999
Old Pasadena: 88 W. Colorado Blvd. (626) 568-9310
San Diego: 7007 Friars Rd. (619) 297-3247
Santa Monica: 101 Santa Monica Blvd. (310) 394-4783

OAKWOOD GRILLED FRESH SALMON – SPECIAL REQUEST ☺

Topped with tomato mango relish and guajillo sauce. Served with fresh vegetables and garlic mashed potatoes. Request vegetables steamed. Mashed potatoes not included in analysis. See analysis below.

✓✓ CALORIES: Excellent Choice (375)
✓ FAT: Good Choice (17 g)*
✓ CHOLESTEROL: Good Choice (105 mg)
✓✓ SODIUM: Excellent Choice (210 mg)**
PROTEIN: 42 g, CARBOHYDRATE: 12 g, FIBER: 4 g   EXCHANGES: 5 Meat, 1¼ Veg, ¼ Fruit, 1 Fat

PACIFIC RIM CHICKEN SALAD – SPECIAL REQUEST ☺

Grilled chicken, bok choy, snow peas, marinated cucumbers, water chestnuts, sweet peppers, sesame seeds, peanuts, with a coriander honey mustard dressing. Request dressing on the side and no wontons. Wontons and dressing (30 cal, 2½ g fat per Tbs.) not included in analysis.

✓✓ CALORIES: Excellent Choice (280)
✓✓ FAT: Excellent Choice (9 g)
✓✓ CHOLESTEROL: Excellent Choice (65 mg)
✓✓ SODIUM: Excellent Choice (155 mg)**
PROTEIN: 31 g, CARBOHYDRATE: 20 g, FIBER: 5 g   EXCHANGES: 3¾ Meat, ½ Bread, 1¾ Veg, 1 Fat

HERB CRUSTED SALMON AND TIGER SHRIMP – SPECIAL REQUEST ☺

Grilled salmon and sautéed shrimp with asparagus, red onions and tomatoes on baby field greens. Request shrimp poached and balsamic vinaigrette dressing on the side. Dressing not included in analysis (60 cal, 6 g fat/Tbs).

✓ CALORIES: Excellent Choice (310)
✓✓ FAT: Excellent Choice (11 g)*
CHOLESTEROL: Moderate (210 mg)
SODIUM: High (1305 mg)
PROTEIN: 38 g, CARBOHYDRATE: 12 g, FIBER: 4 g   EXCHANGES: 4¾ Meat, 1½ Veg, 1 Fat

SMOKED TURKEY BREAST SANDWICH – SPECIAL REQUEST ☺

Thinly sliced and served "double-decker" style on whole wheat toast with dried cranberries, sunflower sprouts, cucumbers & roma tomatoes. Request no mayo (not incl. in analysis) and fresh fruit, salad or black beans instead of fries (see below).

✓ CALORIES: Good Choice (560)
✓✓ FAT: Excellent Choice (6 g)
✓✓ CHOLESTEROL: Excellent Choice (60 mg)
SODIUM: High (2200 mg)
PROTEIN: 43 g, CARBOHYDRATE: 92 g, FIBER: 14 g   EXCHANGES: 4½ Meat, 3 Bread, ½ Veg, 2 Fruit, 1 Fat

GRILLED AHI TUNA SANDWICH – SPECIAL REQUEST ☺

Oakwood grilled fresh ahi tuna with roma tomatoes, baby lettuces, grilled onions on a pan rustique roll. Request no mayo and substitute fresh fruit, salad or black beans instead of fries (see below).

✓ CALORIES: Good Choice (575)
✓ FAT: Good Choice (16 g)*
✓✓ CHOLESTEROL: Excellent Choice (55 mg)
SODIUM: Moderate (910 mg)**
PROTEIN: 41 g, CARBOHYDRATE: 64 g, FIBER: 1g   EXCHANGES: 4 Meat, 4 Bread, ¾ Veg, 2¾ Fat

GRILLED PORTABELLO MUSHROOM SANDWICH – SPECIAL REQUEST ☺

With arugula, roasted peppers and grilled red onions on an onion roll. Request no mayo and substitute fresh fruit, salad or black beans instead of fries (see below).

✓✓ CALORIES: Excellent Choice (410)
✓✓ FAT: Excellent Choice (7 g)*
✓✓ CHOLESTEROL: Excellent Choice (0 mg)
SODIUM: Moderate (685 mg)**
PROTEIN: 15 g, CARBOHYDRATE: 73 g, FIBER: 3 g   EXCHANGES: 4 Bread, 2¼ Veg, 1¼ Fat

FRESH FRUIT (4 OZ) - CAL: 35, FAT: 0 g, CHOL: 0 mg, SOD: 0 mg, PROT: 1 g, CARB: 8 g, FIB: 2 g; EXCH: ½ Fruit
BLACK BEANS - CAL: 160, FAT: 6g, CHOL: 15 mg, SOD: 265 mg; PROT: 7g, CARB: 20g, FIB: 4g; EXCH: 1¼ Br, ¼ Veg, 1¼ Fat
GARLIC MASHED POTATOES - CAL: 205, FAT: 8 g, CHOL: 25 mg, SOD: 540 mg; PROT: 3 g, CARB: 32 g, FIB: 4 g; EXCH: 2 Bread, ¼ Veg, 1½ Fat

☺ at least 2 fruit/vegetable servings
✓ Good Choice   ✓✓ Excellent Choice

It is the unique mix of classical Vietnamese and French cultures that inspires the cuisine at Crustacean. Our food doesn't represent the "typical" Vietnamese style of cooking, but rather the cuisine that was served to Vietnamese royalty and the international elite of French Colonial Vietnam. Crustacean's cuisine is healthy, incorporating Vietnamese herbs and spices that have been used in traditional Eastern healing. We look forward to having the honor and pleasure of welcoming you often in our "home!" $$

Crustacean 9646 Little Santa Monica Blvd., Beverly Hills, CA 90210 (310) 205-8990

STEAMED GINGER SEABASS

✓✓ CALORIES: Excellent Choice (255)   ✓ CHOLESTEROL: Good Choice (105 mg)
✓✓ FAT: Excellent Choice (5 g)*   ✓✓ SODIUM: Excellent Choice (170 mg)**
EXCHANGES: 4½ Meat (extra lean), ¼ Veg
PROTEIN: 47 g, CARBOHYDRATE: 3 g

TRADITIONAL VIETNAMESE SALAD ☺

with chicken cucumbers, cabbage, carrots and vinegar salsify.
✓✓ CALORIES: Excellent Choice (385)   ✓ CHOLESTEROL: Good Choice (150 mg)
✓✓ FAT: Excellent Choice (9 g)   ✓✓ SODIUM: Excellent Choice (185 mg)**
EXCHANGES: 8 Meat (extra lean), 2¾ Veg, ¼ Fat
PROTEIN: 59 g, CARBOHYDRATE: 15 g

BREAST OF CHICKEN IN 5 SPICE ☺

Breast of chicken marinated in five spice and served with grilled Japanese eggplant.
✓ CALORIES: Good Choice (500)   ✓ CHOLESTEROL: Good Choice (150 mg)
✓ FAT: Good Choice (16 g)   ✓ SODIUM: Good Choice (490 mg)**
EXCHANGES: 7¾ Meat (extra lean), 5½ Veg, 1¾ Fat
PROTEIN: 60 g, CARBOHYDRATE: 29 g

VEGETARIAN DELIGHT ☺

✓✓ CALORIES: Excellent Choice (225)   ✓✓ CHOLESTEROL: Excellent Choice (0 mg)
✓✓ FAT: Excellent Choice (11 g)*   ✓✓ SODIUM: Excellent Choice (70 mg)**
EXCHANGES: 5½ Veg, 1¾ Fat
PROTEIN: 8 g, CARBOHYDRATE: 30 g

SALMON TARTARE

✓✓ CALORIES: Excellent Choice (145)   ✓✓ CHOLESTEROL: Excellent Choice (55 mg)
✓✓ FAT: Excellent Choice (6 g)*   ✓✓ SODIUM: Excellent Choice (185 mg)**
EXCHANGES: 2½ Meat
PROTEIN: 19 g, CARBOHYDRATE: 1 g

WARM CHICKEN SALAD ☺

with mixed greens, Roma tomatoes, and raspberry vinaigrette.
✓✓ CALORIES: Excellent Choice (410)   ✓ CHOLESTEROL: Good Choice (150 mg)
✓ FAT: Good Choice (16 g)   ✓✓ SODIUM: Excellent Choice (150 mg)**
EXCHANGES: 7¾ Meat (extra lean), 1¼ Veg, 1¾ Fat
PROTEIN: 57 g, CARBOHYDRATE: 7 g

* Primarily unsaturated fat
** If you request no added salt

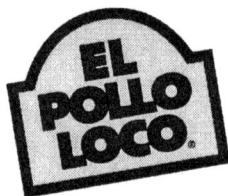

El Pollo Loco offers a fresh, wholesome alternative to traditional fast food with real food you can feel good eating. Our chicken is marinated in a special blend of herbs, spices and fruit juices and then flame-grilled right before your eyes for flavor you won't find anywhere else. We serve our chicken with warm tortillas, fresh salsas and a wide variety of healthful sides, from fresh vegetables and salads to our famous pinto beans and Spanish rice. Complimenting our meals are signature entrees such as our famous Pollo Bowl®, that enable you to satisfy your appetite without sacrifice. Treat yourself to the delicious taste of El Pollo Loco, any way you like it.

El Pollo Loco has over 150 Los Angeles County locations to serve you. For the one nearest you, call 1-888-EPL-TOGO. $

FLAME-GRILLED SKINLESS CHICKEN BREAST – SPECIAL REQUEST
Request chicken skinless.
- ✓✓ CALORIES: Excellent Choice (155)
- ✓✓ FAT: Excellent Choice (4 g)
- ✓ CHOLESTEROL: Good Choice (95 mg)
- ✓ SODIUM: Good Choice (540 mg)

EXCHANGES: 4 Meat
PROTEIN: 29 g, CARBOHYDRATE: 0 g, FIBER: 0 g

POLLO CHOICE SKINLESS BREAST MEAL – SPECIAL REQUEST ☺
Flame-grilled skinless chicken breast with vegetable blend, garden salad & house salsa.
Salad dressing not included in analysis. Request chicken skinless.
- ✓✓ CALORIES: Excellent Choice (345)
- ✓ FAT: Good Choice (16 g)
- ✓ CHOLESTEROL: Good Choice (110 mg)
- SODIUM: High (1065 mg)

EXCHANGES: 4½ Meat, ¼ Bread, 2¼ Veg, 1¼ Fat
PROTEIN: 38 g, CARBOHYDRATE: 16 g, FIBER: 7 g

BRC BURRITO
Pinto beans, rice and cheese in a flour tortilla.
- ✓ CALORIES: Good Choice (530)
- ✓✓ FAT: Excellent Choice (15 g)
- ✓✓ CHOLESTEROL: Excellent Choice (15 mg)
- SODIUM: High (1395 mg)

EXCHANGES: ½ Meat, 5¼ Bread, 2½ Fat
PROTEIN: 17 g, CARBOHYDRATE: 79 g, FIBER: 6 g

POLLO BOWL®
Flame-grilled boneless skinless chicken breast with pinto beans, Spanish rice, pico de gallo, onion & cilantro.
- ✓ CALORIES: Good Choice (545)
- ✓✓ FAT: Excellent Choice (10 g)
- ✓✓ CHOLESTEROL: Excellent Choice (40 mg)
- SODIUM: High (2160 mg)

EXCHANGES: 2¾ Meat, 5¼ Bread, ½ Veg, 1 Fat
PROTEIN: 31 g, CARBOHYDRATE: 84 g, FIBER: 12 g

INDIVIDUAL SIDES:

FRESH VEGETABLES ☺
CAL: 70, FAT: 4 g, CHOL: 0, SOD: 80 mg, PROT: 3 g, CARB: 6 g, FIB: 4 g; EXCH: 1¼ Veg, ¾ Fat

PINTO BEANS
CAL: 165, FAT: 4 g, CHOL: 0, SOD: 715 mg, PROT: 8 g, CARB: 26 g, FIB: 10 g; EXCH: ¼ Meat, 1½ Br, ½ Fat

SPANISH RICE
CAL: 165, FAT: 1 g, CHOL: 0, SOD: 425 mg, PROT: 3 g, CARB: 34 g, FIB: 1 g; EXCH: 2¼ Br, ¼ Fat

GARDEN SALAD (SMALL) ☺
CAL: 110, FAT: 7 g, CHOL: 15, SOD: 270 mg, PROT: 5 g, CARB: 8 g, FIB: 2 g; EXCH: ½ Meat, ¼ Bread, ½ Veg, ½ Fat

☺ at least 2 fruit/vegetable servings for entrees, 1 for side dishes

Nobody else makes Mexican food taste this good. Come to El Torito where we serve traditional Mexican cuisine as well as unique specialties made only with the freshest ingredients. In addition to our Mexican favorites, like sizzling fajitas and Mexican caesar salad, our chefs have prepared a variety of healthy and delicious items prepared daily to meet your nutritional needs. Join us at El Torito for lunch, dinner or Sunday brunch at any of our Southern California locations. $

El Torito Restaurants

with greater Los Angeles area locations in Buena Park, Burbank, Encino, Granada Hills, Hacienda Heights, Hawthorne, Lakewood, Long Beach, Marina del Rey, Northridge, Ontario, Pasadena, Redondo Beach, Sherman Oaks, Simi Valley, Tarzana, Thousand Oaks, Torrance, Upland, Valencia, Ventura, Woodland Hills & West Covina, as well as in Riverside, San Bernardino & Orange County locations.

Visit www.eltorito.com for a complete list of all El Torito locations.

GRILLED CHICKEN QUESADILLA LITE

Seasoned, tender chicken breast, reduced-fat jack cheese, fresh fruit relish and mild green chiles are all wrapped in a soft flour tortilla and lightly grilled. Served with fresh fruit.

- ✓ CALORIES: Good Choice (585)
- ✓ FAT: Good Choice (22 g)

CHOLESTEROL: High (480 mg)
SODIUM: High (1195 mg)

EXCHANGES: 6¼ Meat (extra lean), 1¾ Bread, ½ Veg, 1 Fruit, 2½ Fat
PROTEIN: 50 g, CARBOHYDRATE: 48 g, FIBER: 4 g

SONORA BURRITO LITE

Tender, grilled chicken breast, pico de gallo, mild chiles and reduced-fat jack cheese are all wrapped in a large flour tortilla and topped with roasted tomatillo sauce. Served with fresh fruit and frijoles de la olla (see analysis below).

- ✓ CALORIES: Good Choice (700)
- ✓ FAT: Good Choice (21 g)

CHOLESTEROL: High (330 mg)
SODIUM: High (2330 mg)

EXCHANGES: 8 Meat (extra lean), 2¼ Bread, 2¼ Veg, ¾ Fruit, 2¼ Fat
PROTEIN: 64 g, CARBOHYDRATE: 63 g, FIBER: 8 g

SPINACH ENCHILADAS – SPECIAL REQUEST

Two corn tortillas filled with sautéed spinach, mushrooms, mild chiles and melted cheese – then topped with our zesty fire-roasted tomatillo sauce. Served with fresh fruit relish, Mexican-style rice and frijoles de la olla (see separate analysis for rice and beans below). Request frijoles de la olla (instead of Sonora beans). Sweet corn cake not included in analysis.

- ✓ CALORIES: Good Choice (470)
- ✓ FAT: Good Choice (25 g)

✓✓ CHOLESTEROL: Excellent Choice (45 mg)
SODIUM: High (1665 mg)

EXCHANGES: 1 Meat, 1½ Bread, 2½ Veg, ¼ Fruit, 4 Fat
PROTEIN: 16 g, CARBOHYDRATE: 44 g, FIBER: 7 g

GRILLED SOFT CHICKEN TACOS – SPECIAL REQUEST

Three freshly prepared soft tacos featuring grilled, fresh chicken breast. Accompanied by frijoles de la olla and Mexican-style rice (see separate analysis below). Request frijoles de la olla (instead of Sonora beans). Guacamole, tortilla strips and sweet corn cake not included in analysis.

- ✓ CALORIES: Good Choice (675)
- ✓ FAT: Good Choice (24 g)

CHOLESTEROL: Moderate (155 mg)
SODIUM: High (1555 mg)

EXCHANGES: 7¾ Meat, 2¾ Bread, 1 Veg, 3 Fat
PROTEIN: 63 g, CARBOHYDRATE: 51 g, FIBER: 4 g

FRIJOLES DE LA OLLA (4 OZ) †

- ✓ CALORIES: Good Choice (155)
- ✓✓ FAT: Excellent Choice (1 g)*

✓✓ CHOLESTEROL: Excellent Choice (0 mg)
SODIUM: Moderate (400 mg)

PROTEIN: 9 g, CARBOHYDRATE: 29 g, FIBER: 8 g   EXCHANGES: ½ Meat, 2 Bread

MEXICAN – STYLE RICE (4 OZ.) †

- ✓ CALORIES: Good Choice (150)
- ✓✓ FAT: Excellent Choice (1 g)*

✓✓ CHOLESTEROL: Excellent Choice (0 mg)
SODIUM: Moderate (540 mg)

PROTEIN: 3 g, CARBOHYDRATE: 32 g, FIBER: 0 g   EXCHANGES: 2 Bread, ¼ Veg

Reduced fat cheese and/or fresh fruit available upon request.

* Primarily unsaturated fat

** If you request no added salt

† Side dish guidelines are 1/3 of entree guidelines

Healthy Dining in Los Angeles **73**

The Empress Harbor Restaurant is a new and exciting restaurant offering delicious culinary dishes of the Orient in a warm and comfortable atmosphere. The restaurant offers a tasteful blend of Chinese tradition and contemporary comfort for the ultimate dining experience. Our professional staff awaits to pamper you as you dine in the grandeur of our dining room. Our award-winning chefs have created diversified menus for you to enjoy. If you have any special requests, you can be assured that our entire staff will work with you to accommodate your every need and wish. $-$$

Empress Harbor Seafood

111 North Atlantic Blvd., Ste. 350, Monterey Park 91754 (626) 300-8833
www.EmpressHarbor.com

All analyses is based on ½ of plate (i.e., two people sharing one dish).

STIR-FRIED SHRIMP, SCALLOPS & CHICKEN ☺
in garlic chili sauce.

✓✓ CALORIES: Excellent Choice (330)   CHOLESTEROL: Moderate (175 mg)
✓✓ FAT: Excellent Choice (11 g)   SODIUM: High (1470 mg)**
EXCHANGES: 5¼ Meat (extra lean), ¼ Bread, 1¼ Veg, 1½ Fat
PROTEIN: 38 g, CARBOHYDRATE: 16 g, FIBER: 1 g

ASSORTED MUSHROOMS IN CLAY POT ☺

✓✓ CALORIES: Excellent Choice (180)   ✓✓ CHOLESTEROL: Excellent Choice (25 mg)
✓✓ FAT: Excellent Choice (10 g)*   SODIUM: High (1975 mg)**
EXCHANGES: 2¼ Veg, ¾ Fruit, 1½ Fat
PROTEIN: 10 g, CARBOHYDRATE: 20 g, FIBER: 3 g

EGGPLANT AND RAINBOW DICE – SPECIAL REQUEST ☺
Request cashew nuts on the side (not included in analysis).

✓✓ CALORIES: Excellent Choice (225)   ✓✓ CHOLESTEROL: Excellent Choice (0 mg)
✓✓ FAT: Excellent Choice (14 g)   SODIUM: Moderate (605 mg)**
EXCHANGES: ¾ Bread, 1 Veg, 2¾ Fat
PROTEIN: 6 g, CARBOHYDRATE: 22 g, FIBER: 5 g

STIR-FRIED BEANCURD ABALONE AND ASPARAGUS ☺

✓✓ CALORIES: Excellent Choice (185)   ✓✓ CHOLESTEROL: Excellent Choice (5 mg)
✓✓ FAT: Excellent Choice (12 g)*   SODIUM: Moderate (675 mg)**
EXCHANGES: ¾ Meat, ¼ Bread, 1½ Veg, 1½ Fat
PROTEIN: 12 g, CARBOHYDRATE: 11 g, FIBER: 3 g

VEGETABLE RAINBOW ON RICE ☺

✓✓ CALORIES: Excellent Choice (245)   ✓✓ CHOLESTEROL: Excellent Choice (25 mg)
✓✓ FAT: Excellent Choice (10 g)*   SODIUM: High (2330 mg)**
EXCHANGES: 1¾ Bread, 1 Veg, 1½ Fat
PROTEIN: 11 g, CARBOHYDRATE: 34 g, FIBER: 3 g

☺ at least 2 fruit/vegetable servings
✓ Good Choice   ✓✓ Excellent Choice

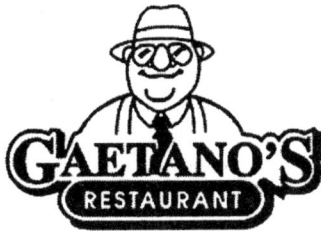

South Bay's best kept secret – Gaetano's Restaurant. Come & experience the pleasure of dining where good friends meet! Gaetano's has been pleasing palates for over 8 years with homemade pastas, fresh seafood, veal, chicken, gourmet pizzas and salads. We offer cocktails, live entertainment, full service catering and a private patio that can seat up to 30 guests. Open Monday – Thursday 11 am to 9 pm, Friday & Saturday 11 am to 10 pm and Sunday 11 am to 8 pm. $$

Gaetano's Restaurant

25345 Crenshaw Blvd., Torrance 90505 (310) 326-3354

CHICKEN AL FORNO ᚪ

Baked chicken breast with garlic, lemon and spices.
Served with assorted vegetables and pasta. See separate analysis below for pasta.

✓✓ CALORIES: Excellent Choice (380) ✓ CHOLESTEROL: Good Choice (115 mg)
  ✓ FAT: Good Choice (20 g) ✓✓ SODIUM: Excellent Choice (135 mg)**
EXCHANGES: 5¾ Meat, 1 Veg, ¼ Fruit, 3 Fat
PROTEIN: 43 g, CARBOHYDRATE: 8 g, FIBER: 3 g

SCAMPI ALLA DIAVOLA ᚪ

Scampi sautéed with fresh tomatoes and herbs.
Served with assorted vegetables and pasta. See separate analysis below for pasta.

✓ CALORIES: Good Choice (475) CHOLESTEROL: High (335 mg)
✓ FAT: Good Choice (22 g)* SODIUM: Moderate (865 mg)**
EXCHANGES: 5 Meat, 3¼ Veg, 3¾ Fat
PROTEIN: 41 g, CARBOHYDRATE: 24 g, FIBER: 6 g

CHECCA BOWTIES ᚪ

Bowtie pasta, Roma tomatoes, fresh basil, garlic and romano cheese in olive oil.

✓ CALORIES: Good Choice (475) ✓✓ CHOLESTEROL: Excellent Choice (5 mg)
✓ FAT: Good Choice (17 g)* ✓✓ SODIUM: Excellent Choice (105 mg)**
EXCHANGES: ¼ Meat, 3¼ Bread, 1¾ Veg, 2¾ Fat
PROTEIN: 12 g, CARBOHYDRATE: 63 g, FIBER: 5 g

SWORDFISH - CATCH OF THE DAY ᚪ

Fresh swordfish grilled with garlic, olive oil and lemon juice.
Served with assorted vegetables and pasta. See separate analysis below for pasta.

✓✓ CALORIES: Excellent Choice (445) ✓ CHOLESTEROL: Good Choice (115 mg)
  ✓ FAT: Good Choice (18 g)* ✓✓ SODIUM: Excellent Choice (300 mg)**
EXCHANGES: 6¼ Meat (extra lean), 1 Veg, ¼ Fruit, 1¼ Fat
PROTEIN: 59 g, CARBOHYDRATE: 9 g, FIBER: 3 g

LINGUINI PESCATORE ᚪ

Linguini with shrimp, mussels, calamari, and clams in a marinara sauce with a seafood flair.

CALORIES: Moderate (800) CHOLESTEROL: High (530 mg)
✓ FAT: Good Choice (24 g)* SODIUM: Moderate (830 mg)**
EXCHANGES: 6¾ Meat (extra lean), 3¼ Bread, 2¼ Veg, 3½ Fat
PROTEIN: 62 g, CARBOHYDRATE: 76 g, FIBER: 6 g

SIDE OF PASTA †

CALORIES: Moderate (260) ✓✓ CHOLESTEROL: Excellent Choice (0 mg)
✓ FAT: Good Choice (8 g)* ✓✓ SODIUM: Excellent Choice (50 mg)**
EXCHANGES: 2½ Bread, ¼ Veg, 1¼ Fat
PROTEIN: 7 g, CARBOHYDRATE: 41 g, FIBER: 2 g

---

* Primarily unsaturated fat † Side dish guidelines are 1/3 of entree guidelines
** If you request no added salt *Healthy Dining in Los Angeles* **75**

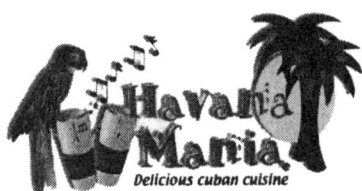

Havana Mania

3615 Inglewood Ave. (at Manhattan Beach Blvd.), Redondo Beach, CA 90278 (310) 725-9075

HALIBUT EN SALSA CRIOLLA ☖

Grilled halibut in our own garlic, cilantro, onions and tomato sauce. Served with black beans and steamed rice (see separate analyses below). Fried plantain not included in analysis.

✓ CALORIES: Good Choice (495) ✓✓ CHOLESTEROL: Excellent Choice (75 mg)
✓ FAT: Good Choice (21 g)* SODIUM: Moderate (775 mg)**
EXCHANGES: 4½ Meat (extra lean), 4¾ Veg, 3 Fat
PROTEIN: 51 g, CARBOHYDRATE: 25 g, FIBER: 5 g

SALTADO DE CAMERONES ☖

Sautéed shrimp in garlic, tomatoes, onions and bell peppers. Served with black beans and steamed rice (see separate analyses below). Fried plantain not included in analysis.

✓✓ CALORIES: Excellent Choice (450) CHOLESTEROL: High (330 mg)
✓ FAT: Good Choice (18 g)* SODIUM: High (1035 mg)
EXCHANGES: 5 Meat (extra lean), 5¼ Veg, 3 Fat
PROTEIN: 40 g, CARBOHYDRATE: 28 g, FIBER: 5 g

FILETE DE POLLO

Chicken breast (boneless) grilled in our own garlic sauce and sautéed onions. Served with black beans and steamed rice (see separate analyses below). Fried plantain not included in analysis.

✓✓ CALORIES: Excellent Choice (405) CHOLESTEROL: Moderate (175 mg)
✓✓ FAT: Excellent Choice (11 g) ✓✓ SODIUM: Excellent Choice (195 mg)**
EXCHANGES: 9 Meat (extra lean), ¾ Veg, ¼ Fruit, ¾ Fat
PROTEIN: 65 g, CARBOHYDRATE: 11 g, FIBER: 1 g

BISTEC CON CEBOLLAS

Grilled top sirloin choice, marinated with garlic and onions. Served with black beans and steamed rice (see separate analyses below). Fried plantain not included in analysis.

✓ CALORIES: Good Choice (570) ✓ CHOLESTEROL: Good Choice (125 mg)
✓ FAT: Good Choice (24 g) ✓✓ SODIUM: Excellent Choice (170 mg)**
EXCHANGES: 9 Meat, ¾ Veg, ¼ Fruit, ¾ Fat
PROTEIN: 76 g, CARBOHYDRATE: 11 g, FIBER: 1 g

FILETE DE POLLO CON CAMERONES

Boneless chicken breast and shrimp grilled to perfection. Served with black beans and steamed rice (see separate analyses below). Fried plantain not included in analysis.

✓ CALORIES: Good Choice (510) CHOLESTEROL: High (340 mg)
✓✓ FAT: Excellent Choice (12 g) ✓ SODIUM: Good Choice (390 mg)**
EXCHANGES: 11½ Meat (extra lean), ¾ Veg, ¼ Fruit, ¾ Fat
PROTEIN: 83 g, CARBOHYDRATE: 11 g, FIBER: 1 g

BLACK BEANS
CAL: 185, FAT: 1 g*, CHOL: 0 mg, SOD: 265 mg, PROT: 13 g, CARB: 34 g, FIBER: 6 g; EXCH: 2¼ Bread

STEAMED RICE
CAL: 295, FAT: 1 g*, CHOL: 0 mg, SOD: <5 mg, PROT: 6 g, CARB: 64 g, FIBER: 2 g; EXCH: 4¼ Bread, ¼ Fat

☖ at least 2 fruit/vegetable servings

✓ Good Choice ✓✓ Excellent Choice

HOTEL *Bel-Air*

LOS ANGELES

Offering a rich history that extends over 50 years, the Hotel Bel-Air has been a favored hideaway of discriminating travelers. The hotel is nestled on 12 acres, which include beautiful gardens, streams and a swan lake. Named "The Most Popular Hotel Restaurant in Los Angeles" by the Zagat Restaurant Guide in 2001, the Restaurant is a popular setting for breakfast, lunch, afternoon tea, dinner and Sunday brunch. It features French-California cuisine seasonally prepared with fresh ingredients and flavored with the hotel's very own garden herbs. $$-$$$

The Restaurant at Hotel Bel Air

701 Stone Canyon Road, Los Angeles 90077 (310) 472-1211

www.hotelbelair.com

POACHED BREAST OF CHICKEN ☺
in spiced consommé with pearl barley and a variety of vegetables.

✓ CALORIES: Good Choice (525)   ✓ CHOLESTEROL: Good Choice (150 mg)
✓✓ FAT: Excellent Choice (9 g)   SODIUM: Moderate (795 mg)**
EXCHANGES: 8 Meat, 2 Bread, 2½ Veg, ½ Fat
PROTEIN: 61 g, CARBOHYDRATE: 47 g, FIBER: 11 g

FILLET OF WHITEFISH
served on a bed of ratatouille, surrounded with tomato-fennel sauce, and topped with a smoked tomato marmalade.

✓✓ CALORIES: Excellent Choice (265)   ✓ CHOLESTEROL: Good Choice (80 mg)
✓✓ FAT: Excellent Choice (12 g)*   ✓✓ SODIUM: Excellent Choice (290 mg)**
EXCHANGES: 1½ Meat, 1½ Veg, 1½ Fat
PROTEIN: 29 g, CARBOHYDRATE: 10 g, FIBER: 2 g

MAINE SCALLOP SALAD
with fennel, frisee and orange segments.

✓✓ CALORIES: Excellent Choice (215)   ✓✓ CHOLESTEROL: Excellent Choice (30 mg)
✓✓ FAT: Excellent Choice (8 g)*   ✓✓ SODIUM: Excellent Choice (195 mg)**
EXCHANGES: 1¼ Meat (extra lean), ¼ Veg, 1 Fruit, 1¼ Fat
PROTEIN: 17 g, CARBOHYDRATE: 23 g, FIBER: 3 g

PENNE PASTA ☺
with a medley of vegetables and tomato basil sauce.

✓ CALORIES: Good Choice (540)   ✓✓ CHOLESTEROL: Excellent Choice (0 mg)
✓✓ FAT: Excellent Choice (9 g)*   ✓ SODIUM: Good Choice (325 mg)**
EXCHANGES: 5¼ Bread, 4 Veg, 1 Fat
PROTEIN: 19 g, CARBOHYDRATE: 100 g, FIBER: 11 g

CHICKEN & SHRIMP SALAD WITH PAPAYA ☺
with a honey-poppy seed yogurt dressing.

✓ CALORIES: Good Choice (550)   CHOLESTEROL: Moderate (295 mg)
✓✓ FAT: Excellent Choice (12 g)   SODIUM: Moderate (625 mg)**
EXCHANGES: 9¼ Meat (extra lean), ¾ Veg, ¼ Milk, 2 Fruit, 1 Fat
PROTEIN: 69 g, CARBOHYDRATE: 38 g, FIBER: 6 g

* Primarily unsaturated fat
** If you request no added salt

Il Forno is a Northern Italian restaurant with the flavor of California and a warm, welcoming atmosphere where each diner is treated with friendly hospitality. Superior and innovative food includes creations by Chef Domenico Salvatore, a highly respected culinary artist. The "Spa Cuisine" caters to many southern Californians' interest in lighter, healthier eating. $$

il Forno

2901 Ocean Park Blvd., Santa Monica 90405 (310) 450-1241

POLLO ALLA ERBE

Served over baby greens with balsamic vinaigrette.

✓✓ CALORIES: Excellent Choice (410)   CHOLESTEROL: Moderate (175 mg)
✓✓ FAT: Excellent Choice (14 g)   ✓✓ SODIUM: Excellent Choice (160 mg)**
EXCHANGES: 9 Meat, ¼ Veg, 1¼ Fat
PROTEIN: 64 g, CARBOHYDRATE: 3 g, FIBER: 1 g

SPA PIZZA ALLA IL FORNO ☙

Fresh dough baked to crispy perfection and topped with low-fat cheeses, fresh tomatoes and other assorted vegetables. Seasoned with garlic and herbs. This can also be cheeseless.

✓ CALORIES: Good Choice (590)   ✓✓ CHOLESTEROL: Excellent Choice (30 mg)
✓✓ FAT: Excellent Choice (13 g)   SODIUM: High (1415 mg)**
EXCHANGES: 1¾ Meat, 5 Bread, 1½ Veg, ¾ Fat
PROTEIN: 27 g, CARBOHYDRATE: 91 g, FIBER: 6 g

SPAGHETTI VECCHIO STYLE ☙

Spaghetti with eggplant, mushrooms, parsley, basil and radicchio in homemade tomato sauce.

✓ CALORIES: Good Choice (495)   ✓✓ CHOLESTEROL: Excellent Choice (0 mg)
✓✓ FAT: Excellent Choice (3 g)*   ✓✓ SODIUM: Excellent Choice (30 mg)**
EXCHANGES: 5½ Bread, 2¾ Veg
PROTEIN: 18 g, CARBOHYDRATE: 100 g, FIBER: 9 g

SPAGHETTI INTEGRALI PRIMAVERA ☙

Wheat pasta with assorted vegetables, garlic, fresh tomatoes and crushed pepper.

✓ CALORIES: Good Choice (470)   ✓✓ CHOLESTEROL: Excellent Choice (0 mg)
✓✓ FAT: Excellent Choice (7 g)*   ✓✓ SODIUM: Excellent Choice (75 mg)**
EXCHANGES: 5 Bread, 3 Veg, 1 Fat
PROTEIN: 22 g, CARBOHYDRATE: 90 g, FIBER: 17 g

SCAMPI MEDITERRANEA ☙

Scampi baked in the oven with a touch of brandy, fresh grapefruit juice, green peppercorn and Dijon mustard. Served with seasonal vegetables.

✓✓ CALORIES: Excellent Choice (280)   CHOLESTEROL: Moderate (280 mg)
✓✓ FAT: Excellent Choice (8 g)*   ✓ SODIUM: Good Choice (385 mg)**
EXCHANGES: 4¼ Meat, 1¼ Veg, ¼ Fruit, 1 Fat
PROTEIN: 34 g, CARBOHYDRATE: 11 g, FIBER: 4 g

PESCE BIANCO ALL ADRIATICA ☙

White fish sautéed with fresh tomatoes, zucchini, herbs and spices. Served with seasonal vegetables.

✓✓ CALORIES: Excellent Choice (365)   ✓ CHOLESTEROL: Good Choice (120 mg)
✓ FAT: Good Choice (18 g)*   ✓✓ SODIUM: Excellent Choice (150 mg)**
EXCHANGES: 2¼ Meat, 2¼ Veg, 2 Fat
PROTEIN: 42 g, CARBOHYDRATE: 12 g, FIBER: 5 g

☙ at least 2 fruit/vegetable servings
✓ Good Choice   ✓✓ Excellent Choice

Il Moro serves exquisite fresh, wholesome, Italian food. Our goal is to ensure a remarkable dining experience for all our guests. Il Moro restaurant is the perfect place for a power lunch or a relaxing romantic dinner. The floor-to-ceiling dining room windows allow our beautiful pepper trees, waterfall and stream to be part of the indoor décor. Our warm and stylish private rooms are the perfect place to host any special event while enjoying Italian cooking at its very best. And now Il Moro can come to your door; if you need food delivery or full catering service, we will be there for you. Il Moro restaurant has launched a late night menu on Fridays and Saturdays after 10 pm. If you are looking for a light, fun supper with an incredible rare beer list to compliment your food choices, come to Il Moro and enjoy yourself on our beautiful garden patio. $$

Il Moro   11400 W. Olympic Blvd., Los Angeles, CA 90064   (310) 575-3530

MARE CALDO
A warm seafood platter of baby clams, shrimp and sea scallops, served with Italian cannelloni beans in a sage, lemon, and olive oil dressing.

✓✓ CALORIES: Excellent Choice (355) CHOLESTEROL: Moderate (165 mg)
✓ FAT: Good Choice (16 g)* SODIUM: Moderate (615 mg)**
EXCHANGES: 5½ Meat (extra lean), ¾ Bread, 2¾ Fat
PROTEIN: 40 g, CARBOHYDRATE: 16 g, FIBER: 4 g

TRANCIO DI TONNO
Tartare of ahi tune (raw), mixed with anchovies, onions and garlic, in a lemon and olive oil dressing on a bed of baby lettuces and julienne of leeks.

✓✓ CALORIES: Excellent Choice (205) ✓✓ CHOLESTEROL: Excellent Choice (35 mg)
✓✓ FAT: Excellent Choice (9 g)* ✓✓ SODIUM: Excellent Choice (120 mg)**
EXCHANGES: 2¾ Meat (extra lean), 1¼ Veg, 1 Fat
PROTEIN: 22 g, CARBOHYDRATE: 9 g, FIBER: 2 g

INSALATA DI GAMBERI – SPECIAL REQUEST ⌘
Grilled shrimp salad with Belgium endive, arugula and diced tomatoes in a mustard vinegar dressing.
<u>Request dressing on the side</u> (50 calories, 4 g fat for 2 Tbs).

✓✓ CALORIES: Excellent Choice (180) CHOLESTEROL: Moderate (220 mg)
✓✓ FAT: Excellent Choice (4 g)* ✓✓ SODIUM: Excellent Choice (300 mg)**
EXCHANGES: 3¼ Meat (extra lean), 1¼ Veg, ½ Fat
PROTEIN: 27 g, CARBOHYDRATE: 10 g, FIBER: 5 g

SALMONE GRIGLIA ⌘
King wild Alaskan salmon, charcoal broiled, with a side of vegetables and roasted potatoes.

✓✓ CALORIES: Excellent Choice (400) ✓ CHOLESTEROL: Good Choice (105 mg)
✓✓ FAT: Excellent Choice (15 g)* ✓ SODIUM: Good Choice (380 mg)**
EXCHANGES: 5 Meat, 1¼ Bread, ¾ Veg, ½ Fat
PROTEIN: 42 g, CARBOHYDRATE: 23 g, FIBER: 5 g

PICCHIATELLI AI RAGU
Short pasta sautéed with a ragu of vegetables.

✓✓ CALORIES: Excellent Choice (380) ✓✓ CHOLESTEROL: Excellent Choice (20 mg)
✓✓ FAT: Excellent Choice (15 g) SODIUM: Moderate (605 mg)**
EXCHANGES: 1¾ Meat, 2½ Bread, ¾ Veg, 2 Fat
PROTEIN: 19 g, CARBOHYDRATE: 44 g, FIBER: 4 g

SPAGHETTINO AL POMODORO FRESCO ⌘
Spaghetti with fresh diced Roma tomatoes, a touch of tomato sauce, basil, garlic and extra virgin olive oil.

✓✓ CALORIES: Excellent Choice (290) ✓✓ CHOLESTEROL: Excellent Choice (0 mg)
✓✓ FAT: Excellent Choice (9 g)* ✓✓ SODIUM: Excellent Choice (210 mg)**
EXCHANGES: 2 Bread, 2½ Veg, 1¼ Fat
PROTEIN: 9 g, CARBOHYDRATE: 48 g, FIBER: 6 g

* Primarily unsaturated fat
** If you request no added salt

JACK SPRAT'S
· G R I L L E ·

Jack Sprat's Grille is widely known for its delectable and healthful food at moderate prices. The vast variety of selections includes casual and dinner items and offers something for every palate. According to Bon Appetit magazine, "Jack Sprat and his wife had opposite eating habits but both of them would be satisfied at Jack Sprat's Grille." Most dishes are accompanied by a choice of exciting salsas and sauces which add a burst of flavor. Lunch & dinner daily, dinner only on Sunday. Free parking in the rear after 5:30 pm. $$

Jack Sprat's Grille
10668 W. Pico Blvd. (at Overland), Los Angeles, CA 90064 (310) 837-6662

FIRE ROASTED TOMATO SOUP WITH CHICKEN - SPECIAL REQUEST 🍎
Bell peppers, roasted corn and cilantro, topped with guacamole, fat-free sour cream.
Request no tortilla chips (chips not included in analysis).
✓✓ CALORIES: Excellent Choice (165)   ✓✓ CHOLESTEROL: Excellent Choice (50 mg)
✓✓ FAT: Excellent Choice (4 g)   ✓✓ SODIUM: Excellent Choice (75 mg)**
EXCHANGES: 2½ Meat (extra lean), ¼ Bread, 1 Veg, ¼ Fat
PROTEIN: 20 g, CARBOHYDRATE: 14 g, FIBER: 3 g

CHARBROILED AHI TUNA SALAD WITH FRESH MANGO KIWI SALSA 🍎
with shredded jicama and mango kiwi salsa. Tortilla strips not included in analysis.
✓✓ CALORIES: Excellent Choice (310)   ✓✓ CHOLESTEROL: Excellent Choice (45 mg)
✓✓ FAT: Excellent Choice (5 g)*   SODIUM: High (1205 mg)
EXCHANGES: 3¼ Meat (extra lean), 3 Veg, 1¼ Fruit, ¾ Fat
PROTEIN: 26 g, CARBOHYDRATE: 41 g, FIBER: 4 g

JACK'S CHARBROILED BONELESS SKINLESS CHICKEN BREAST
Marinated in fresh rosemary, sage & garlic and topped with mango kiwi salsa.
✓✓ CALORIES: Excellent Choice (390)   ✓ CHOLESTEROL: Good Choice (150 mg)
✓✓ FAT: Excellent Choice (14 g)   ✓✓ SODIUM: Excellent Choice (295 mg)**
EXCHANGES: 8 Meat (extra lean), ½ Fruit, 1½ Fat
PROTEIN: 56 g, CARBOHYDRATE: 8 g, FIBER: 1 g

GRILLED TIGER SHRIMP WITH FIERY PINEAPPLE SALSA 🍎
Served on a bed of shredded jicama.
✓✓ CALORIES: Excellent Choice (270)   CHOLESTEROL: Moderate (250 mg)
✓✓ FAT: Excellent Choice (6 g)*   SODIUM: High (1105 mg)
EXCHANGES: 3¾ Meat (extra lean), 2½ Veg, ½ Fruit, 1 Fat
PROTEIN: 29 g, CARBOHYDRATE: 27 g, FIBER: 1 g

AHI TUNA BURGER
with guacamole and chipotle chile mayonnaise and topped with fiery pineapple salsa.
✓✓ CALORIES: Excellent Choice (420)   ✓✓ CHOLESTEROL: Excellent Choice (50 mg)
✓✓ FAT: Excellent Choice (12 g)*   SODIUM: Moderate (610 mg)**
EXCHANGES: 3½ Meat (extra lean), 2¼ Bread, ¾ Veg, ¼ Fruit, 2¼ Fat
PROTEIN: 33 g, CARBOHYDRATE: 46 g, FIBER: 8 g

LINGUINI WITH FRESH ARUGULA, SUNDRIED TOMATOES & PINE NUTS - SPECIAL REQUEST 🍎
with roasted garlic, fresh arugula, sundried tomatoes and pine nuts. Request less oil (¼ oz).
✓ CALORIES: Good Choice (660)   ✓✓ CHOLESTEROL: Excellent Choice (0 mg)
✓ FAT: Good Choice (16 g)*   SODIUM: Moderate (955 mg)**
EXCHANGES: 4¼ Bread, 7 Veg, 2½ Fat
PROTEIN: 26 g, CARBOHYDRATE: 115 g, FIBER: 11 g

🍎 at least 2 fruit/vegetable servings

✓ Good Choice   ✓✓ Excellent Choice

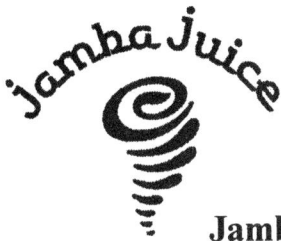

Jamba Juice is a leading retail purveyor of blended-to-order smoothies and fresh squeezed juices. Our mission is to enrich the daily experience of our customers, community & team members through the life-nourishing qualities of fruits & vegetables. All smoothies include one FREE Juice Boost & can be made non-dairy! Also, try our nutritious breads that are perfect with a smoothie. $

Jamba Juice with over 50 Los Angeles county locations in: Beverly Hills, Brentwood, Burbank, Cerritos, Culver City, Encino, Glendale, Hermosa Beach, Lakewood, Larchmont, Long Beach, Los Angeles, Loyola, Manhattan Beach, Marina Del Rey, Melrose, Northridge, Palmdale, Pasadena, Redondo Beach, Rolling Hills Estates, Santa Monica, Sherman Oaks, Studio City, Tarzana, Torrence, USC, Valencia, W. Hollywood, W. Los Angeles, Westlake Village, Westminster & Woodland Hills. **Call 1-888-JAMBA12 or visit www.jambajuice.com for your nearest location.**

THE JAMBA POWERBOOST™ SMOOTHIE _(24 oz.)_

Powered from all 6 Juice Boosts, fresh squeezed orange juice, strawberries, raspberries, banana, nonfat Jamba sorbet and ice.

✓✓ CALORIES: Excellent Choice (440) ✓✓ CHOLESTEROL: Excellent Choice (0 mg)
✓✓ FAT: Excellent Choice (1 g)* ✓✓ SODIUM: Excellent Choice (40 mg)
PROTEIN: 6 g, CARBOHYDRATE: 105 g, FIBER: 7 g

THE COLDBUSTER™ SMOOTHIE _(24 oz.)_

Orange juice, peaches, banana, orange sherbet, immunity boost and ice.

✓✓ CALORIES: Excellent Choice (430) ✓✓ CHOLESTEROL: Excellent Choice (5 mg)
✓✓ FAT: Excellent Choice (2½ g) ✓✓ SODIUM: Excellent Choice (35 mg)
PROTEIN: 5 g, CARBOHYDRATE: 100 g, FIBER: 5 g

KIWI BERRY BURNER™ SMOOTHIE _(24 oz.)_

Kiwi juice, strawberries, peaches, nonfat Jamba sorbet, nonfat frozen yogurt, Burner Boost and ice.

✓ CALORIES: Good Choice (470) ✓✓ CHOLESTEROL: Excellent Choice (0 mg)
✓✓ FAT: Excellent Choice (½ g) ✓✓ SODIUM: Excellent Choice (85 mg)
PROTEIN: 4 g, CARBOHYDRATE: 112 g, FIBER: 5 g

PROTEIN BERRY PIZZAZZ SMOOTHIE _(24 oz.)_

Protein Berry Pizzazz is packed with over 20 grams of protein, or over 50% of your daily recommended protein, and is high in calcium & phosphorus. Dreamy-creamy with soy protein, strawberries and bananas.

✓✓ CALORIES: Excellent Choice (440) ✓✓ CHOLESTEROL: Excellent Choice (0 mg)
✓✓ FAT: Excellent Choice (1½ g)* ✓✓ SODIUM: Excellent Choice (240 mg)
PROTEIN: 20 g, CARBOHYDRATE: 92 g, FIBER: 6 g

CARIBBEAN PASSION™ SMOOTHIE _(24 oz.)_

Passionfruit mango juice, peaches, strawberries, orange sherbet and ice.

✓✓ CALORIES: Excellent Choice (440) ✓✓ CHOLESTEROL: Excellent Choice (5 mg)
✓✓ FAT: Excellent Choice (2 g) ✓✓ SODIUM: Excellent Choice (60 mg)
PROTEIN: 4 g, CARBOHYDRATE: 102 g, FIBER: 5 g

RAZZMATAZZ™ SMOOTHIE _(24 oz.)_

Raspberry juice, strawberries, banana, orange sherbet and ice.

✓ CALORIES: Good Choice (480) ✓✓ CHOLESTEROL: Excellent Choice (5 mg)
✓✓ FAT: Excellent Choice (2 g) ✓✓ SODIUM: Excellent Choice (70 mg)
PROTEIN: 3 g, CARBOHYDRATE: 112 g, FIBER: 4 g

GRIN & CARROT BREAD _(1 mini loaf) Packed with shreds of carrots, raisins, walnuts, pineapple & hints of cinnamon._
CAL: 250, FAT: 10 g*, CHOL: 25 mg, SOD: 250 mg; PROT: 5 g, CARB: 36 g, FIBER: 1 g

HONEY BERRY BRAN BREAD _(1 mini loaf) with raisins, blueberries & spices. Good source of protein, fiber & iron!_
CAL: 320, FAT: 12 g*, CHOL: 30 mg, SOD: 360 mg; PROT: 6 g, CARB: 48 g, FIBER: 6 g

Nutrition information supplied by Jamba Juice.

* Primarily unsaturated fat
** If you request no added salt

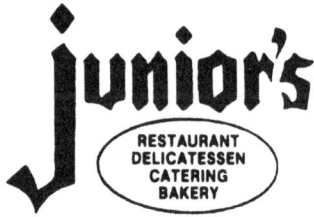

Junior's, run by David and Jon Saul, is a warm, fun, family restaurant, established in 1959. We offer an expansive menu featuring a wide variety of freshly prepared cuisines. All foods are prepared on the premises. We have an award-winning bakery and a large deli. We offer eat-in as well as take-out and a great "u-call we-haul" delivery service. We have catering for all occasions and make unbelievable wedding cakes. Valet service available. Open weekdays 6:30 am – 11:00pm & weekends 7:00am – midnight. $-$$

Junior's

2379 Westwood Blvd., Los Angeles 90064 (310) 839-8085

NOVA LOX AND EGG WHITES – SPECIAL REQUEST ☙
Scrambled with onions. Served with fresh fruit and toasted rye bread. Request egg whites.
✓✓ CALORIES: Excellent Choice (345)   ✓✓ CHOLESTEROL: Excellent Choice (15 mg)
✓✓ FAT: Excellent Choice (4 g)*   SODIUM: High (1070 mg)**
EXCHANGES: 5 Meat (extra lean), 1 Bread, ½ Veg, 1 Fruit, ¼ Fat
PROTEIN: 41 g, CARBOHYDRATE: 35 g, FIBER: 2 g

VEGETABLE OMELETTE WITH EGG WHITES – SPECIAL REQUEST ☙
Served with fresh fruit and toasted rye bread. Request egg whites.
✓✓ CALORIES: Excellent Choice (295)   ✓✓ CHOLESTEROL: Excellent Choice (0 mg)
✓✓ FAT: Excellent Choice (2 g)*   SODIUM: Moderate (655 mg)**
EXCHANGES: 3¾ Meat (extra lean), 1 Bread, 1¼ Veg, 1 Fruit, ¼ Fat
PROTEIN: 33 g, CARBOHYDRATE: 37 g, FIBER: 5 g

CALIFORNIA SALAD – SPECIAL REQUEST ☙
Chicken breast, hard-boiled egg, tomatoes, red onion, and cucumber over romaine and iceberg lettuce. Served with choice of dressing on the side (dressing not included in analysis). Fat free thousand island available. Request cheese on the side and use sparingly (not included in analysis).
✓✓ CALORIES: Excellent Choice (340)   CHOLESTEROL: High (310 mg)
✓✓ FAT: Excellent Choice (10 g)   ✓✓ SODIUM: Excellent Choice (170 mg)**
EXCHANGES: 6 Meat (extra lean), 2 Veg, ½ Fat
PROTEIN: 46 g, CARBOHYDRATE: 15 g, FIBER: 6 g

BREAST OF ROASTED TURKEY DINNER ☙
Served with vegetables, boiled potatoes and stuffing. Gravy served on the side (not included in analysis).
✓ CALORIES: Good Choice (520)   ✓ CHOLESTEROL: Good Choice (95 mg)
✓✓ FAT: Excellent Choice (11 g)   SODIUM: Moderate (805 mg)**
EXCHANGES: 5 Meat (extra lean), 3½ Bread, 1¼ Veg, 2 Fat
PROTEIN: 43 g, CARBOHYDRATE: 61 g, FIBER: 7 g

TURKEY STEAK ☙
Skinless and marinated in Junior's special sauce, served with fresh fruit and boiled potatoes.
✓ CALORIES: Good Choice (470)   CHOLESTEROL: Moderate (165 mg)
✓✓ FAT: Excellent Choice (2 g)   SODIUM: High (1010 mg)**
EXCHANGES: 8¾ Meat (extra lean), 2 Bread, 1 Fruit
PROTEIN: 65 g, CARBOHYDRATE: 47 g, FIBER: 5 g

GARDEN BURGER ☙
A vegetarian burger served with fresh fruit. French fries not included in analysis.
✓ CALORIES: Good Choice (600)   ✓✓ CHOLESTEROL: Excellent Choice (20 mg)
✓✓ FAT: Excellent Choice (15 g)*   SODIUM: High (1510 mg)**
EXCHANGES: ¾ Meat, 5½ Bread, ¼ Veg, 1 Fruit, 3 Fat
PROTEIN: 19 g, CARBOHYDRATE: 100 g, FIBER: 10 g

☙ at least 2 fruit/vegetable servings
✓ Good Choice   ✓✓ Excellent Choice

KHOURY'S

RESTAURANT

Enjoy waterfront dining and surround yourself with fresh flowers, lush greenery and elegant watercolor art. The best restaurant for innovative seafood, chicken and beef entrees, fresh salads, savory soups and delightful desserts. We present healthy gourmet dining at reasonable prices. Patio dining, full bar, and great entertainment. $

Khoury's 110 Marina Drive, Long Beach, CA 90803 (562) 598-6800

CHICKEN BOLOGNAISE ☺

Chicken tenders cooked in tomato sauce with garlic, fresh basil, mushrooms and celery. Served with rice or pasta (not included in analysis).

✓✓ CALORIES: Excellent Choice (375)
✓✓ FAT: Excellent Choice (11 g)
✓ CHOLESTEROL: Good Choice (130 mg)
SODIUM: Moderate (695 mg)**

EXCHANGES: 6¾ Meat (extra lean), 1¼ Veg, 1 Fat
PROTEIN: 53 g, CARBOHYDRATE: 15 g, Fiber: 3g

CHICKEN DILL - SPECIAL REQUEST ☺

Chicken tenders sautéed with baby dill, mushrooms and lemon butter sauce. Served with rice or pasta (not included in analysis). Request vegetables steamed and less butter (1 Tbs.).

✓✓ CALORIES: Excellent Choice (420)
✓ FAT: Good Choice (20 g)
✓ CHOLESTEROL: Good Choice (130 mg)
✓✓ SODIUM: Excellent Choice (190 mg)**

EXCHANGES: 6¾ Meat (extra lean), 1 Veg, ¼ Fruit, 2¾ Fat
PROTEIN: 50 g, CARBOHYDRATE: 9 g, Fiber: 2g

CHICKEN TARRAGON - SPECIAL REQUEST

Chicken tenders sautéed and served with fresh tarragon and lemon butter sauce. Served with rice pilaf or pasta (not included in analysis). Request vegetables steamed and less butter (1 Tbs.).

✓✓ CALORIES: Excellent Choice (415)
✓ FAT: Good Choice (20 g)
✓ CHOLESTEROL: Good Choice (130 mg)
✓✓ SODIUM: Excellent Choice (185 mg)**

EXCHANGES: 6¾ Meat (extra lean), ½ Veg, ¼ Fruit, 2¾ Fat
PROTEIN: 49 g, CARBOHYDRATE: 7 g, Fiber: 1g

CHICKEN THYME - SPECIAL REQUEST ☺

Sautéed chicken tenders served with fresh thyme, diced tomato, mushrooms, and lemon butter sauce. Served with rice pilaf or pasta (not included in analysis). Request vegetables steamed and less butter (1 Tbs.).

✓✓ CALORIES: Excellent Choice (435)
✓ FAT: Good Choice (20 g)
✓ CHOLESTEROL: Good Choice (130 mg)
✓✓ SODIUM: Excellent Choice (195 mg)**

EXCHANGES: 6¾ Meat (extra lean), 1½ Veg, ¼ Fruit, 2¾ Fat
PROTEIN: 51 g, CARBOHYDRATE: 12 g, Fiber: 2g

CHICKEN BASIL - SPECIAL REQUEST ☺

Sautéed chicken tenders topped with fresh basil, diced tomato, mushrooms and lemon butter sauce. Served with rice or pasta (not included in analysis). Request vegetables steamed and less butter (1 Tbs.).

✓✓ CALORIES: Excellent Choice (435)
✓ FAT: Good Choice (20 g)
✓ CHOLESTEROL: Good Choice (130 mg)
✓✓ SODIUM: Excellent Choice (195 mg)**

EXCHANGES: 6¾ Meat (extra lean), 1½ Veg, ¼ Fruit, 2¾ Fat
PROTEIN: 51 g, CARBOHYDRATE: 11 g, Fiber: 2g

CHICKEN PICCATA - SPECIAL REQUEST

Sautéed chicken tenders served with the classic capers and lemon butter sauce. Served with rice or pasta (not included in analysis). Request vegetables steamed and less butter (1 Tbs.).

✓✓ CALORIES: Excellent Choice (410)
✓ FAT: Good Choice (20 g)
✓ CHOLESTEROL: Good Choice (130 mg)
SODIUM: Moderate (820 mg)**

EXCHANGES: 6¾ Meat (extra lean), ½ Veg, ¼ Fruit, 2¾ Fat, Fiber: 1g
PROTEIN: 49 g, CARBOHYDRATE: 6 g

* Primarily unsaturated fat
** If you request no added salt

Kincaid's Bay House

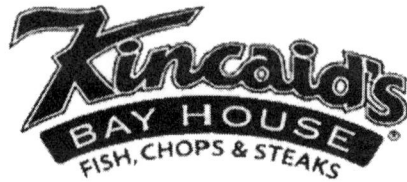

A classic "Fish, Chop & Steak House," Kincaid's has a menu that elicits tradition, yet shows a modern flair of its own. Celebrating the best of American products, Kincaid's Executive Chef James Nalu Miller features fresh Pacific finfish and shellfish, premium Nebraska Select beef steaks, chops and roasts and carefully selected pork, game, poultry and lamb entrees.

Kincaid's offers spectacular ocean views with an outdoor patio and large operable windows surrounding all dining and bar areas. The unique setting is complemented by a warm and traditional design featuring rich wood tabletops, mahogany accents, dramatic chandeliers, an old-fashioned saloon-style mirrored back bar and marble tile floors. $$$

Kincaid's Bay House
500 The Pier, Redondo Beach 90277 (310) 318-6080

REQUEST HEALTHY DINING PREPARATION FOR THE FOLLOWING ENTREES:

CAJUN SEARED AHI – HEALTHY DINING ☺

Fresh steak cut of sashimi-grade Hawaiian yellowfin tuna seasoned with Cajun spices, flash-seared medium-rare. Served with sweet sushi jasmine rice and steamed fresh, seasonal vegetables.
- ✓ CALORIES: Good Choice (540)
- ✓✓ FAT: Excellent Choice (9 g)
- ✓ CHOLESTEROL: Good Choice (115 mg)
- SODIUM: High (1775 mg)**

EXCHANGES: 6¼ Meat, 3¼ Bread, 1¾ Veg, 1¼ Fat
PROTEIN: 56 g, CARBOHYDRATE: 59 g, FIBER: 7 g

GRILLED SALMON – HEALTHY DINING ☺

Fresh Atlantic salmon hardwood grilled to perfection. Served with sweet sushi jasmine rice and steamed fresh, seasonal vegetables.
- ✓ CALORIES: Good Choice (580)
- ✓ FAT: Good Choice (19 g)
- ✓ CHOLESTEROL: Good Choice (130 mg)
- ✓ SODIUM: Good Choice (450 mg)**

EXCHANGES: 5 Meat, 3 Bread, 1¾ Veg, 1¼ Fat
PROTEIN: 48 g, CARBOHYDRATE: 55 g, FIBER: 7 g

PAN SEARED SCALLOPS – HEALTHY DINING ☺

Tender scallops pan-seared with a sweet Cabernet reduction and garnished with toasted macadamia nuts. Accompanied by sushi jasmine rice and steamed fresh, seasonal vegetables.
- ✓ CALORIES: Good Choice (630)
- ✓ FAT: Good Choice (18 g)*
- ✓ CHOLESTEROL: Good Choice (120 mg)
- SODIUM: Moderate (850 mg)**

EXCHANGES: 6¼ Meat, 3½ Bread, 1¾ Veg, 2¾ Fat
PROTEIN: 56 g, CARBOHYDRATE: 65 g, FIBER: 8 g

GRILLED AUSTRALIAN ROCK LOBSTER TAIL – HEALTHY DINING ☺

Australian cold-water rock lobster is superior in texture and flavor. Grilled and served with sweet sushi jasmine rice and steamed fresh, seasonal vegetables.
- ✓ CALORIES: Good Choice (595)
- ✓✓ FAT: Excellent Choice (11 g)*
- CHOLESTEROL: Moderate (205 mg)
- SODIUM: High (1330 mg)**

EXCHANGES: 4¾ Meat, 3 Bread, 1¾ Veg, 1¾ Fat
PROTEIN: 64 g, CARBOHYDRATE: 58 g, FIBER: 7 g

☺ at least 2 fruit/vegetable servings
✓ Good Choice   ✓✓ Excellent Choice

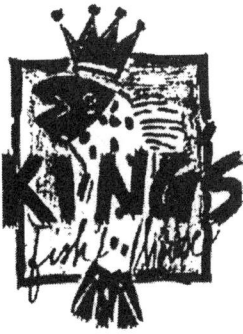
PINE AVENUE

A fish is a fish is a fish, so they say. But King's Pine Avenue Fish House excels in resourcing only the freshest, highest quality fish and shellfish available. Located in downtown Long Beach and Calabasas, King's Pine Avenue Fish House provides the most extensive variety of daily changing seafood west of the Mississippi, serving more than 35 varieties of fresh seafood prepared in 10 different ways. The menu also offers expertly prepared chicken, steak, and pasta, all at prices guests from far and near find attractive. Lunch is served 11 am to 4 pm; dinner until 10 pm Sunday through Thursday, until 11 pm Friday and Saturday. $$

King's Fish House

100 W. Broadway, Long Beach 90802 (562) 432-7463
1798 Commons Way, The Commons at Calabasas 91302 (818) 225-1979

CHARBROILED ATLANTIC SALMON – SPECIAL REQUEST ☺
Served with house salad and garden vegetables. Request no butter on fish and steamed vegetables. Salad dressing not included in analysis.
- ✓✓ CALORIES: Excellent Choice (390)
- ✓ FAT: Good Choice (17 g)*
- ✓ CHOLESTEROL: Good Choice (110 mg)
- ✓✓ SODIUM: Excellent Choice (190 mg)**

EXCHANGES: 5 Meat (extra lean), ½ Bread, 1¼ Veg, ¾ Fat
PROTEIN: 43 g, CARBOHYDRATE: 14 g, FIBER: 3 g

NORTHERN HALIBUT – SPECIAL REQUEST ☺
Served with house salad and garden vegetables. Request no butter on fish and steamed vegetables. Salad dressing not included in analysis.
- ✓✓ CALORIES: Excellent Choice (350)
- ✓✓ FAT: Excellent Choice (10 g)*
- ✓✓ CHOLESTEROL: Excellent Choice (75 mg)
- ✓✓ SODIUM: Excellent Choice (225 mg)**

EXCHANGES: 4½ Meat (extra lean), ½ Bread, 1¼ Veg, ¾ Fat
PROTEIN: 51 g, CARBOHYDRATE: 14 g, FIBER: 3 g

ANGEL HAIR PASTA WITH SHRIMP – SPECIAL REQUEST ☺
Angel hair pasta with fresh tomatoes, garlic and basil. Request less oil (½ oz.). Also served vegetarian.
- ✓ CALORIES: Good Choice (595)
- ✓ FAT: Good Choice (17 g)*
- CHOLESTEROL: Moderate (220 mg)
- ✓ SODIUM: Good Choice (480 mg)**

EXCHANGES: 3¼ Meat (extra lean), 3¾ Bread, 2¾ Veg, 2¾ Fat
PROTEIN: 36 g, CARBOHYDRATE: 74 g, FIBER: 6 g

KING'S SEAFOOD COMBO – SPECIAL REQUEST ☺
Brochettes of ahi, swordfish and yellowtail. Served with house salad and garden vegetables. Request vegetables steamed. Salad dressing not included in analysis.
- ✓ CALORIES: Good Choice (490)
- ✓✓ FAT: Excellent Choice (15 g)*
- ✓✓ CHOLESTEROL: Excellent Choice (65 mg)
- SODIUM: High (1170 mg)**

EXCHANGES: 6 Meat (extra lean), ½ Bread, 1¼ Veg, ½ Fruit, 1 Fat
PROTEIN: 57 g, CARBOHYDRATE: 30 g, FIBER: 4 g

SHRIMP & CRAB LOUIE COMBO – SPECIAL REQUEST ☺
Bay shrimp and King crab meat with onion, cucumber, tomato, carrot, celery and avocado. Request dressing on the side (not included in analysis).
- ✓✓ CALORIES: Excellent Choice (450)
- ✓ FAT: Good Choice (23 g)
- CHOLESTEROL: Moderate (265 mg)
- SODIUM: High (1100 mg)**

EXCHANGES: 5 Meat (extra lean), 5¾ Veg, 6¼ Fat
PROTEIN: 44 g, CARBOHYDRATE: 21 g, FIBER: 8 g

CIOPPINO ☺
Dungeness crab, shrimp, calamari, mussels, clams and fresh fish.
- ✓ CALORIES: Good Choice (625)
- ✓ FAT: Good Choice (24 g)*
- CHOLESTEROL: High (370 mg)
- SODIUM: High (1320 mg)**

EXCHANGES: 7½ Meat (extra lean), 2½ Veg, 3¼ Fat
PROTEIN: 74 g, CARBOHYDRATE: 22 g, FIBER: 3 g

☺ at least 2 fruit/vegetable servings

* Primarily unsaturated fat

** If you request no added salt

Healthy Dining in Los Angeles **85**

KOO·KOO·ROO
GOOD FOR YOO.

Koo Koo Roo California Kitchen features Original Skinless Flame-Broiled Chicken,™ fresh oven-roasted turkey breast, garlic & country herb rotisserie chicken, salads, and a wide assortment of freshly prepared gourmet side dishes. Food is made fresh throughout the day and appeals to those who appreciate delicious, high quality, fresh food that can be enjoyed on the premises or as a home meal replacement. Take out and catering available. $

Koo Koo Roo locations in:

Beverly Hills, Brentwood, Burbank, Canoga Park, Downtown LA, Encino, Larchmont, Los Angeles, Manhattan Beach, Marina del Rey, Monrovia, Pasadena, Redondo Beach, Santa Monica, Studio City, Toluca Lake, Torrance, Venice, West Hollywood, West Los Angeles & Woodland Hills.

KOO KOO ROO SKINLESS CHICKEN BREAST *(4.2 oz.)*

✓✓ CALORIES: Excellent Choice (195)   ✓ CHOLESTEROL: Good Choice (120 mg)
✓✓ FAT: Excellent Choice (6 g)   ✓ SODIUM: Good Choice (435 mg)
EXCHANGES: 5 Meat (extra lean)
PROTEIN: 35 g, CARBOHYDRATE: 0 g, FIBER: 0 g

ORIGINAL CHICKEN SANDWICH – SPECIAL REQUEST
Request no dressing.

✓✓ CALORIES: Excellent Choice (375)   ✓ CHOLESTEROL: Good Choice (90 mg)
✓✓ FAT: Excellent Choice (6 g)   SODIUM: Moderate (710 mg)
EXCHANGES: 3¾ Meat (extra lean), 2¾ Bread, ½ Veg, ¼ Fat
PROTEIN: 35 g, CARBOHYDRATE: 45 g, FIBER: 3 g

TURKEY SANDWICH – SPECIAL REQUEST
Request no mayo.

✓ CALORIES: Good Choice (445)   ✓ CHOLESTEROL: Good Choice (120 mg)
✓✓ FAT: Excellent Choice (3 g)   ✓✓ SODIUM: Excellent Choice (270 mg)
EXCHANGES: 6¼ Meat (extra lean), 3¼ Bread, ¼ Veg, ½ Fat
PROTEIN: 49 g, CARBOHYDRATE: 52 g, FIBER: 3 g

Side Dishes:

VEGETABLE SOUP† *(8 oz.)* ☺

✓✓ CALORIES: Excellent Choice (120)   ✓✓ CHOLESTEROL: Excellent Choice (0 mg)
✓✓ FAT: Excellent Choice (3 g)*   SODIUM: High (620 mg)
EXCHANGES: ½ Bread, 1¾ Veg, ½ Fat; PROTEIN: 3 g, CARBOHYDRATE: 21 g, FIBER: 4 g

BUTTERNUT SQUASH† *(6 oz.)* ☺

✓✓ CALORIES: Excellent Choice (65)   ✓✓ CHOLESTEROL: Excellent Choice (0 mg)
✓✓ FAT: Excellent Choice (0 g)   ✓✓ SODIUM: Excellent Choice (5 mg)
EXCHANGES: ¾ Bread, 2½ Veg; PROTEIN: 2 g, CARBOHYDRATE: 17 g, FIBER: 4 g

STEAMED VEGETABLES† *(4 oz.)* ☺

✓✓ CALORIES: Excellent Choice (35)   ✓✓ CHOLESTEROL: Excellent Choice (0 mg)
✓✓ FAT: Excellent Choice (0 g)   ✓✓ SODIUM: Excellent Choice (30 mg)
EXCHANGES: 1½ Veg; PROTEIN: 2 g, CARBOHYDRATE: 7 g, FIBER: 2 g

GREEN BEANS† *(4 oz.)* ☺

✓✓ CALORIES: Excellent Choice (60)   ✓✓ CHOLESTEROL: Excellent Choice (5 mg)
✓✓ FAT: Excellent Choice (3 g)   ✓ SODIUM: Good Choice (170 mg)
EXCHANGES: 1½ Veg, ½ Fat; PROTEIN: 2 g, CARBOHYDRATE: 8 g, FIBER: 2 g

ROASTED GARLIC POTATOES† *(5 oz.)* ☺

✓✓ CALORIES: Excellent Choice (145)   ✓✓ CHOLESTEROL: Excellent Choice (5 mg)
✓✓ FAT: Excellent Choice (3 g)   ✓ SODIUM: Good Choice (145 mg)
EXCHANGES: 1¾ Bread, ½ Fat; PROTEIN: 2 g, CARBOHYDRATE: 28 g, FIBER: 2 g

☺ at least 2 fruit/vegetable servings for entrees, 1 for side dishes

† Side dish guidelines are 1/3 of entree guidelines

La Salsa

FRESH MEXICAN GRILL®

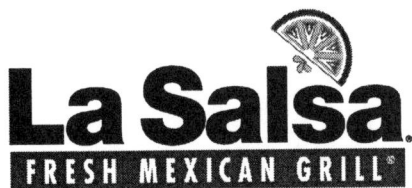

The Original Made-to-Order Fresh Mexican Restaurant! At La Salsa you'll find a variety of delicious Mexican recipes and tastes all prepared individually to your order and liking. A fresh salsa bar also allows you to garnish with a wide variety of salsas and trimmings. No prepackaged burritos, no MSG, no microwaves. Tell us what you want...we'll make it fresh! For more info & locations, visit www.lasalsa.com. $

La Salsa Los Angeles locations in: Beverly Hills, Brentwood, Calabasas, Canoga Park, Cerritos, Downtown, Glendale, Lakewood, LAX, Malibu, Northridge, Pico, Redondo Beach, Rolling Hills Estates, Santa Monica, Sherman Oaks, Studio City, Tarzana, Torrance, USC, Vinci Plaza, Westlake Village, Westside Pavilion, and Westwood.

Chips not included in analyses below.

CHICKEN TACO LA SALSA

Two soft corn tortillas filled with charbroiled chicken, Jack and Cheddar cheeses, lettuce and tomatoes.

✓✓ CALORIES: Excellent Choice (270) ✓✓ CHOLESTEROL: Excellent Choice (65 mg)
✓✓ FAT: Excellent Choice (8 g) ✓ SODIUM: Good Choice (330 mg)
PROTEIN: 17 g, CARBOHYDRATE: 32 g, FIBER: 2 g

SONORA MAHI MAHI TACO

Flour tortilla taco filled with grilled Mahi Mahi, lettuce, tomatoes, Jack and Cheddar cheeses and topped with our Sonora sauce and a squeeze of lime.

✓✓ CALORIES: Excellent Choice (200) ✓✓ CHOLESTEROL: Excellent Choice (30 mg)
✓✓ FAT: Excellent Choice (8 g) SODIUM: Moderate (640 mg)
PROTEIN: 13 g, CARBOHYDRATE: 17 g, FIBER: 0 g

VEGGIE TACO

Two soft corn tortillas filled with fajita vegetables, black beans, Jack & Cheddar cheeses, lettuce & tomatoes.

✓✓ CALORIES: Excellent Choice (280) ✓✓ CHOLESTEROL: Excellent Choice (25 mg)
✓✓ FAT: Excellent Choice (10 g) ✓ SODIUM: Good Choice (420 mg)
PROTEIN: 12 g, CARBOHYDRATE: 37 g, FIBER: 4 g

CHILE-LIME SALAD – SPECIAL REQUEST

Chicken, Romaine, Cotija cheese, tomatoes & avocado, with our own Chile–Lime dressing. Request no tortilla strips and dressing on the side (neither included in analysis). Mango Salsa is an excellent dressing alternative.

✓ CALORIES: Good Choice (495) ✓ CHOLESTEROL: Good Choice (95 mg)
✓✓ FAT: Excellent Choice (15 g) SODIUM: Moderate (820 mg)
PROTEIN: 29 g, CARBOHYDRATE: 19 g, FIBER: 5 g

LOS CABOS SHRIMP BURRITO – SPECIAL REQUEST

Grilled shrimp, Sonora sauce, fire-roasted fajita veggies, rice, cabbage, crema & avocado in a flour tortilla. Request no cheese.

✓ CALORIES: Good Choice (555) ✓✓ CHOLESTEROL: Excellent Choice (60 mg)
✓ FAT: Good Choice (21 g) SODIUM: High (1995 mg)
PROTEIN: 21 g, CARBOHYDRATE: 77 g, FIBER: 4 g

CHICKEN, BEAN & CHEESE BURRITO

With freshly made beans and Jack and Cheddar cheese in a flour tortilla.

✓ CALORIES: Good Choice (725) ✓ CHOLESTEROL: Good Choice (100 mg)
✓ FAT: Good Choice (22 g) SODIUM: High (1545 mg)
PROTEIN: 43 g, CARBOHYDRATE: 88 g, FIBER: 9 g

½ **RICE & ½ BEANS:** CAL: 235, FAT: 4 g*, CHOL: 0 mg, SOD: 775 mg; PROT: 10 g, CARB: 45 g, FIBER: 9 g

Nutrition information supplied by La Salsa.

* Primarily unsaturated fat

We specialize in social and corporate catering, but have also found a lot of success and fulfillment from our Cafe, which we cordially invite you to visit. Our philosophy and goal is to provide our customers with the best-tasting, freshest and most interesting food, at an affordable price. Our aim is to make you feel well taken care of, as you are important to us. We are proud that our company is an integral part of the community. Please visit our website at www.lisasbonappetit.com. $

Lisa's Bon Appétit 3511 Pacific Coast Highway, Torrance, CA (310) 784-1070

VIETNAMESE ROLLS†
An appetizer made with ground chicken, julienned vegetables, cellophane noodles, Hoisin, green onions, fresh lettuce and basil, wrapped in rice paper, and served cold with a tamarind dipping sauce.
- ✓ CALORIES: Good Choice (165)
- ✓ FAT: Good Choice (6 g)
- ✓✓ CHOLESTEROL: Excellent Choice (20 mg)
- SODIUM: High (530 mg)**

EXCHANGES: ¾ Meat, ¾ Bread, ¼ Veg, ½ Fruit, ½ Fat
PROTEIN: 6 g, CARBOHYDRATE: 21 g, FIBER: 0 g

GREEK SALAD – SPECIAL REQUEST ✿
Crisp romaine lettuce with Kalamata olives, crumbled feta cheese, cucumbers, tomatoes, and red onions. Request dressing on the side (58 cal, 6 g fat per Tbs., not included in analysis).
- ✓✓ CALORIES: Excellent Choice (275)
- ✓ FAT: Good Choice (19 g)
- ✓✓ CHOLESTEROL: Excellent Choice (50 mg)
- SODIUM: High (1135 mg)

EXCHANGES: 1 Meat, 1½ Veg, 1¾ Fat
PROTEIN: 12 g, CARBOHYDRATE: 18 g, FIBER: 5 g

CITRUS CHICKEN SALAD – SPECIAL REQUEST ✿
Grilled chicken breast glazed with an achiote marinade served with baby greens, mandarin sections, peppers, and pecans, with lo-fat orange dressing. Request less pecans (½ oz).
- ✓ CALORIES: Good Choice (525)
- ✓ FAT: Good Choice (25 g)
- ✓ CHOLESTEROL: Good Choice (95 mg)
- ✓ SODIUM: Good Choice (555 mg)**

EXCHANGES: 5 Meat (extra lean), ¼ Bread, 1¼ Veg, 1¼ Fruit, 4 Fat
PROTEIN: 41 g, CARBOHYDRATE: 36 g, FIBER: 5 g

BBQ CHICKEN SALAD – SPECIAL REQUEST ✿
BBQ chicken, cucumber, bell peppers, pepperoncini, and red cabbage, served on a bed of iceberg lettuce and romaine. Request dressing on the side (58 cal, 6 g fat per Tbs., not incl. in analysis) and no fried onions.
- ✓✓ CALORIES: Excellent Choice (265)
- ✓✓ FAT: Excellent Choice (4 g)
- ✓ CHOLESTEROL: Good Choice (95 mg)
- SODIUM: High (1175 mg)

EXCHANGES: 7½ Meat (extra lean), 3½ Bread, 1 Veg, 6 Fat
PROTEIN: 37 g, CARBOHYDRATE: 17 g, FIBER: 4 g

VEGGIE SANDWICH – SPECIAL REQUEST ✿
Choice of cheese with avocado, cucumber, tomato and sprouts. Request no mayo or mayo on the side (not included in analysis).
- ✓ CALORIES: Good Choice (455)
- ✓ FAT: Good Choice (21 g)
- ✓✓ CHOLESTEROL: Excellent Choice (30 mg)
- SODIUM: Moderate (635 mg)**

EXCHANGES: 1 Meat, 3 Bread, ½ Veg, 3¼ Fat
PROTEIN: 17 g, CARBOHYDRATE: 51 g, FIBER: 3 g

ORTEGA TURKEY SANDWICH – SPECIAL REQUEST
Breast of turkey, ortega chilies and pepper Jack cheese on grilled sourdough. Request bread toasted without butter and no mayo.
- ✓ CALORIES: Good Choice (515)
- ✓ FAT: Good Choice (16 g)
- ✓ CHOLESTEROL: Good Choice (125 mg)
- SODIUM: High (2200 mg)

EXCHANGES: 5 Meat, 3 Bread, ¼ Veg, 2 Fat
PROTEIN: 42 g, CARBOHYDRATE: 48 g, FIBER: 0 g

† Side dish guidelines are 1/3 of entree guidelines
✿ at least 2 fruit/vegetable servings

The name "Malvasia" comes from Monemvasia, hometown of the owner's father. Monemvasia exported a sweet white wine (called Malvasia or Malmsey) throughout Europe until the 16th century, when production was destroyed after the Turkish conquest of Greece. Monemvasia's turbulent history and the countries where the green-gold Malvasia grape eventually spread (Spain, Italy, France) have inspired this pan-Mediterranean menu. The extensive menu offers hot and cold meze/antipasti/tapas, soups, salads, pastas, risotto and paella. Grilled whole and fillet fish, lamb, veal and chicken dishes prepared in the style of your favorite Mediterranean country will give you plenty of reasons to return. Nicely priced beer and wine list. $$

Malvasia
5316 E. 2nd Street, Long Beach 90803 (562) 433-5005

INSALATE MALVASIA – SPECIAL REQUEST ☺
Mixed baby greens, broiled chicken breast, sliced red onions, fire roasted red peppers, fresh mozzarella, kalamata olives, roma tomatoes, capers and artichoke hearts.
<u>*Request dressing and cheese served on the side (not included in analysis).*</u>
✓ CALORIES: Good Choice (580)   CHOLESTEROL: Moderate (215 mg)
✓✓ FAT: Excellent Choice (13 g)   SODIUM: High (1325 mg)**
EXCHANGES: 11¼ Meat, 3¼ Veg
PROTEIN: 86 g, CARBOHYDRATE: 24 g, FIBER: 9 g

FRESH HALIBUT ☺
Grilled and brushed with extra virgin olive oil, lemon and fresh herbs.
Served with vegetables of the day and roast potatoes (potatoes not included in analysis).
✓ CALORIES: Good Choice (510)   ✓ CHOLESTEROL: Good Choice (90 mg)
✓ FAT: Good Choice (25 g)*   ✓✓ SODIUM: Excellent Choice (180 mg)**
EXCHANGES: 5½ Meat (extra lean), 1 Veg, ½ Fruit, 3½ Fat
PROTEIN: 62 g, CARBOHYDRATE: 10 g, FIBER: 4 g

NEW ZEALAND SEABASS WITH MANGO SALSA – SPECIAL REQUEST ☺
Grilled and brushed with extra virgin olive oil, lemon and fresh herbs. Served with vegetables of the day and roast potatoes (potatoes not included in analysis). Request less oil (1/2 Tbs.).
✓✓ CALORIES: Excellent Choice (450)   ✓ CHOLESTEROL: Good Choice (120 mg)
✓ FAT: Good Choice (20 g)*   ✓✓ SODIUM: Excellent Choice (220 mg)**
EXCHANGES: 5 Meat (extra lean), 1 Veg, ¼ Fruit, 2¾ Fat
PROTEIN: 56 g, CARBOHYDRATE: 11 g, FIBER: 4 g

ALLA GURGUGLIONE – SPECIAL REQUEST ☺
Sauteed Japanese eggplant with garlic, onions, zucchini, red and green peppers in a fresh basil sauce.
<u>*Request less oil (1 Tbs.).*</u>
✓ CALORIES: Good Choice (655)   ✓✓ CHOLESTEROL: Excellent Choice (0 mg)
✓ FAT: Good Choice (23 g)*   ✓✓ SODIUM: Excellent Choice (25 mg)**
EXCHANGES: 4¼ Bread, 5 Veg, 4 Fat
PROTEIN: 15 g, CARBOHYDRATE: 98 g, FIBER: 9 g

SPAGHETTI AL CARTOCCIO – SPECIAL REQUEST ☺
Spaghetti cooked in parchment paper with clams, mussels, scallops and shrimp in a fresh tomato herb sauce.
<u>*Request less oil (1 Tbs.).*</u>
✓ CALORIES: Good Choice (735)   CHOLESTEROL: Moderate (175 mg)
✓ FAT: Good Choice (25 g)*   ✓ SODIUM: Good Choice (445 mg)**
EXCHANGES: 4 Meat (extra lean), 4¼ Bread, 1¾ Veg, 4 Fat
PROTEIN: 47 g, CARBOHYDRATE: 80 g, FIBER: 6 g

* Primarily unsaturated fat
** If you request no added salt

MCCORMICK&SCHMICK'S
S E A F O O D   R E S T A U R A N T

McCormick & Schmick's Seafood Restaurant is one of Los Angeles' most popular dining and gathering spots. Our menu features fresh seafood from the Pacific Northwest and other regional favorites. Salads, pastas, poultry and steak entrees are also available. Enjoy the timeless and traditional presentation and decor. Happy hour 3 - 7 pm Monday thru Friday. Dinner served daily from 5 pm. Reservations recommended. $$

McCormick & Schmick's Seafood Restaurant

111 N. Los Robles, Pasadena, CA 91101	(626) 405-0064
633 West 5th St. 4th Level, Los Angeles, CA 90071	(213) 629-1929
206 North Rodeo Drive, Beverly Hills, CA 90210	(310) 859-0434
2101 Rosecrans Ave., El Segundo, CA 90245	(310) 416-1123

GRILLED HALIBUT WITH FRESH SALSA – SPECIAL REQUEST ☙
served with Chefs special salsa of the day. Request steamed vegetables.

✓✓ CALORIES: Excellent Choice (300)   ✓✓ CHOLESTEROL: Excellent Choice (65 mg)
✓✓ FAT: Excellent Choice (9 g)*   ✓✓ SODIUM: Excellent Choice (195 mg)**
EXCHANGES: 4 Meat, 1 Veg, ½ Fruit, ¾ Fat
PROTEIN: 44 g, CARBOHYDRATE: 11 g, FIBER: 4 g

SEARED BLACKENED AHI
served rare with Cajun spices, pickled ginger and wasabi.

✓✓ CALORIES: Excellent Choice (255)   ✓✓ CHOLESTEROL: Excellent Choice (75 mg)
✓✓ FAT: Excellent Choice (4 g)*   SODIUM: High (2905 mg)**
EXCHANGES: 5½ Meat, ¼ Fat
PROTEIN: 44 g, CARBOHYDRATE: 15 g, FIBER: 1 g

NICOISE SALAD – SPECIAL REQUEST ☙
with seared rare ahi tuna. Request dressing on the side and use sparingly (dressing not included in ananlysis)

✓✓ CALORIES: Excellent Choice (290)   ✓ CHOLESTEROL: Good Choice (105 mg)
✓✓ FAT: Excellent Choice (5 g)   SODIUM: High (1400 mg)
EXCHANGES: 3¾ Meat, ¾ Bread, 1¾ Veg
PROTEIN: 33 g, CARBOHYDRATE: 31 g, FIBER: 3 g

ATLANTIC SALMON – SPECIAL REQUEST ☙
Baked on a cedar plank and served with a Pinot Noir sauce.
Request steamed vegetables and sauce on the side (sauce not included in analysis).

✓✓ CALORIES: Excellent Choice (360)   ✓ CHOLESTEROL: Good Choice (105 mg)
✓ FAT: Good Choice (19 g)*   ✓✓ SODIUM: Excellent Choice (110 mg)**
EXCHANGES: 5 Meat, 1 Veg, 1¼ Fat
PROTEIN: 41 g, CARBOHYDRATE: 5 g, FIBER: 3 g

HAWAIIAN ALBACORE WITH CITRUS TERIYAKI GLAZE ☙
Served with stir-fry vegetables and rice.

✓ CALORIES: Good Choice (630)   ✓ CHOLESTEROL: Good Choice (115 mg)
✓✓ FAT: Excellent Choice (15 g)*   ✓ SODIUM: Good Choice (440 mg)**
EXCHANGES: 8½ Meat, 3¼ Bread, 1½ Veg, 2¼ Fat
PROTEIN: 68 g, CARBOHYDRATE: 55 g, FIBER: 6 g

PACIFIC SEAFOOD STEW
Mussels, crab, clams and prawns.

✓✓ CALORIES: Excellent Choice (415)   CHOLESTEROL: Moderate (260 mg)
✓✓ FAT: Excellent Choice (14 g)   SODIUM: High (1305 mg)**
EXCHANGES: 6½ Meat, 2 Veg, 1¼ Fat

☙ at least 2 fruit/vegetable servings
✓ Good Choice   ✓✓ Excellent Choice

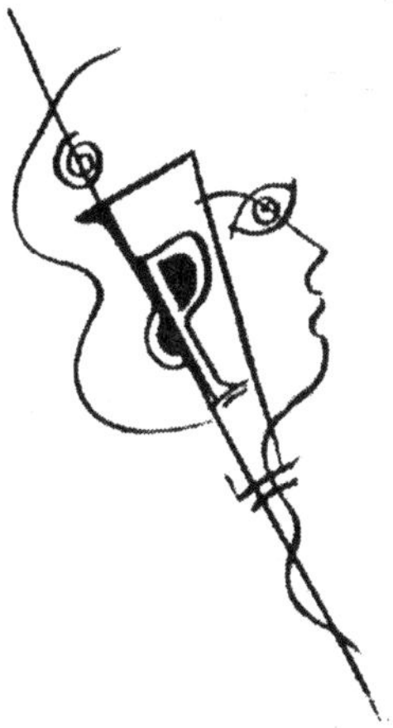

Mi Piace means "I like it" in Italian. That is just how the owners Armen Shirvanian and Takis Markoutsis make you feel about their restaurant. You'll receive the warmest greeting at the door, the friendliest servers at your table, and great food with moderate prices for your pocket. People walk out saying, "I like it." Mi Piace in Pasadena has been voted "Best Italian Restaurant" for 10 consecutive years. Mi Piace in Burbank has been voted "Best Gourmet Restaurant" from 1999-2000 and "Best Continental Restaurant" in 2001. In 2001, both restaurants received the "Award of Excellence" from Wine Spectator Magazine. $$

Mi Piace

25 E. Colorado Blvd., Old Town Pasadena 91105 (626) 795-3131
801 N. San Fernando Rd., Burbank 91502 (818) 843-1111
4799 Commons Way, Calabasas 91302 (818) 591-8822

PESCATORE
Rustic seafood stew with spinach linguine, calamari, shrimp, scallops, clams, mussels and white fish in red sauce.
- ✓ CALORIES: Good Choice (630)
- ✓ FAT: Good Choice (25 g)*

CHOLESTEROL: Moderate (265 mg)
- ✓ SODIUM: Good Choice (595 mg)**

EXCHANGES: 5½ Meat (extra lean), 2 Bread, 3½ Fat, 1¼ Veg
PROTEIN: 51 g, CARBOHYDRATE: 44 g, FIBER: 3 g

PEPPERONATA CON FETTUCCINI E GAMBERI
Fettuccine with fresh water prawns, bell peppers and roasted eggplant fondue.
- ✓ CALORIES: Good Choice (600)
- ✓ FAT: Good Choice (19 g)*

CHOLESTEROL: High (445 mg)
SODIUM: Moderate (720 mg)**

EXCHANGES: 6¾ Meat (extra lean), 2¾ Bread, 1¼ Veg, 3 Fat
PROTEIN: 55 g, CARBOHYDRATE: 48 g, FIBER: 3 g

LINGUINI CAPESANTE – SPECIAL REQUEST
Linguine with seared sea scallops and broccoli rabe. *Request no butter.*
- ✓✓ CALORIES: Excellent Choice (415)
- ✓ FAT: Good Choice (16 g)*

✓✓ CHOLESTEROL: Excellent Choice (30 mg)
✓✓ SODIUM: Excellent Choice (175 mg)**

EXCHANGES: 1¼ Meat (extra lean), 2¾ Bread, 1¼ Veg, 2¾ Fat
PROTEIN: 22 g, CARBOHYDRATE: 47 g, FIBER: 4 g

CAPPELLINI PRIMAVERA – SPECIAL REQUEST ♨
Pasta with fresh seasonal julienned vegetables. *Request less oil (½ oz.) and no butter.*
- ✓ CALORIES: Good Choice (505)
- ✓ FAT: Good Choice (22 g)*

✓✓ CHOLESTEROL: Excellent Choice (10 mg)
✓ SODIUM: Good Choice (530 mg)**

EXCHANGES: ½ Meat, 3¼ Bread, 3 Veg, 3¾ Fat
PROTEIN: 16 g, CARBOHYDRATE: 64 g, FIBER: 7 g

PENNE ALL'ARRABBIATA – SPECIAL REQUEST
Pasta with crushed red pepper, fresh garlic and housemade marinara sauce. *Request less oil (¼ oz.) and no butter.*
- ✓ CALORIES: Good Choice (565)
- ✓ FAT: Good Choice (22 g)

✓✓ CHOLESTEROL: Excellent Choice (5 mg)
✓ SODIUM: Good Choice (550 mg)**

EXCHANGES: ¼ Meat, 3¾ Bread, 3¼ Veg, 3¾ Fat
PROTEIN: 15 g, CARBOHYDRATE: 78 g, FIBER: 6 g

SPAGHETTI ALLA CHECCA – SPECIAL REQUEST ♨
Spaghetti with freshly chopped tomatoes in a basil, garlic and extra virgin olive oil sauce. *Request less oil (½ oz.)*
- ✓ CALORIES: Good Choice (490)
- ✓ FAT: Good Choice (16 g)

✓✓ CHOLESTEROL: Excellent Choice (0 mg)
✓✓ SODIUM: Excellent Choice (20 mg)**

EXCHANGES: 3¾ Bread, 3 Veg, 2¾ Fat
PROTEIN: 13 g, CARBOHYDRATE: 75 g, FIBER: 6 g

* Primarily unsaturated fat
** If you request no added salt

OCEAN AVE SEAFOOD

Dining at Ocean Avenue Seafood is an experience in healthy dining! All of our seafood is the freshest <u>and</u> safest available. Whether broiled or grilled, sautéed or baked, any of our menu items can be prepared to suit your special dietary needs. Visit Ocean Avenue Seafood and dine on your favorite shellfish and seafood while enjoying a spectacular view of the Pacific Ocean! Open 7 days a week for lunch and dinner. Brunch served on Sunday. $$

Ocean Avenue Seafood

1401 Ocean Avenue, Santa Monica, CA 90401 (310) 394-5669

www.oceanave.com

ALASKAN KING CRAB DINNER ☺

served with red potatoes and vegetables. Butter served on the side is not included in analysis.

✓✓ CALORIES: Excellent Choice (345)   ✓ CHOLESTEROL: Good Choice (95 mg)
✓✓ FAT: Excellent Choice (6 g)   SODIUM: High (1865 mg)
EXCHANGES: 2¾ Meat (extra lean), 1¾ Bread, 1¼ Veg, ¾ Fat
PROTEIN: 38 g, CARBOHYDRATE: 35 g

SEARED AHI - SPECIAL REQUEST ☺

Seared rare ahi with Asian vinaigrette, served with jasmine rice and vegetables. <u>Request less oil</u> (¼ oz.).

✓ CALORIES: Good Choice (590)   ✓ CHOLESTEROL: Good Choice (80 mg)
✓ FAT: Good Choice (19 g)   SODIUM: Moderate (805 mg)**
EXCHANGES: 5½ Meat (extra lean), 2¾ Bread, 2 Veg, 2 Fat
PROTEIN: 51 g, CARBOHYDRATE: 53 g

CHILEAN SEABASS

with sake-kasu, teriyaki and seaweed salad..

✓ CALORIES: Good Choice (555)   ✓✓ CHOLESTEROL: Excellent Choice (75 mg)
✓ FAT: Good Choice (18 g)*   SODIUM: High (1710 mg)**
EXCHANGES: 3 Meat (extra lean), 3¼ Bread, ¼ Veg, ½ Fruit, 2¾ Fat
PROTEIN: 37 g, CARBOHYDRATE: 60 g

AVOCADO SWORDFISH

with grilled vegetables.

✓✓ CALORIES: Excellent Choice (340)   ✓ CHOLESTEROL: Good Choice (90 mg)
✓✓ FAT: Excellent Choice (14 g)*   ✓✓ SODIUM: Excellent Choice (220 mg)**
EXCHANGES: 5 Meat, ½ Veg, 1 Fat
PROTEIN: 46 g, CARBOHYDRATE: 5 g

STEAMED CLAMS OR MUSSELS - SPECIAL REQUEST

with white wine and garlic. <u>Request less herb butter</u> (½ oz.).

✓✓ CALORIES: Excellent Choice (310)   ✓ CHOLESTEROL: Good Choice (85 mg)
✓✓ FAT: Excellent Choice (12 g)   ✓✓ SODIUM: Excellent Choice (245 mg)**
EXCHANGES: 4¼ Meat (extra lean), 4 Veg, 2¼ Fat
PROTEIN: 29 g, CARBOHYDRATE: 13 g

☺ at least 2 fruit/vegetable servings, 1 for side dish

✓ Good Choice   ✓✓ Excellent Choice

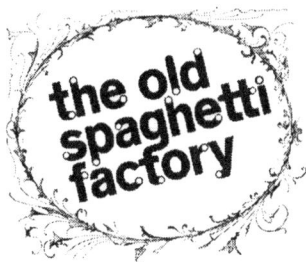

For more than a generation, families and friends have been coming to Old Spaghetti Factories, located across the United States, to enjoy our delicious food, charming atmosphere and friendly service. We invite you to dine amidst old world antiques, collected from around the world, while savoring perfectly cooked pasta and spaghetti sauces, freshly made using only the finest ingredients. $

The Old Spaghetti Factory

Hollywood: 5939 Sunset Blvd., 90028 (323) 469-7149
Duarte: 1431 Buena Vista, 91010 (626) 358-2115

Analyses below do not include bread, salad and ice cream served with the entrée.

SPAGHETTI WITH TOMATO SAUCE
Italians would say "Marinara."

✓✓ CALORIES: Excellent Choice (450)   ✓✓ CHOLESTEROL: Excellent Choice (0 mg)
✓✓ FAT: Excellent Choice (6 g)*   SODIUM: Moderate (820 mg)**
EXCHANGES: 5 Bread, 1¾ Veg, ¾ Fat
PROTEIN: 14 g, CARBOHYDRATE: 85 g, FIBER: 7 g

SPAGHETTI WITH MUSHROOM SAUCE
Fresh tender mushrooms, swimming in authentic Italian tomato sauce.

✓ CALORIES: Good Choice (455)   ✓✓ CHOLESTEROL: Excellent Choice (0 mg)
✓✓ FAT: Excellent Choice (7 g)*   SODIUM: Moderate (625 mg)**
EXCHANGES: 4¾ Bread, 1¾ Veg, 1 Fat
PROTEIN: 14 g, CARBOHYDRATE: 84 g, FIBER: 6 g

SPINACH & CHEESE RAVIOLI
Tender pillows of pasta stuffed with spinach and three kinds of cheese, topped with our savory tomato sauce.

✓✓ CALORIES: Excellent Choice (450)   ✓✓ CHOLESTEROL: Excellent Choice (60 mg)
✓✓ FAT: Excellent Choice (13 g)   SODIUM: Moderate (935 mg)**
EXCHANGES: 2 Meat, 3¾ Bread, 1 Veg, 2½ Fat
PROTEIN: 21 g, CARBOHYDRATE: 63 g, FIBER: 4 g

SPINACH TORTELLINI WITH MUSHROOM SAUCE – SPECIAL REQUEST
Hat shaped pasta, stuffed with a delicious blend of meat & cheese. Request Mushroom Sauce instead of Alfredo.

✓ CALORIES: Good Choice (560)   ✓✓ CHOLESTEROL: Excellent Choice (55 mg)
✓✓ FAT: Excellent Choice (14 g)   SODIUM: High (1420 mg)
EXCHANGES: 1 Meat, 5¼ Bread, 1 Veg, 2 Fat
PROTEIN: 24 g, CARBOHYDRATE: 84 g, FIBER: 4 g

SPAGHETTI WITH RICH MEAT SAUCE
For purists – our recipe comes straight from Naples.

✓ CALORIES: Good Choice (505)   ✓✓ CHOLESTEROL: Excellent Choice (25 mg)
✓✓ FAT: Excellent Choice (10 g)   SODIUM: Moderate (955 mg)**
EXCHANGES: ¾ Meat, 5 Bread, 1¼ Veg, 1¼ Fat
PROTEIN: 19 g, CARBOHYDRATE: 83 g, FIBER: 6 g

HOUSE SALAD WITH HONEY MUSTARD FAT FREE DRESSING†

✓✓ CALORIES: Excellent Choice (50)   ✓✓ CHOLESTEROL: Excellent Choice (0 mg)
✓✓ FAT: Excellent Choice (0 g)*   ✓ SODIUM: Good Choice (170 mg)**
EXCHANGES: ½ Veg, ½ Fruit
PROTEIN: 1 g, CARBOHYDRATE: 11, FIBER: 1 g

---

* Primarily unsaturated fat   † Side dish guidelines are 1/3 of entree guidelines
** If you request no added salt

Shutters On The Beach, a member of The Leading Hotels of the World, is the only luxury hotel in Los Angeles nestled right on the sand. One Pico is the hotel's signature restaurant with magnificent windows which wrap around three sides of the dining room, affording one of the most scenic restaurant experiences in Los Angeles. Sunset views along the beach provide a stunning backdrop for the chef's menu, which features modern American cuisine. The restaurant elicits the perfect California experience, with warm woods, monolithic limestone fireplace, amber-colored wood floor and clean, contemporary lines. $$

One Pico
at Shutters On The Beach
One Pico Blvd., Santa Monica, CA 90405 (310) 587-1717

WARM POACHED SALMON, TOMATO AND HERB SALAD
with dill dressing. Featured on lunch menu.

✓✓ CALORIES: Excellent Choice (330) ✓ CHOLESTEROL: Good Choice (110 mg)
✓✓ FAT: Excellent Choice (13 g)* ✓✓ SODIUM: Excellent Choice (115 mg)**
EXCHANGES: 5 Meat, ½ Veg
PROTEIN: 42 g, CARBOHYDRATE: 9 g, FIBER: 1 g

WARM LOBSTER SALAD - SPECIAL REQUEST 🍎
with mango, avocado and tarragon vinaigrette. Featured on lunch menu. Request no butter.

✓ CALORIES: Good Choice (455) ✓ CHOLESTEROL: Good Choice (100 mg)
✓ FAT: Good Choice (18 g)* SODIUM: Moderate (935 mg)**
EXCHANGES: 3½ Meat (extra lean), 1½ Veg, 1¼ Fruit, 3¼ Fat
PROTEIN: 35 g, CARBOHYDRATE: 40 g, FIBER: 9 g

SEARED AHI TUNA WITH SPICY GREENS
Featured on dinner menu.

✓✓ CALORIES: Excellent Choice (165) ✓✓ CHOLESTEROL: Excellent Choice (40 mg)
✓✓ FAT: Excellent Choice (4 g)* ✓✓ SODIUM: Excellent Choice (115 mg)**
EXCHANGES: 2¾ Meat (extra lean), 1 Veg, ½ Fat
PROTEIN: 24 g, CARBOHYDRATE: 9 g, FIBER: 2 g

ROAST CHILEAN SEABASS
with black bean sauce and scallions. Featured on dinner menu.

✓✓ CALORIES: Excellent Choice (315) ✓ CHOLESTEROL: Good Choice (100 mg)
✓✓ FAT: Excellent Choice (10 g) ✓ SODIUM: Good Choice (585 mg)**
EXCHANGES: 4 Meat (extra lean), ¾ Veg, 1 Fat
PROTEIN: 45 g, CARBOHYDRATE: 8 g, FIBER: 2 g

GRILLED AHI TUNA WITH SHITTAKE MUSHROOMS
and bok choy. Featured on dinner menu.

✓✓ CALORIES: Excellent Choice (445) ✓ CHOLESTEROL: Good Choice (90 mg)
✓ FAT: Good Choice (17 g)* SODIUM: High (1115 mg)
EXCHANGES: 6¼ Meat (extra lean), ¾ Bread, ¾ Veg, 3 Fat
PROTEIN: 50 g, CARBOHYDRATE: 16 g, FIBER: 3 g

🍎 at least 2 fruit/vegetable servings

✓ Good Choice ✓✓ Excellent Choice

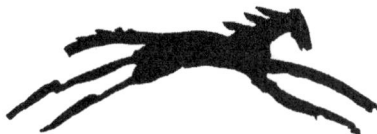

PALOMINO
RESTAURANT · ROTISSERIA · BAR

Palomino is conveniently located in Westwood Village between Santa Monica and Beverly Hills. Executive Chef Jeff Marino's menu showcases an eclectic variety of American cuisine inspired by the flavors and technologies of Italy, Spain and France. He has taken his favorite flavors from southern Europe and combined them with the unique taste of California cuisine to create delicious salads, pizzas, smoked meats and seafood with intense flavor and depth. A stylish nightspot and neighborhood bar, Palomino's lounge is always alive with a festive cosmopolitan feel. Palomino is great for pre-and post-theater dining. Reservations recommended. $$-$$$

Palomino
10877 Wilshire Blvd., Los Angeles 90024 (310) 208-1960

GRILLED CHICKEN BREAST WITH APRICOT CILANTRO SAUCE – SPECIAL REQUEST ✆
With fresh ginger, onion and plum tomatoes. Request steamed vegetables & couscous (see analysis below).
- ✓✓ CALORIES: Excellent Choice (420)
- ✓ FAT: Good Choice (16 g)
- ✓ CHOLESTEROL: Good Choice (130 mg)
- ✓ SODIUM: Good Choice (460 mg)**

EXCHANGES: 6¾ Meat (extra lean), 1¼ Veg, ¼ Fruit, 2 Fat
PROTEIN: 51 g, CARBOHYDRATE: 18 g, FIBER: 4 g

OVEN ROASTED SALMON – SPECIAL REQUEST ✆
with honey peppercorn crust. Fresh salmon rubbed with cracked peppercorns, brushed with honey and oven roasted. Request sauce on the side (not included in analysis) and steamed vegetables and couscous (see analysis below).
- ✓✓ CALORIES: Excellent Choice (365)
- ✓✓ FAT: Excellent Choice (13 g)*
- ✓ CHOLESTEROL: Good Choice (105 mg)
- SODIUM: Moderate (740 mg)**

EXCHANGES: 5 Meat (extra lean), ¼ Bread, ¾ Veg
PROTEIN: 41 g, CARBOHYDRATE: 21 g, FIBER: 3 g

SEARED AHI – SPECIAL REQUEST ✆
with mushrooms, asparagus and artichoke hearts. Request less butter (1½ Tbs.) and couscous (see analysis below).
- ✓ CALORIES: Good Choice (460)
- ✓ FAT: Good Choice (20 g)
- ✓ CHOLESTEROL: Good Choice (135 mg)
- ✓ SODIUM: Good Choice (325 mg)**

EXCHANGES: 6¼ Meat, 3½ Veg, 3½ Fat
PROTEIN: 55 g, CARBOHYDRATE: 19 g, FIBER: 8 g

BRICK OVEN-ROASTED VEGETABLES – SPECIAL REQUEST ✆
Balsamic-shallot marinade, almond wood-charred vegetables, romaine greens. Also available with garlic prawns or wood-grilled chicken. Request dressing served on the side (not included in analysis).
- ✓✓ CALORIES: Excellent Choice (330)
- ✓ FAT: Good Choice (24 g)
- ✓✓ CHOLESTEROL: Excellent Choice (25 mg)
- ✓ SODIUM: Good Choice (430 mg)**

EXCHANGES: ½ Meat, ½ Bread, 2¾ Veg, 4¼ Fat
PROTEIN: 11 g, CARBOHYDRATE: 22 g, FIBER: 6 g

CINNAMON COUS COUS †
- ✓ CALORIES: Good Choice (160)
- ✓✓ FAT: Excellent Choice (3 g)
- ✓✓ CHOLESTEROL: Excellent Choice (0 mg)
- SODIUM: Moderate (220 mg)

EXCHANGES: 1¾ Bread, ¼ Veg, ¼ Fruit, ½ Fat
PROTEIN: 4 g, CARBOHYDRATE: 29 g, FIBER: 6 g

---

* Primarily unsaturated fat

** If you request no added salt

† Side dish guidelines are 1/3 of entree guidelines

Pane e Vino

TRATTORIA

Even with the craze of Italian cooking sweeping the nation, it is still hard to find an authentic Italian trattoria. Well, look no further. Pane e Vino is the quintessential example and has one of the most dynamic and romantic settings in L.A. Chef and co-owner Claudio Marchesan can rightly claim credit for bringing this style of cooking to L.A. Together with his partner, graphic designer Rod Dyer, they have created elegant yet homey restaurants in L.A., San Francisco, and Santa Barbara. The patio dining and the main room with frescos are chic yet unintimidating. Open Mon.-Sat. 11:30 am to 11:30 pm, Sun. 5 pm to 10:30 pm. $$

Pane e Vino

8265 Beverly Boulevard, Los Angeles, CA 90048   (323) 651-4600

ZITI ALLA PUTTANESCA
Short tube pasta, capers, olives, oregano, and tomato sauce.
- ✓ CALORIES: Good Choice (475)
- ✓✓ CHOLESTEROL: Excellent Choice (0 mg)
- ✓ FAT: Good Choice (16 g)*
- SODIUM: Moderate (835 mg)**

EXCHANGES: 4 Bread, 1¼ Veg, 2¼ Fat
PROTEIN: 12 g, CARBOHYDRATE: 67 g, FIBER: 5 g

RIGATONI AL POMODORO E BASILICO
Short tubes, fresh tomato sauce and basil.
- ✓✓ CALORIES: Excellent Choice (365)
- ✓✓ CHOLESTEROL: Excellent Choice (0 mg)
- ✓✓ FAT: Excellent Choice (6 g)*
- ✓ SODIUM: Good Choice (465 mg)**

EXCHANGES: 4 Bread, 1 Veg, 1 Fat
PROTEIN: 11 g, CARBOHYDRATE: 65 g, FIBER: 4 g

CAPELLINI AL POMODORO NATURALE - SPECIAL REQUEST
Angel hair pasta, fresh tomatoes, basil, garlic, and extra virgin olive oil. <u>Request less oil (1 Tbs.)</u>.
- ✓✓ CALORIES: Excellent Choice (445)
- ✓✓ CHOLESTEROL: Excellent Choice (0 mg)
- ✓✓ FAT: Excellent Choice (15 g)*
- ✓✓ SODIUM: Excellent Choice (205 mg)**

EXCHANGES: 4 Bread, 1 Veg, 2¾ Fat
PROTEIN: 11 g, CARBOHYDRATE: 66 g, FIBER: 5 g

PIATTO DI VEGETALI AL FORNO ♨
Mixed vegetables and herbs cooked in a clay pot.
- ✓✓ CALORIES: Excellent Choice (230)
- ✓✓ CHOLESTEROL: Excellent Choice (15 mg)
- ✓✓ FAT: Excellent Choice (10 g)*
- ✓✓ SODIUM: Excellent Choice (150 mg)**

EXCHANGES: 5¾ Veg, 1¼ Fat
PROTEIN: 18 g, CARBOHYDRATE: 29 g, FIBER: 14 g

PESCE FRESCO ♨
Fresh fish served with seasonal vegetables. Analysis for ahi & Dover sole.
Roasted potatoes not included in analysis.
- ✓✓ CALORIES: Excellent Choice (350)
- ✓ CHOLESTEROL: Good Choice (100 mg)
- ✓✓ FAT: Excellent Choice (9 g)*
- ✓✓ SODIUM: Excellent Choice (120 mg)**

EXCHANGES: 7¼ Meat (extra lean), 1¾ Veg, 1¼ Fat
PROTEIN: 57 g, CARBOHYDRATE: 8 g, FIBER: 5 g

PAILLARD DI POLLO CON ARUGULA ♨
Chicken breast with arugula and parmesan cheese, served with seasonal vegetables.
Roasted potatoes not included in analysis.
- ✓ CALORIES: Good Choice (545)
- CHOLESTEROL: Moderate (215 mg)
- ✓ FAT: Good Choice (18 g)
- ✓ SODIUM: Good Choice (485 mg)**

EXCHANGES: 11½ Meat (extra lean), 1½ Veg, 1¼ Fat
PROTEIN: 85 g, CARBOHYDRATE: 9 g, FIBER: 5 g

♨ at least 2 fruit/vegetable servings

✓ Good Choice   ✓✓ Excellent Choice

PATINA
RESTAURANT

| | | | | | | | | |

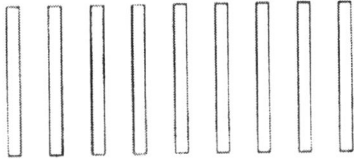

"In a town full of great restaurants, this may be the finest of them all," raves Los Angeles Magazine about Patina Restaurant. This understated jewel located in the heart of Hollywood's studio district has offered Joachim Splichal's inspired Franco-California cuisine since 1989. Rated Number One for seven consecutive years by the popular Los Angeles Zagat Survey, Patina has earned Joachim numerous awards and great loyalty among L.A.'s food aficionados. Patina was also rated one of the "Top Restaurants" in Los Angeles in Gourmet magazine's October 1996 and 1997 restaurant issue. Menu changes seasonally. $$$

Patina
5955 Melrose Ave., Los Angeles, CA 90038
(323) 467-1108

GRILLED PEPPERED AHI TUNA ♻
with baby bok choy, shiitake mushrooms and a grilled scallion ponzu.

✓✓ CALORIES: Excellent Choice (300)
✓✓ FAT: Excellent Choice (7 g)*
✓ CHOLESTEROL: Good Choice (85 mg)
SODIUM: High (1135 mg)

EXCHANGES: 5¾ Meat (extra lean), 1¾ Veg, ¾ Fat
PROTEIN: 45 g, CARBOHYDRATE: 15 g

SEARED WHITEFISH - SPECIAL REQUEST ♻
with French fries "not fried," and roasted garlic cloves. Request no brandade sauce and less oil (½ oz.).

✓ CALORIES: Good Choice (510)
✓ FAT: Good Choice (22 g)*
✓ CHOLESTEROL: Good Choice (80 mg)
✓✓ SODIUM: Excellent Choice (135 mg)**

EXCHANGES: 1¾ Meat , 2½ Bread, 1½ Veg, 3¼ Fat
PROTEIN: 30 g, CARBOHYDRATE: 52 g

AHI TUNA TOWER ♻
with avocado, plum tomato and yellow bell pepper.

✓✓ CALORIES: Excellent Choice (225)
✓ FAT: Good Choice (16 g)*
✓✓ CHOLESTEROL: Excellent Choice (20 mg)
✓✓ SODIUM: Excellent Choice (30 mg)**

EXCHANGES: 1¼ Meat (extra lean), 1½ Veg, 3 Fat
PROTEIN: 12 g, CARBOHYDRATE: 10 g

SANTA BARBARA SHRIMP - SPECIAL REQUEST ♻
with sundried tomatoes and leeks. Request less oil (¼ oz).

✓✓ CALORIES: Excellent Choice (355)
✓✓ FAT: Excellent Choice (13 g)*
CHOLESTEROL: Moderate (260 mg)
SODIUM: Moderate (950 mg)

EXCHANGES: 3¾ Meat (extra lean), 2½ Veg, 2½ Fat
PROTEIN: 32 g, CARBOHYDRATE: 26 g

* Primarily unsaturated fat
** If you request no added salt

Pick Up Stix prepares food with minimal oil in exhibition kitchens using only the finest ingredients. These Chinese bistros freshly *wok each order without MSG or the usual heavy and/or salty sauces. Pick Up Stix specializes in take out but also offers casual service dining rooms for your enjoyment.* $

Pick Up Stix

Chinese Wok'd Fresh

Locations in: Calabasas, Granada Hills, Hermosa Beach, Long Beach, Long Beach Marketplace, Newbury Park, Porter Ranch (Northridge), San Pedro, Santa Monica, Studio City, Torrance, Valencia and Westlake. Please visit www.pickupstix.com/lacounty.html for details.

CHICKEN WITH VEGETABLES (½ SERVING) ♉

Chicken breast meat with broccoli, carrots, zucchini, mushrooms and water chestnuts in a sauce of white wine, garlic and soy. Analysis for ½ serving.

✓✓ CALORIES: Excellent Choice (315) ✓ CHOLESTEROL: Good Choice (85 mg)
✓✓ FAT: Excellent Choice (5 g) ✓ SODIUM: Good Choice (305 mg)**
EXCHANGES: 4½ Meat (extra lean), 1 Bread, 2½ Veg, ¼ Fat
PROTEIN: 34 g, CARBOHYDRATE: 33 g, FIBER: 5 g

GARLIC SHRIMP (½ SERVING) ♉

Plump shrimp stir-fried with zucchini, broccoli, onions, mushrooms, and water chestnuts in our special garlic sauce. Analysis for ½ serving.

✓✓ CALORIES: Excellent Choice (300) CHOLESTEROL: Moderate (175 mg)
✓✓ FAT: Excellent Choice (7 g*) ✓ SODIUM: Good Choice (405 mg)**
EXCHANGES: 2½ Meat (extra lean), 1½ Bread, 1¾ Veg, 1¼ Fat
PROTEIN: 21 g, CARBOHYDRATE: 37 g, FIBER: 5 g

SZECHWAN VEGETABLES (½ SERVING) ♉

Seared red chili peppers are wok'd with fresh broccoli, zucchini, carrots, celery, mushrooms, water chestnuts and green and white onions, in a zesty Szechwan sauce. Analysis for ½ serving.

✓✓ CALORIES: Excellent Choice (165) ✓✓ CHOLESTEROL: Excellent Choice (0 mg)
✓✓ FAT: Excellent Choice (2 g*) ✓✓ SODIUM: Excellent Choice (295 mg)**
EXCHANGES: 1 Bread, 2¾ Veg, ¼ Fat
PROTEIN: 5 g, CARBOHYDRATE: 34 g, FIBER: 6 g

CHINESE CHICKEN SALAD WITH FAT FREE SPICY LIME CILANTRO DRESSING ♉

Oven roasted chicken breast over fresh greens, sprinkled with sunflower seeds and topped with Chinese croutons. Analysis includes 4 oz. fat-free Spicy Lime Cilantro dressing served on the side.

✓ CALORIES: Good Choice (675) ✓ CHOLESTEROL: Good Choice (80 mg)
✓ FAT: Good Choice (20 g) SODIUM: High (1330 mg)
EXCHANGES: 4½ Meat (extra lean), 3¼ Bread, 2¼ Veg, 3 Fat
PROTEIN: 43 g, CARBOHYDRATE: 83 g, FIBER: 3 g

SZECHWAN SHRIMP (½ SERVING) ♉

Seared red chili peppers are wok'd with shrimp, celery, carrots and green and white onions. Analysis for ½ serving.

✓✓ CALORIES: Excellent Choice (290) CHOLESTEROL: Moderate (175 mg)
✓✓ FAT: Excellent Choice (8 g*) ✓ SODIUM: Good Choice (470 mg)**
EXCHANGES: 2½ Meat (extra lean), 1¼ Bread, 2½ Veg, 1¼ Fat
PROTEIN: 21 g, CARBOHYDRATE: 34 g, FIBER: 3 g

♉ at least 2 fruit/vegetable servings
✓ Good Choice....✓✓ Excellent Choice

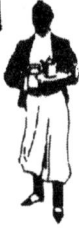

PINOT

RESTAURANTS

Since launching Patina Restaurant in 1989, Joachim and Christine Splichal have opened five acclaimed French bistros. Rather than create a prototype that is applied to each new location equally, the Pinot Restaurants are unique to each particular neighborhood. The consistent theme is high quality and imaginative presentation of food, and a gracious style of service. As a result, each Pinot restaurant offers a "unique familiarity" – you know you're in a Splichal restaurant, but you also notice the touches that make each a singular dining experience. $$

Pinot Bistro 12969 Ventura Blvd., Studio City	(818) 990-0500
Cafe Pinot 700 West Fifth Street, Los Angeles	(213) 239-6500
Pinot Hollywood 1448 N. Gower St., Los Angeles	(323) 461-8800

MIDDLE EASTERN RED LENTIL SOUP †
with yogurt and lemon.
✓✓ CALORIES: Excellent Choice (140)   ✓✓ CHOLESTEROL: Excellent Choice (5 mg)
✓✓ FAT: Excellent Choice (2 g)   ✓✓ SODIUM: Excellent Choice (15 mg)**
EXCHANGES: ¾ Meat, 1¼ Bread, ¼ Veg, ¼ Milk, ¼ Fat
PROTEIN: 9 g, CARBOHYDRATE: 22 g

JAPANESE SOBA NOODLES WITH GINGERED CHICKEN AND SHIITAKE BROTH
✓✓ CALORIES: Excellent Choice (405)   ✓ CHOLESTEROL: Good Choice (80 mg)
✓✓ FAT: Excellent Choice (6 g)   ✓✓ SODIUM: Excellent Choice (165 mg)**
EXCHANGES: 3¾ Meat (extra lean), 3¼ Bread, 3¼ Veg
PROTEIN: 36 g, CARBOHYDRATE: 53 g

CHILLED CUCUMBER SOUP WITH KUMOMOTO OYSTER AND FRESH CORIANDER
✓✓ CALORIES: Excellent Choice (240)   ✓✓ CHOLESTEROL: Excellent Choice (10 mg)
✓ FAT: Good Choice (20 g)*   ✓✓ SODIUM: Excellent Choice (235 mg)**
EXCHANGES: ¼ Meat, ¾ Veg, ¼ Fruit, 3¾ Fat
PROTEIN: 5 g, CARBOHYDRATE: 15 g

GRILLED BREAST OF CHICKEN AND MASHED ROOT VEGETABLES - SPECIAL REQUEST ♻
with mustard greens and a horseradish sauce. Request less oil (½ Tbs.).
✓ CALORIES: Good Choice (580)   CHOLESTEROL: Moderate (215 mg)
✓ FAT: Good Choice (17 g)   ✓ SODIUM: Good Choice (415 mg)**
EXCHANGES: 11 Meat (extra lean), 1 Bread, 1¼ Veg, 1¼ Fat
PROTEIN: 83 g, CARBOHYDRATE: 21 g

BAKED SALMON WITH BRAISED FENNEL - SPECIAL REQUEST ♻
with stewed tomatoes and fresh bay leaves. Request less oil (½ Tbs.).
✓✓ CALORIES: Excellent Choice (385)   ✓ CHOLESTEROL: Good Choice (90 mg)
✓ FAT: Good Choice (18 g)*   ✓✓ SODIUM: Excellent Choice (265 mg)**
EXCHANGES: 4¼ Meat, 2½ Veg, 1½ Fat
PROTEIN: 36 g, CARBOHYDRATE: 16 g

WARM SALAD OF ACORN SQUASH, ROASTED SHALLOTS AND CITRUS VINAIGRETTE ♻
✓✓ CALORIES: Excellent Choice (340)   ✓✓ CHOLESTEROL: Excellent Choice (0 mg)
✓ FAT: Good Choice (22 g)*   ✓✓ SODIUM: Excellent Choice (15 mg)**
EXCHANGES: 1 Bread, ¼ Veg, ¾ Fruit, 4¼ Fat
PROTEIN: 8 g, CARBOHYDRATE: 33 g

---

* Primarily unsaturated fat

** If you request no added salt

† Side dish guidelines are 1/3 of entree guidelines

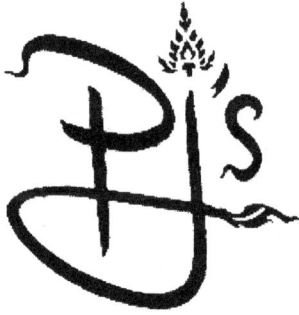

Come and enjoy the finest in authentic Thai cuisine. We are located in the beautiful Belmont Shores in Long Beach. A private room is available for you and your guests. Open daily. $

PJ's Thai Restaurant
5372 East 2nd Street, Long Beach, CA 90803
(562) 434-3565

SPICY CHICKEN SOUP (TOM YUM KAI) ☺
Chicken soup with lemon juice, chili paste and mushroom. Analysis for medium size.
✓✓ CALORIES: Excellent Choice (320)   ✓✓ CHOLESTEROL: Excellent Choice (60 mg)
✓✓ FAT: Excellent Choice (7 g)   SODIUM: High (1930 mg)
EXCHANGES: 3¼ Meat (extra lean), 1 Bread, ¾ Veg, 1¼ Fruit, ¾ Fat
PROTEIN: 27 g, CARBOHYDRATE: 39 g, FIBER: 3 g

CHICKEN - SPICY MINT WITH GREEN CHILE PEPPER & ONION ☺
✓✓ CALORIES: Excellent Choice (350)   ✓✓ CHOLESTEROL: Excellent Choice (60 mg)
✓✓ FAT: Excellent Choice (13 g)   SODIUM: High (1675 mg)
EXCHANGES: 3 Meat, ¼ Bread, 5¼ Veg, 1¾ Fat
PROTEIN: 26 g, CARBOHYDRATE: 33 g, FIBER: 8 g

SPICY BEEF SALAD ☺
Sliced beef with spicy sauce and vegetables.
✓ CALORIES: Good Choice (490)   ✓ CHOLESTEROL: Good Choice (100 mg)
✓ FAT: Good Choice (17 g)   SODIUM: High (1290 mg)
EXCHANGES: 4¾ Meat, ¼ Bread, 3 Veg, 2 Fruit, 1¼ Fat
PROTEIN: 39 g, CARBOHYDRATE: 50 g, FIBER: 7 g

ASSORTED VEGETABLES WITH TOFU ☺
Stir fried mixed vegetables and tofu.
✓✓ CALORIES: Excellent Choice (300)   ✓✓ CHOLESTEROL: Excellent Choice (0 mg)
✓✓ FAT: Excellent Choice (14 g)*   SODIUM: High (1045 mg)
EXCHANGES: 1¼ Meat, ½ Bread, 4¼ Veg, 1¾ Fat
PROTEIN: 16 g, CARBOHYDRATE: 32 g, FIBER: 8 g

GARLIC SHRIMP
Stir fried shrimp with garlic, black pepper and cilantro.
✓✓ CALORIES: Excellent Choice (300)   CHOLESTEROL: High (350 mg)
✓✓ FAT: Excellent Choice (13 g)*   SODIUM: High (2345 mg)
EXCHANGES: 5 Meat(extra lean), ¼ Bread, ¼ Veg, 1¾ Fat
PROTEIN: 40 g, CARBOHYDRATE: 7 g, FIBER: 0 g

HOUSE SPECIAL NOODLES
Stir fried noodles with shrimp, chicken, egg, vegetables and ground peanuts.
✓ CALORIES: Good Choice (685)   CHOLESTEROL: High (315 mg)
✓ FAT: Good Choice (18 g)   SODIUM: Moderate (835 mg)**
EXCHANGES: 4½ Meat, 4½ Bread, 1½ Veg, 2½ Fat
PROTEIN: 42 g, CARBOHYDRATE: 88 g, FIBER: 3 g

☺ at least 2 fruit/vegetable servings
✓ Good Choice   ✓✓ Excellent Choice

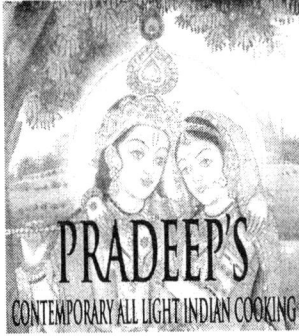

We are pleased to feature a new concept in Indian cuisine for Californians. Our philosophy answers the continuing trend for healthier dining without sacrificing flavor. Our focus is on preparing high quality, low fat, low cholesterol, and high fiber cuisine. Chef Pradeep, who has worked in India and Europe, creates all of our delicious dishes. You will notice an emphasis of freshness on every plate. We offer regional Indian food that has never before been presented in this part of the world. We welcome you to have a great dining or take-out experience at Pradeep's – Enjoy! $-$$

Pradeep's www.pradeepsindiancuisine.com
1405 Montana Avenue, Santa Monica 90403   (310) 393-1467

ALOO GOBI ⏾
Potato and cauliflower cooked with onions, tomatoes, ginger, garlic and curry spices.

✓✓ CALORIES: Excellent Choice (175)   ✓✓ CHOLESTEROL: Excellent Choice (0 mg)
✓✓ FAT: Excellent Choice (5 g)*   ✓ SODIUM: Good Choice (305 mg)**
EXCHANGES: 1¼ Bread, 1¾ Veg, 1 Fat
PROTEIN: 4 g, CARBOHYDRATE: 30 g, FIBER: 3 g

SAAG AND ORGANIC TOFU CURRY
Slowly cooked spinach with organic tofu.

✓✓ CALORIES: Excellent Choice (140)   ✓✓ CHOLESTEROL: Excellent Choice (0 mg)
✓✓ FAT: Excellent Choice (7 g)*   ✓ SODIUM: Good Choice (395 mg)**
EXCHANGES: 1 Meat, ¼ Bread, 1½ Veg, 1 Fat
PROTEIN: 10 g, CARBOHYDRATE: 12 g, FIBER: 4 g

BAIGAN KA BHURTA ⏾
Roughly chopped roasted eggplant cooked with red onions, tomatoes, ginger, garlic, curry spices and cilantro.

✓✓ CALORIES: Excellent Choice (130)   ✓✓ CHOLESTEROL: Excellent Choice (0 mg)
✓✓ FAT: Excellent Choice (5 g)*   ✓✓ SODIUM: Excellent Choice (280 mg)**
EXCHANGES: ¾ Bread, 1 Veg, 1 Fat
PROTEIN: 3 g, CARBOHYDRATE: 21 g, FIBER: 4 g

TANDOORI MARINATED CHICKEN – SPECIAL REQUEST
Breast of chicken served over fluffy basmati rice, curry infused lentils and California greens.
Request chicken breast meat.

✓ CALORIES: Good Choice (465)   ✓ CHOLESTEROL: Good Choice (130 mg)
✓✓ FAT: Excellent Choice (8 g)   ✓ SODIUM: Good Choice (395 mg)**
EXCHANGES: 6¾ Meat, 2 Bread, 1¼ Veg, ½ Fat
PROTEIN: 55 g, CARBOHYDRATE: 40 g, FIBER: 5 g

PRADEEP'S SALMON
Tandoori marinated salmon served over turmeric and cilantro flavored mashed potatoes, California organic greens, balsamic and mint chutney.

✓✓ CALORIES: Excellent Choice (370)   ✓ CHOLESTEROL: Good Choice (90 mg)
✓✓ FAT: Excellent Choice (14 g)*   ✓ SODIUM: Good Choice (390 mg)**
EXCHANGES: 4¼ Meat, ¾ Bread, ¼ Veg, ½ Milk, ¾ Fat
PROTEIN: 38 g, CARBOHYDRATE: 21 g, FIBER: 3 g

CARROT & CORIANDER SOUP † ⏾
A unique blend of organically-grown carrots and dry coriander from the fields of Punjab, with a scent of cilantro and lime.

✓✓ CALORIES: Excellent Choice (110)   ✓✓ CHOLESTEROL: Excellent Choice (0 mg)
✓✓ FAT: Excellent Choice (2 g)*   ✓✓ SODIUM: Excellent Choice (50 mg)
EXCHANGES: ½ Bread, 2¾ Veg
PROTEIN: 3 g, CARBOHYDRATE: 25 g, FIBER: 5 g

---

* Primarily unsaturated fat   † Side dish guidelines are 1/3 of entree guidelines, 1 for side dishes
** If you request no added salt

Healthy Dining in Los Angeles **101**

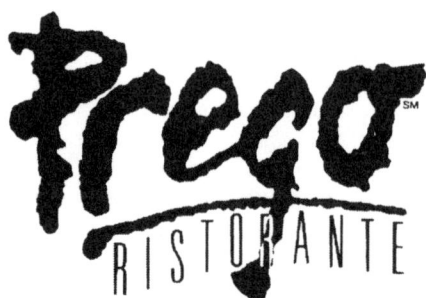

A warm, rustic Tuscan trattoria with the energy and vibrancy of a big-city restaurant, Prego is a unique and inviting experience in the heart of the Beverly Hills shopping district. Prego bustles with excitement both from its busy exhibition kitchen and its frequent famous guests. Prego can serve your needs for most any event, with a private dining room that seats 85. Valet parking available at dinner. Dinner nightly; lunch Mondays through Saturdays. $$

Prego Ristorante   362 N. Camden Drive, Beverly Hills, CA 90210 (310) 277-7346

ZITI AL POMODORO E BASILICO
Short tube pasta with fresh tomato sauce and basil.
- ✓ CALORIES: Good Choice (505)
- ✓ FAT: Good Choice (16 g)
- ✓✓ CHOLESTEROL: Excellent Choice (30 mg)
- SODIUM: Moderate (730 mg)**

EXCHANGES: 4½ Bread, 1½ Veg, 3 Fat
PROTEIN: 14 g, CARBOHYDRATE: 77 g, FIBER: 5 g

PESCE SPADA ALL'ISOLANA - SPECIAL REQUEST
Swordfish topped with a tomato basil sauce. <u>*Request less oil (½ Tbs.)*</u>
- ✓✓ CALORIES: Excellent Choice (375)
- ✓ FAT: Good Choice (16 g)*
- ✓ CHOLESTEROL: Good Choice (90 mg)
- ✓ SODIUM: Good Choice (375 mg)**

EXCHANGES: 5 Meat, 1¼ Veg, 1¼ Fat
PROTEIN: 47 g, CARBOHYDRATE: 9 g, FIBER: 2 g

PIZZA VEGETARIANA ♉
with fresh tomatoes, zucchini, mushrooms, garlic, basil and no cheese.
- ✓ CALORIES: Good Choice (685)
- ✓ FAT: Good Choice (19 g)*
- ✓✓ CHOLESTEROL: Excellent Choice (0 mg)
- SODIUM: High (1275 mg)

EXCHANGES: 5½ Bread, 4¼ Veg, 3¼ Fat
PROTEIN: 18 g, CARBOHYDRATE: 115 g, FIBER: 10 g

CAPELLINI ALLA CHECCA - SPECIAL REQUEST ♉
Angel hair pasta with chopped tomato, basil, garlic and extra virgin olive oil. <u>*Request less oil (1 Tbs.)*</u>
- ✓ CALORIES: Good Choice (525)
- ✓ FAT: Good Choice (16 g)*
- ✓✓ CHOLESTEROL: Excellent Choice (0 mg)
- ✓✓ SODIUM: Excellent Choice (25 mg)**

EXCHANGES: 4½ Bread, 2 Veg, 2¾ Fat
PROTEIN: 14 g, CARBOHYDRATE: 82 g, FIBER: 7 g

RIGATONI AL POLLO
Pasta tubes, grilled chicken breast, broccoli, sun-dried tomatoes, extra virgin olive oil and garlic.
- ✓ CALORIES: Good Choice (680)
- ✓ FAT: Good Choice (19 g)
- ✓✓ CHOLESTEROL: Excellent Choice (65 mg)
- SODIUM: Moderate (665 mg)**

EXCHANGES: 3½ Meat (extra lean), 4½ Bread, 1¾ Veg, 2¾ Fat
PROTEIN: 41 g, CARBOHYDRATE: 88 g, FIBER: 5 g

♉ at least 2 fruit/vegetable servings
✓ Good Choice   ✓✓ Excellent Choice

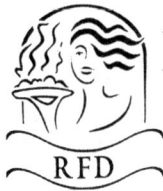

REAL FOOD DAILY

ORGANIC VEGETARIAN COOKING

RFD

L.A.'s premier organic vegetarian restaurant. This hip, eclectic hot spot attracts vegetarians, celebrities, trendsetting young eaters with sophisticated palates, and the mature diner seeking gourmet health-promoting cuisine. Ann Gentry, the creator of Real Food Daily, has taken two different California trends – vegetarian and the organic seasonal cooking – and has come up with a cuisine that is as interesting and delicious as it is healthful. Please visit www.realfood.com. $

514 Santa Monica Blvd., Santa Monica 90401   (310) 451-7544
414 N. La Cienega Blvd., West Hollywood 90048   (310) 289-9910

RAW ROCK 'N' ROLL ☺

Rice paper wrapped around julienned carrots, peppers, daikon, cabbages, mango, fresh mint and cilantro, served with a raw mango ponzu dipping sauce. Two spring rolls per order; analysis for one roll and ½ portion of sauce.

✓✓ CALORIES: Excellent Choice (130)
✓✓ FAT: Excellent Choice (0 g)*
✓ CHOLESTEROL: Excellent Choice (0 mg)
✓ SODIUM: Good Choice (585 mg)**
EXCHANGES: ½ Bread, 1 Veg, 1 Fruit
PROTEIN: 2 g, CARBOHYDRATE: 31 g, FIBER: 4 g

TOTAL REUBEN

Baked marinated tempeh on toasted caraway rye bread with our house-made tofu "cheese," thousand island dressing and sauerkraut.

✓ CALORIES: Good Choice (530)
✓ FAT: Good Choice (20 g)*
✓✓ CHOLESTEROL: Excellent Choice (0 mg)
SODIUM: High (1630 mg)**
EXCHANGES: 3½ Meat, 3¼ Bread, ¾ Veg, 1¾ Fat
PROTEIN: 35 g, CARBOHYDRATE: 55 g, FIBER: 9 g

R & B BURRITO ☺

Spanish rice, refried black beans and guacamole rolled in a whole wheat tortilla, topped with ranchero sauce and tofu "sour cream," served with a salad and carrot salsa.

CALORIES: Moderate (805)
✓ FAT: Good Choice (18 g)
✓✓ CHOLESTEROL: Excellent Choice (0 mg)
SODIUM: High (1770 mg)**
EXCHANGES: ¼ Meat, 6¾ Bread, 4¼ Veg, 2¾ Fat
PROTEIN: 34 g, CARBOHYDRATE: 132 g, FIBER: 21 g

REAL FOOD MEAL ☺

Whole grains in the center of the plate surrounded by an array of sea and seasonal land vegetables, a small amount of plant based protein and condiments.

✓✓ CALORIES: Excellent Choice (395)
✓✓ FAT: Excellent Choice (4 g)
✓✓ CHOLESTEROL: Excellent Choice (0 mg)
✓ SODIUM: Good Choice (585 mg)**
EXCHANGES: ½ Meat, 4 Bread, 2½ Veg, ¼ Fat
PROTEIN: 15 g, CARBOHYDRATE: 77 g, FIBER: 8 g

FARM CHOP – SPECIAL REQUEST ☺

A potpourri of chopped fresh seasonal vegetables served on a bed of shredded cabbage.
<u>*Request dressing on the side.*</u> *Dressing not included in analysis. Oil free dressing available.*

✓✓ CALORIES: Excellent Choice (225)
✓✓ FAT: Excellent Choice (9 g)
✓✓ CHOLESTEROL: Excellent Choice (0 mg)
✓✓ SODIUM: Excellent Choice (160 mg)**
EXCHANGES: ¾ Bread, 4¼ Veg, 1½ Fat
PROTEIN: 6 g, CARBOHYDRATE: 37 g, FIBER: 9 g

TOFU CHEESECAKE

Delicious tofu cheesecake served with fresh fruit topping.

✓✓ CALORIES: Excellent Choice (405)
✓ FAT: Good Choice (18 g)
✓✓ CHOLESTEROL: Excellent Choice (0 mg)
✓✓ SODIUM: Excellent Choice (55 mg)**
EXCHANGES: 1 Meat, 1¼ Bread, 3 Fat, ½ Fruit
PROTEIN: 10 g, CARBOHYDRATE: 53 g, FIBER: 6 g

* Primarily unsaturated fat
** If you request no added salt

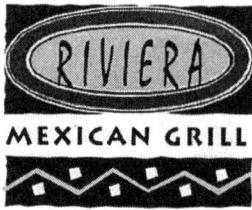

Welcome to the new Riviera Mexican Grill; just the place for people who think life's a little bit better splashed with salsa. When you pull up a chair, we want you to know that our food is always going to be fresh and good and that this is one place where the sun shines and the surf's up every day of the year! So, eat, drink and be mellow, amigos, you're in the Riviera! $-$$

Riviera Mexican Grill

1615 Pacific Coast Hwy., Redondo Beach 90277 (310) 540-2501

PAPAYA & GRILLED CHICKEN SALAD ⌁

Field greens, sliced avocado and ripe papaya with charbroiled chicken breast and mango vinaigrette.

✓✓ CALORIES: Excellent Choice (390)   ✓ CHOLESTEROL: Good Choice (110 mg)
✓ FAT: Good Choice (19 g)   ✓✓ SODIUM: Excellent Choice (170 mg)**
EXCHANGES: 5¾ Meat (extra lean), ¼ Veg, ½ Fruit, 2¾ Fat
PROTEIN: 42 g, CARBOHYDRATE: 13 g, FIBER: 3 g

GRILLED FRESH FISH TACOS ⌁

Grilled fresh catch wrapped in warm flour tortillas and served with chili tartar sauce, pico de gallo salsa and tequila-marinated cabbage. Served with zuni chopped salad and black beans (separate analysis for beans below).

✓ CALORIES: Good Choice (510)   ✓ CHOLESTEROL: Good Choice (85 mg)
✓ FAT: Good Choice (22 g)*   SODIUM: Moderate (960 mg)**
EXCHANGES: 4½ Meat, 2 Bread, 1¼ Veg, 2¾ Fat
PROTEIN: 38 g, CARBOHYDRATE: 40 g, FIBER: 4 g

SHRIMP FAJITAS ⌁

Seasoned shrimp with tomatoes, bell peppers and onions, served on a sizzling platter with four corn tortillas, salsa and guacamole. Served with Zuni chopped salad and black beans (see separate analysis for beans below). Sour cream not included in analysis.

✓ CALORIES: Good Choice (530)   CHOLESTEROL: Moderate (275 mg)
✓✓ FAT: Excellent Choice (14 g)*   SODIUM: Moderate (690 mg)**
EXCHANGES: 4¼ Meat (extra lean), 3 Bread, 2½ Veg, 1¾ Fat
PROTEIN: 37 g, CARBOHYDRATE: 61 g, FIBER: 7 g

VEGGIE BURRITO ⌁

Grilled red and yellow bell peppers, avocado, red onion, roasted chilies, black beans and rice with two salsas and guacamole. Cheese by request (not included in analysis). Served with Zuni chopped salad and black beans (see separate analysis for beans below).

✓ CALORIES: Good Choice (630)   ✓✓ CHOLESTEROL: Excellent Choice (5 mg)
✓ FAT: Good Choice (19 g)*   SODIUM: Moderate (655 mg)**
EXCHANGES: 5 Bread, 3¾ Veg, 3½ Fat
PROTEIN: 18 g, CARBOHYDRATE: 102 g, FIBER: 14 g

SHRIMP TACOS DEL MAR

Grilled marinated shrimp served open face with pickled onion, cilantro, tomatillo salsa and avocado. Served with Zuni chopped salad and black beans (see separate analysis for beans below).

✓✓ CALORIES: Excellent Choice (370)   CHOLESTEROL: Moderate (275 mg)
✓✓ FAT: Excellent Choice (9 g)*   SODIUM: Moderate (620 mg)**
EXCHANGES: 4¼ Meat, 1¾ Bread, 1¼ Veg, 1 Fat
PROTEIN: 34 g, CARBOHYDRATE: 37 g, FIBER: 4 g

BLACK BEANS †

CALORIES: Moderate (250)   ✓✓ CHOLESTEROL: Excellent Choice (0 mg)
✓✓ FAT: Excellent Choice (5 g)   ✓✓ SODIUM: Excellent Choice (45 mg)
EXCHANGES: 2½ Bread, ¾ Fat
PROTEIN: 9 g, CARBOHYDRATE: 26 g, FIBER: 7 g

† Side dish guidelines are 1/3 of entree guidelines
⌁ at least 2 fruit/vegetable servings

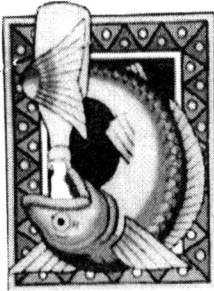

Feel the flavor at one of Manhattan Beach pier's hottest restaurants. This incredible dining experience will take you coast to coast, from Louisiana-style gumbo to Chicago-style steak, and the freshest California seafood. Upbeat jazz and blues provide a wonderful atmosphere for enjoying a specialty martini or a bottle from the fine list of wines. Join your friends at the bar, mezzanine, or on the patio. Sat. thru Thur. 11:30 am – midnight. Fri thru Sat. 11:30 am – 2 am.
$$

Rock'N Fish

120 Manhattan Beach Blvd., Manhattan Beach (310) 379-9900

AUSTRALIAN COLD WATER LOBSTER TAIL ☸
Served with oak grilled vegetables and steamed spinach. Butter on side not included in analysis.
- ✓✓ CALORIES: Excellent Choice (320)
- ✓✓ FAT: Excellent Choice (7 g)*
- ✓ CHOLESTEROL: Good Choice (135 mg)
- SODIUM: Moderate (805 mg)**

EXCHANGES: 3¼ Meat (extra lean), 3½ Veg, ¼ Fruit, 1 Fat
PROTEIN: 45 g, CARBOHYDRATE: 23 g, FIBER: 7 g

FRESH SEARED AHI TUNA
Served with steamed spinach, wasabi and sticky rice (see separate analysis for rice below).
- ✓ CALORIES: Good Choice (535)
- ✓ FAT: Good Choice (23 g)*
- ✓ CHOLESTEROL: Good Choice (100 mg)
- ✓✓ SODIUM: Excellent Choice (175 mg)**

EXCHANGES: 7¼ Meat (extra lean), ¾ Veg, 4¼ Fat
PROTEIN: 64 g, CARBOHYDRATE: 20 g, FIBER: 8 g

TUNA NICOISE SALAD – SPECIAL REQUEST ☸
Ahi tuna, marinated green beans, carrots, Kalamata olives, potato, hard boiled egg, onion and tomato with spring lettuce. Request dressing on the side (75 calories, 8 g fat per Tbs).
- ✓ CALORIES: Good Choice (475)
- ✓ FAT: Good Choice (16 g)
- CHOLESTEROL: Moderate (265 mg)
- SODIUM: Moderate (650 mg)**

EXCHANGES: 4½ Meat, ¾ Bread, 4¾ Veg, 1 Fat
PROTEIN: 42 g, CARBOHYDRATE: 45 g, FIBER: 12 g

NAPA SONOMA SALAD – SPECIAL REQUEST ☸
Pine nuts, fresh mozzarella, sun dried tomatoes, Roma tomato, cucumber, red onion and spring lettuce. Request less pine nuts (2 Tbs.) and dressing on the side (dressing not included in analysis).
- ✓ CALORIES: Good Choice (475)
- ✓ FAT: Good Choice (20 g)
- ✓✓ CHOLESTEROL: Excellent Choice (30 mg)
- ✓ SODIUM: Good Choice (355 mg)**

EXCHANGES: 1¾ Meat, 4¼ Veg, 2½ Fat
PROTEIN: 30 g, CARBOHYDRATE: 56 g, FIBER: 9 g

LINGUINI DEL MAR – SPECIAL REQUEST
Assorted seafood with marinara sauce over pasta. Request less oil (½ oz).
- ✓ CALORIES: Good Choice (695)
- ✓ FAT: Good Choice (19 g)*
- CHOLESTEROL: Moderate (275 mg)
- SODIUM: Moderate (850 mg)**

EXCHANGES: 4½ Meat (extra lean), 4¼ Bread, 1¼ Veg, 3 Fat
PROTEIN: 49 g, CARBOHYDRATE: 76 g, FIBER: 5 g

OAK GRILLED SHRIMP & GARLIC BROCHETTES ☸
Served with steamed spinach & sticky rice with teriyaki sauce (see separate analyses for rice & sauce below).
- ✓✓ CALORIES: Excellent Choice (410)
- ✓✓ FAT: Excellent Choice (13 g)
- CHOLESTEROL: High (470 mg)
- SODIUM: Moderate (995 mg)**

EXCHANGES: 6¾ Meat (extra lean), ¼ Bread, 3¼ Veg, 2 Fat
PROTEIN: 54 g, CARBOHYDRATE: 21 g, FIBER: 4 g

STICKY RICE: CAL: 220, FAT: <1, CHOL: 0, SOD: <5 mg; EXCH: 3¼ Bread; PROT: 5 g, CARB: 48 g, FIBER: 1 g
TERIYAKI SAUCE *(1 Tbs.):* CAL: 20, FAT: 0, CHOL: 0, SOD: 215 mg; EXCH: ¼ Br; PROT: 1 g, CARB: 5 g, FIB: 0

---

* Primarily unsaturated fat
** If you request no added salt

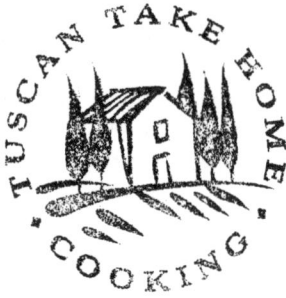

Our mission is to provide delicious and healthy food, presented with warmth, imagination, and generosity of spirit. Rosti's hallmark is innovative Tuscan Italian cuisine, made from the freshest seasonal ingredients. Delivery and catering available. Lunch and dinner served 7 days a week. Visit our website at www.RostiTuscanKitchen.com. $-$$

Rosti

233 S. Beverly Drive, Beverly Hills 90212	(310) 275-3285
16403 Ventura Blvd., Encino 91436	(818) 995-7179
931 Montana Ave., Santa Monica 90403	(310) 393-3236
160 Promenade Way, Ste A, Westlake 91362	(805) 370-1939

ROSEMARY GRILLED CHICKEN ☺

Skinless chicken breast, pounded and seasoned with olive oil & rosemary. Served with seasonal vegetables (included in analysis) and your choice of another side dish (not included in analysis).
- ✓ CALORIES: Good Choice (510)
- ✓ FAT: Good Choice (21 g)
- ✓ CHOLESTEROL: Good Choice (150 mg)
- ✓ SODIUM: Good Choice (380 mg)**

EXCHANGES: 8 Meat (extra lean), 3¾ Veg, 2¾ Fat
PROTEIN: 60 g, CARBOHYDRATE: 21 g, FIBER: 7 g

FRESH GRILLED SALMON ☺

Served with checca and seasonal vegetables.
- ✓ CALORIES: Good Choice (485)
- ✓ FAT: Good Choice (25 g)*
- ✓ CHOLESTEROL: Good Choice (90 mg)
- SODIUM: Moderate (615 mg)**

EXCHANGES: 4¼ Meat, 5 Veg, 2½ Fat
PROTEIN: 41 g, CARBOHYDRATE: 29 g, FIBER: 12 g

GOAT CHEESE & GRILLED VEGETABLE SALAD – SPECIAL REQUEST ☺

Served chilled on mixed greens with Rosti dressing. Analysis is for full size salad.
Request dressing on the side (90 calories, 10 g fat per Tbs).
- ✓✓ CALORIES: Excellent Choice (165)
- ✓✓ FAT: Excellent Choice (9 g)
- ✓✓ CHOLESTEROL: Excellent Choice (25 mg)
- ✓✓ SODIUM: Excellent Choice (200 mg)**

EXCHANGES: ¾ Meat, 1¾ Veg, 1¼ Fat
PROTEIN: 10 g, CARBOHYDRATE: 12 g, FIBER: 5 g

INSALATA DI POLLO (HALF SIZE SALAD) – SPECIAL REQUEST ☺

Romaine lettuce, cucumbers and pine nuts, with chopped marinated chicken, checca and Rosti dressing. Analysis is for the half size salad. Request dressing on the side (90 calories, 10 g fat per Tbs).
- ✓✓ CALORIES: Excellent Choice (230)
- ✓✓ FAT: Excellent Choice (11 g)
- ✓✓ CHOLESTEROL: Excellent Choice (60 mg)
- ✓ SODIUM: Good Choice (330 mg)**

EXCHANGES: 3¼ Meat, 1 Veg, 1¾ Fat
PROTEIN: 26 g, CARBOHYDRATE: 8 g, FIBER: 3 g

PENNE ALL'ARRABBIATA – SPECIAL REQUEST ☺

With spicy tomato sauce, garlic and herbs. Request less oil (½ oz). Also available with chicken or shrimp.
- ✓✓ CALORIES: Excellent Choice (420)
- ✓✓ FAT: Excellent Choice (15 g)*
- ✓✓ CHOLESTEROL: Excellent Choice (0 mg)
- ✓ SODIUM: Good Choice (505 mg)**

EXCHANGES: 3¼ Bread, 2½ Veg, 2¾ Fat
PROTEIN: 11 g, CARBOHYDRATE: 61 g, FIBER: 5 g

SPAGHETTINI VONGOLE – SPECIAL REQUEST

Spaghetti with fresh clams in shell with white wine sauce. Request less oil (½ oz).
- ✓ CALORIES: Good Choice (570)
- ✓ FAT: Good Choice (16 g)*
- ✓✓ CHOLESTEROL: Excellent Choice (35 mg)
- SODIUM: Moderate (800 mg)**

EXCHANGES: ½ Meat, 5¼ Bread, ½ Veg, 2¾ Fat
PROTEIN: 18 g, CARBOHYDRATE: 83 g, FIBER: 4 g

☺ at least 2 fruit/vegetable servings

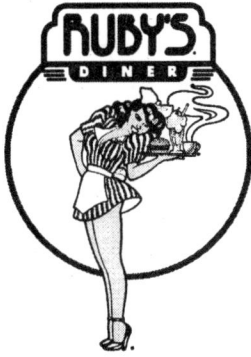

Ruby's Diner is the authentic 1940's diner! Step back in time to 40's memorabilia, gleaming red and white interiors and friendly, courteous service. Ruby's offers items to please every palate, including a variety of salads, sandwiches, and home style breakfasts. Swing into Ruby's today and experience great food and great service with a 40's flair. $

Ruby's Diner

with 10 Los Angeles area locations to serve you!

LA Airport-Term. 6	(310) 646-2480	Redondo Beach	(310) 376-7829
Marina Del Rey	(310) 574-7829	Riverside	(909) 359-7829
Palm Springs	(760) 406-7829	Seal Beach	(562) 431-7829
Pasadena	(626) 796-7829	Whittier	(562) 947-7829
Palos Verde	(310) 544-7829	Woodland Hills	(818) 340-7829

For locations outside LA County, call 1-800 HEY RUBY or visit our website at www.rubys.com.

ROAST TURKEY BREAST SANDWICH – SPECIAL REQUEST
With lettuce and cranberry sauce on a soft RubyRoll. Just like Thanksgiving!
Request no margarine or mayonnaise.

✓ CALORIES: Good Choice (600)   ✓ CHOLESTEROL: Good Choice (120 mg)
✓✓ FAT: Excellent Choice (7 g)   SODIUM: Moderate (610 mg)**
EXCHANGES: 6¼ Meat, 3¾ Bread, 1½ Fruit, 1¼ Fat
PROTEIN: 52 g, CARBOHYDRATE: 80 g, FIBER: 3 g

CHICKEN RUBYBURGER – SPECIAL REQUEST
With a tender boneless, skinless chicken breast. Request no margarine or mayonnaise.

✓ CALORIES: Good Choice (485)   ✓ CHOLESTEROL: Good Choice (130 mg)
✓✓ FAT: Excellent Choice (10 g)   SODIUM: Moderate (950 mg)**
EXCHANGES: 6¾ Meat, 2½ Bread, ¾ Fat
PROTEIN: 55 g, CARBOHYDRATE: 41 g, FIBER: 1 g

TURKEY RUBYBURGER – SPECIAL REQUEST
With a full ⅓ lb. of lean ground turkey. Request no margarine or Ruby sauce.

✓ CALORIES: Good Choice (490)   ✓ CHOLESTEROL: Good Choice (145 mg)
✓ FAT: Good Choice (19 g)*   ✓ SODIUM: Good Choice (485 mg)**
EXCHANGES: 4 Meat, 2¾ Bread, 1½ Fat
PROTEIN: 35 g, CARBOHYDRATE: 43 g, FIBER: 1 g

VEGGIE RUBYBURGER – SPECIAL REQUEST
With a tasty vegetable, rice, oats and wheat Garden Burger patty. Request no margarine or mayonnaise.

✓ CALORIES: Good Choice (500)   ✓✓ CHOLESTEROL: Excellent Choice (5 mg)
✓✓ FAT: Excellent Choice (9 g)*   SODIUM: High (1085 mg)
EXCHANGES: ¼ Meat, 5½ Bread, ¾ Veg, 1¼ Fat
PROTEIN: 19 g, CARBOHYDRATE: 85 g, FIBER: 8 g

VEGGIE SOFT TACOS – SPECIAL REQUEST
Two whole wheat tortillas filled with fresh lettuce, cheese, vegetarian black beans, olives and salsa. Dressing not included in analysis. Request less cheese (½ oz.) and salsa as dressing.

✓ CALORIES: Good Choice (495)   ✓✓ CHOLESTEROL: Excellent Choice (15 mg)
✓ FAT: Good Choice (16 g)   SODIUM: High (1375 mg)
EXCHANGES: ½ Meat, 3¾ Bread, 1¼ Veg, 3¼ Fat
PROTEIN: 13 g, CARBOHYDRATE: 66 g, FIBER: 8 g

* Primarily unsaturated fat
** If you request no added salt

Sammy's Woodfired Pizza

2575 Pacific Coast Highway, Torrance, CA 90505 (310) 257-1333
(across from the AMC Theaters)

HEALTHY DINING VEGETARIAN PIZZA (½ PIZZA) ☙

Grilled eggplant, onions, bell peppers, fontina, garlic, zucchini and Roma tomatoes with fat-free mozzarella. Analysis is for ½ of a pizza.

CALORIES: Moderate (885) ✓✓ CHOLESTEROL: Excellent Choice (20 mg)
✓ FAT: Good Choice (21 g)* SODIUM: High (2110 mg)
EXCHANGES: 2¾ Meat, 7¾ Bread, 1¼ Veg, 3½ Fat
PROTEIN: 38 g, CARBOHYDRATE: 130 g, FIBER: 4 g

HEALTHY DINING TOMATO ANGEL HAIR PASTA ☙

Roma tomatoes, fresh basil and garlic.

✓ CALORIES: Good Choice (650) ✓✓ CHOLESTEROL: Excellent Choice (15 mg)
✓ FAT: Good Choice (18 g)* ✓✓ SODIUM: Excellent Choice (65 mg)**
EXCHANGES: 5¾ Bread, 2 Veg, 2¾ Fat
PROTEIN: 22 g, CARBOHYDRATE: 105 g, FIBER: 3 g

HEALTHY DINING GRILLED VEGETABLE PENNE ☙

Seasonal grilled vegetables with spinach, olive oil, balsamic vinegar and Romano cheese.

✓ CALORIES: Good Choice (610) ✓✓ CHOLESTEROL: Excellent Choice (30 mg)
✓ FAT: Good Choice (21 g)* SODIUM: Moderate (685 mg)**
EXCHANGES: 1 Meat, 4¼ Bread, 2 Veg, 3½ Fat
PROTEIN: 24 g, CARBOHYDRATE: 84 g, FIBER: 3 g

HEALTHY DINING CHINESE CHICKEN SALAD ☙

Individual size salad with Chinese greens, bell peppers, sesame seeds, cilantro, scallions, Mandarin oranges and fat-free Oriental dressing.

✓ CALORIES: Good Choice (480) ✓ CHOLESTEROL: Good Choice (85 mg)
✓✓ FAT: Excellent Choice (13 g) SODIUM: High (2455 mg)
EXCHANGES: 4½ Meat (extra lean), ½ Bread, 3½ Veg, ¾ Fruit, ¾ Fat
PROTEIN: 42 g, CARBOHYDRATE: 49 g, FIBER: 1 g

HEALTHY DINING CHOPPED CHICKEN SALAD ☙

Individual size salad with chicken breast, lettuce, tomatoes, olives, fat-free mozzarella, basil and fat-free dressing.

✓✓ CALORIES: Excellent Choice (395) ✓ CHOLESTEROL: Good Choice (90 mg)
✓✓ FAT: Excellent Choice (11 g) SODIUM: High (3130 mg)
EXCHANGES: 6¾ Meat (extra lean), 1¼ Veg, ¼ Fruit, 1¼ Fat
PROTEIN: 52 g, CARBOHYDRATE: 20 g, FIBER: 1 g

After 60 years in the seafood business, Santa Monica Seafood takes enormous pride in being regarded as Southern California's #1 seafood retailer. Santa Monica Seafood offers oceans of fresh seafood daily, over 30 varieties from all over the world. This guarantees that our customers get the best and freshest of the catch. Santa Monica Seafood also offers fresh produce, fine wines, imported beers, fresh pasta, imported and domestic cheeses, gourmet condiments and fresh bread. Santa Monica Seafood's concern for quality and service to their customers makes visiting this store a truly pleasant experience. $

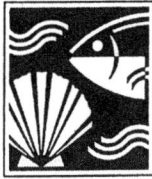

Santa Monica Seafood

1205 Colorado Ave., Santa Monica, CA 90404 (310) 393-5244
424 South Main Street, Suite F, Orange, CA 92868 (714) 921-2632
154 East 17th St., Costa Mesa, CA 92627 (949) 574-8862

SUSHI ROLL COMBINATION
Includes tuna roll, cucumber roll, salmon roll and California roll.

✓✓ CALORIES: Excellent Choice (405)   ✓✓ CHOLESTEROL: Excellent Choice (55 mg)
✓✓ FAT: Excellent Choice (5 g)*   ✓✓ SODIUM: Excellent Choice (125 mg)**
EXCHANGES: 2 Meat (extra lean), 4¼ Bread, ½ Veg, ½ Fat
PROTEIN: 22 g, CARBOHYDRATE: 63 g, FIBER: 4 g

SALMON WITH VEGETABLE MEDLEY ♂
in balsamic sauce.

✓✓ CALORIES: Excellent Choice (350)   ✓ CHOLESTEROL: Good Choice (95 mg)
✓✓ FAT: Excellent Choice (12 g)*   SODIUM: High (2360 mg)**
EXCHANGES: 4¼ Meat (extra lean), 3¼ Veg
PROTEIN: 41 g, CARBOHYDRATE: 22 g, FIBER: 6 g

SOUTHWESTERN SNAPPER
Served with orzo and wild rice.

✓ CALORIES: Good Choice (635)   ✓✓ CHOLESTEROL: Excellent Choice (65 mg)
✓ FAT: Good Choice (23 g)*   SODIUM: High (1910 mg)**
EXCHANGES: 3 Meat (extra lean), 2¾ Bread, 1¼ Veg, 3¼ Fat
PROTEIN: 53 g, CARBOHYDRATE: 56 g, FIBER: 8 g

MUSTARD GLAZED MAHI MAHI WITH SPINACH ♂
Served with new potatoes.

✓ CALORIES: Good Choice (485)   ✓ CHOLESTEROL: Good Choice (125 mg)
✓ FAT: Good Choice (20 g)*   ✓✓ SODIUM: Excellent Choice (270 mg)**
EXCHANGES: 2¾ Meat (extra lean), 2 Bread, ¾ Veg, 3½ Fat
PROTEIN: 37 g, CARBOHYDRATE: 40 g, FIBER: 4 g

MANHATTAN CHOWDER *(8 oz. serving)*

✓✓ CALORIES: Excellent Choice (70)   ✓✓ CHOLESTEROL: Excellent Choice (10 mg)
✓✓ FAT: Excellent Choice (1 g)*   SODIUM: Moderate (700 mg)**
EXCHANGES: ¾ Meat, 1 Veg
PROTEIN: 7 g, CARBOHYDRATE: 11 g, FIBER: 2 g

CEVICHE *(8 oz. serving)*

✓✓ CALORIES: Excellent Choice (105)   ✓✓ CHOLESTEROL: Excellent Choice (20 mg)
✓✓ FAT: Excellent Choice (<1 g)*   ✓✓ SODIUM: Excellent Choice (245 mg)**
EXCHANGES: 1½ Meat (extra lean), ¼ Veg, ¼ Fruit
PROTEIN: 17 g, CARBOHYDRATE: 8 g, FIBER: 1 g

---

* Primarily unsaturated fat

** If you request no added salt

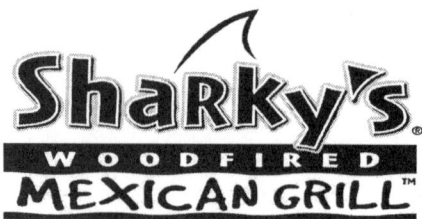

SHARKY'S CHICKEN TACO
Served on our handmade corn tortilla with onions, cilantro and hot or mild salsa.

✓✓ CALORIES: Excellent Choice (160)   ✓✓ CHOLESTEROL: Excellent Choice (25 mg)
✓✓ FAT: Excellent Choice (2 g)   SODIUM: Information not available
PROTEIN: 12 g, CARBOHYDRATE: 22 g, Fiber: 3g

SHARKY'S VEGETARIAN TACO
*Fire roasted vegetables, organic rice, organic beans and cheese
served on a handmade corn tortilla with hot or mild salsa.*

✓✓ CALORIES: Excellent Choice (260)   ✓✓ CHOLESTEROL: Excellent Choice (10 mg)
✓✓ FAT: Excellent Choice (11 g)   SODIUM: Information not available
PROTEIN: 8 g, CARBOHYDRATE: 34 g, Fiber: 5g

SHARKY'S MESQUITE BROILED FISH TACO
*Choice of today's catch, cabbage, pico de gallo, our special blend of
cheeses, achiote sauce and a lime on a flour tortilla.*

✓✓ CALORIES: Excellent Choice (270)   ✓✓ CHOLESTEROL: Excellent Choice (40 mg)
✓✓ FAT: Excellent Choice (15 g)   SODIUM: Information not available
PROTEIN: 15 g, CARBOHYDRATE: 17 g, Fiber: 1g

SHARKY'S SHRIMP TACO
*Tiger shrimp sautéed with fresh garlic and lime juice, topped with ranchero sauce,
shredded cabbage, onions, cilantro, and lime on our handmade corn tortilla.*

✓✓ CALORIES: Excellent Choice (130)   ✓✓ CHOLESTEROL: Excellent Choice (55 mg)
✓✓ FAT: Excellent Choice (1 g)   SODIUM: Information not available
PROTEIN: 8 g, CARBOHYDRATE: 20 g, Fiber: 3g

SHARKY'S CHICKEN SALAD – SPECIAL REQUEST
*Mixed lettuce, tomatoes, roasted peppers, tortilla strips, toasted pepitas, cotija cheese, and red chile croutons,
tossed with our poblano-caesar dressing served in a fresh flour tortilla shell. Request dressing on the side
(Tortilla shell and dressing not included in analysis)*

✓✓ CALORIES: Excellent Choice (420)   ✓ CHOLESTEROL: Excellent Choice (65 mg)
✓✓ FAT: Excellent Choice (12 g)   SODIUM: Information not available
PROTEIN: 31 g, CARBOHYDRATE: 47 g, Fiber: 6g

SHARKY'S CHICKEN FAJITA BOWL – SPECIAL REQUEST
*Layers of organic rice, organic beans, fire roasted vegetables, topped with mesquite
broiled chicken and pico de gallo. Request no sour cream or guacamole.*

✓ CALORIES: Good Choice (500)   ✓✓ CHOLESTEROL: Excellent Choice (35 mg)
✓✓ FAT: Excellent Choice (13 g)   SODIUM: Information not available
PROTEIN: 25 g, CARBOHYDRATE: 70 g, Fiber: 8g

Nutrition information supplied by Sharky's Woodfired Mexican Grill

🍎 at least 2 fruit/vegetable servings

✓ Good Choice   ✓✓ Excellent Choice

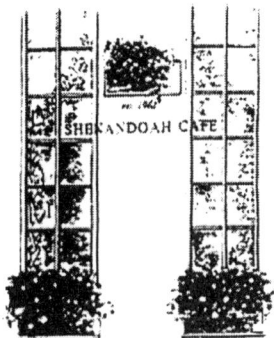

The Shenandoah Cafe offers down-home "American" dishes. Shenandoah Cafe strives to achieve the very best for you by constantly having only the freshest, best quality products available. Most items are cooked with original country style. Quality is never sacrificed. Come enjoy a wonderful meal and unlock the memories of a warm home, country living and family traditions. $$

Shenandoah Cafe (562) 434-3469
4722 East 2nd Street, Long Beach, CA 90803

NEW ORLEANS SPICY ROCK SHRIMP SALAD ☺
Crisp greens served with warm spicy shrimp, black olives, tomatoes and artichoke hearts.
✓✓ CALORIES: Excellent Choice (355)   CHOLESTEROL: Moderate (195 mg)
 ✓ FAT: Good Choice (18 g)*   ✓ SODIUM: Good Choice (520 mg)**
EXCHANGES: 3 Meat (extra lean), 3¾ Veg, 2¾ Fat
PROTEIN: 29 g, CARBOHYDRATE: 24 g, Fiber: 11g

LINGUINI WITH TOMATOES - SPECIAL REQUEST ☺
Fresh basil and garlic. Request no butter.
 ✓ CALORIES: Good Choice (610)   ✓✓ CHOLESTEROL: Excellent Choice (20 mg)
 ✓ FAT: Good Choice (20 g)   ✓✓ SODIUM: Excellent Choice (250 mg)**
EXCHANGES: ¾ Meat, 4¾ Bread, 2¼ Veg, 3 Fat
PROTEIN: 22 g, CARBOHYDRATE: 86 g, Fiber: 6g

ROASTED VEGETABLE PASTA - SPECIAL REQUEST ☺
Assorted fresh flame roasted veggies, combined with fresh garlic, tomato and basil.
Request no pesto and less cheese (1 oz.).
 ✓ CALORIES: Good Choice (595)   ✓✓ CHOLESTEROL: Excellent Choice (30 mg)
✓✓ FAT: Excellent Choice (12 g)   ✓ SODIUM: Good Choice (570 mg)**
EXCHANGES: 1¾ Meat, 4¾ Bread, 3 Veg, ¾ Fat
PROTEIN: 30 g, CARBOHYDRATE: 93 g, Fiber: 10g

BBQ STYLE CHICKEN - SPECIAL REQUEST
A boneless breast, charbroiled and basted with our Texas style sauce. Request no skin and vegetables steamed.
✓✓ CALORIES: Excellent Choice (400)   CHOLESTEROL: Moderate (185 mg)
✓✓ FAT: Excellent Choice (8 g)   ✓✓ SODIUM: Excellent Choice (265 mg)**
EXCHANGES: 9½ Meat (extra lean), 1¼ Veg
PROTEIN: 71 g, CARBOHYDRATE: 8 g, Fiber: 4g

SAN FRANCISCO SWORDFISH - SPECIAL REQUEST
Marinated in soy, dijon, lemon and garlic and charbroiled. Request vegetables steamed.
✓✓ CALORIES: Excellent Choice (370)   ✓ CHOLESTEROL: Good Choice (100 mg)
✓✓ FAT: Excellent Choice (13 g)*   ✓ SODIUM: Good Choice (390 mg)**
EXCHANGES: 5¾ Meat, 1¼ Veg, ½ Fat
PROTEIN: 54 g, CARBOHYDRATE: 6 g, Fiber: 4g

FRESH FISH OF THE DAY - SPECIAL REQUEST ☺
with artichokes, mushrooms, white wine and olive oil and served with vegetables.
Analysis for halibut; other fish slightly higher. Request no butter and vegetables steamed.
✓✓ CALORIES: Excellent Choice (415)   ✓✓ CHOLESTEROL: Excellent Choice (75 mg)
✓✓ FAT: Excellent Choice (13 g)*   ✓ SODIUM: Good Choice (375 mg)**
EXCHANGES: 4½ Meat (extra lean), 3½ Veg, 1¼ Fat
PROTEIN: 55 g, CARBOHYDRATE: 20 g, Fiber: 8g

---

* Primarily unsaturated fat

** If you request no added salt

Healthy Dining in Los Angeles **111**

SISLEY

Home-style cooking speaks to all who love to eat, and at Sisley Italian Kitchen you will find truly memorable food guaranteed to ignite even the most jaded palates. Sisley boasts of an enticing list of pastas, grilled chicken, seafood, gourmet pizzas and more. Come and experience the overwhelming attention we pay to every detail at Sisley Italian Kitchen! Sisley, creating magic. $

Sisley Italian Kitchen   www.sisleykitchen.com

10800 West Pico Boulevard, Los Angeles, CA 90064	(310) 446-3030
24201 West Valencia Boulevard, Valencia, CA 91355	(805) 287-4444
15300 Ventura Blvd., Sherman Oaks, CA 91403	(818) 905-8444
446 W. Hillcrest Dr., Thousand Oaks, CA 91360	(805) 777-7511

BROILED COUNTRY HERB CHICKEN - SPECIAL REQUEST ☺
Chicken breast marinated in white wine, fruit juices, herbs and spices.
Request vegetables steamed. Potatoes not included in analysis.
✓ CALORIES: Good Choice (500)   CHOLESTEROL: Moderate (215 mg)
✓✓ FAT: Excellent Choice (13 g)   ✓✓ SODIUM: Excellent Choice (240 mg)**
EXCHANGES: 11¼ Meat (extra lean), 2 Veg, ¾ Fat
PROTEIN: 82 g, CARBOHYDRATE: 11 g, FIBER: 4 g

CHEESELESS PIZZA (½ PIZZA) ☺
Broccoli, mushrooms, sundried tomatoes, onions and grilled eggplant. Analysis for ½ pizza.
✓✓ CALORIES: Excellent Choice (430)   ✓✓ CHOLESTEROL: Excellent Choice (0 mg)
✓✓ FAT: Excellent Choice (11 g)*   SODIUM: High (1455 mg)
EXCHANGES: 3¼ Bread, 2 Veg, 2 Fat
PROTEIN: 13 g, CARBOHYDRATE: 75 g, FIBER: 3 g

DIJON MUSTARD BOWTIE PASTA - SPECIAL REQUEST ☺
Chicken, garlic, mushrooms and onions with a Dijon and white wine sauce
over bowtie pasta. Request less oil (¼ oz).
✓ CALORIES: Good Choice (675)   ✓ CHOLESTEROL: Good Choice (95 mg)
✓✓ FAT: Excellent Choice (15 g)   ✓✓ SODIUM: Excellent Choice (195 mg)**
EXCHANGES: 4½ Meat, 4¼ Bread, 3 Veg, 1¼ Fat
PROTEIN: 50 g, CARBOHYDRATE: 83 g, FIBER: 7 g

PASTA PRIMAVERA - SPECIAL REQUEST ☺
Sautéed mushrooms, carrots, tomatoes, broccoli, pinenuts, white wine, basil,
olive oil and fresh garlic tossed with penne pasta. Request less oil (¼ oz).
✓ CALORIES: Good Choice (565)   ✓✓ CHOLESTEROL: Excellent Choice (10 mg)
✓✓ FAT: Excellent Choice (15 g)*   ✓✓ SODIUM: Excellent Choice (75 mg)**
EXCHANGES: 4¼ Bread, 4½ Veg, 2½ Fat
PROTEIN: 21 g, CARBOHYDRATE: 89, FIBER: 10 g

☺ at least 2 fruit/vegetable servings

✓ Good Choice   ✓✓ Excellent Choice

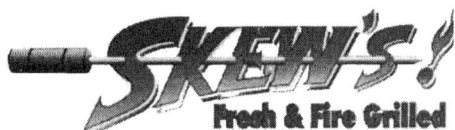

Skew's is a modern food concept for today's busy, health conscious lifestyle... FRESH, FAST and GREAT TASTING. We're a new style of restaurant but we are based on old family traditions of exceptionally consistent food quality, freshness and friendly personal service. Our famous center-cut chicken breast, sirloin steak or shrimp are deliciously prepared before your eyes in the healthiest, tastiest method known... fire grilling. Try our fusion cuisine, featuring Asian, Polynesian, Mediterranean and Western flavors. We know you will be pleased, as Skew's truly does serve great tasting food that is good for you. Enjoy! $

Skew's Fresh & Fire Grilled   300 South Grand Ave., Los Angeles (213) 613-0300

MAUI CHICKEN SKEWER
Aloha! All white chicken marinated in a pineapple teriyaki sauce and fire grilled to perfection. Served with choice of two sides.

✓✓ CALORIES: Excellent Choice (270) ✓ CHOLESTEROL: Good Choice (120 mg)
✓✓ FAT: Excellent Choice (5 g) ✓ SODIUM: Good Choice (525 mg)**
EXCHANGES: 6¼ Meat (extra lean), ¾ Fruit
PROTEIN: 45 g, CARBOHYDRATE: 12 g, FIBER: 0 g

TUSCAN CHICKEN SKEWER
All white chicken breast marinated in zesty herbs and spices. Served with choice of two sides.

✓✓ CALORIES: Excellent Choice (285) ✓ CHOLESTEROL: Good Choice (120 mg)
✓✓ FAT: Excellent Choice (7 g) ✓ SODIUM: Good Choice (435 mg)**
EXCHANGES: 6¼ Meat (extra lean), ¾ Veg, ½ Fat
PROTEIN: 44 g, CARBOHYDRATE: 4 g, FIBER: 0 g

SANTE FE SHRIMP SKEWER
Four jumbo grilled shrimp brushed with our zesty chile marinade. Served with choice of two sides.

✓✓ CALORIES: Excellent Choice (105) CHOLESTEROL: Moderate (165 mg)
✓✓ FAT: Excellent Choice (2 g)* ✓ SODIUM: Good Choice (325 mg)**
EXCHANGES: 2½ Meat (extra lean), ¼ Veg, ¼ Fat
PROTEIN: 18 g, CARBOHYDRATE: 2 g, FIBER: 0 g

CALIFORNIA CHICKEN SKEWER
Fresh grilled chicken breast with no sugar added. Served with choice of two sides.

✓✓ CALORIES: Excellent Choice (235) ✓ CHOLESTEROL: Good Choice (120 mg)
✓✓ FAT: Excellent Choice (5 g) ✓✓ SODIUM: Excellent Choice (105 mg)**
EXCHANGES: 6¼ Meat (extra lean)
PROTEIN: 44 g, CARBOHYDRATE: 1 g, FIBER: 0 g

SAN ANTONIO STEAK
Fresh USDA choice steak marinated in our Texas teriyaki, fire grilled to perfection & served with two sides.

✓✓ CALORIES: Excellent Choice (380) ✓ CHOLESTEROL: Good Choice (125 mg)
✓✓ FAT: Excellent Choice (12 g) SODIUM: High (1010 mg)**
EXCHANGES: 5¾ Meat, 1½ Fruit
PROTEIN: 43 g, CARBOHYDRATE: 22 g, FIBER: 0 g

SUN VALLEY VEGGIE SKEWER ♨
Fresh zucchini, squash, mushrooms, bell peppers & onions steamed al dente. Served with choice of two sides.

✓✓ CALORIES: Excellent Choice (105) ✓✓ CHOLESTEROL: Excellent Choice (0 mg)
✓✓ FAT: Excellent Choice (1 g)* ✓✓ SODIUM: Excellent Choice (15 mg)**
EXCHANGES: 4 Veg
PROTEIN: 6 g, CARBOHYDRATE: 23 g, FIBER: 6 g

FRESH STEAMED VEGGIES - CAL: 30, FAT: 0, CHOL: 0, SOD: 5 mg, PROT: 2g, CARB: 6g, Fiber: 2g; EXCH: 1¼ Veg
BLACK BEANS - CAL: 310, FAT: 1g, CHOL: 0, SOD: 1460 mg, PROT: 20g, CARB: 56g, Fiber: 10g; Ex: 3½ Br, ¼ Veg
GARLIC MASHED POTATOES - CAL: 375, FAT: 0, CHOL: 0, SOD: 365 mg, PROT: 11g, CARB: 85g, Fiber: 9g; EXCH: 5 Bread, ½ Milk
BROWN RICE - CAL: 250, FAT: 2g, CHOL: 0, SOD: 10 mg, PROT: 6g, CARB: 52g, Fiber: 4g; EXCH: 3¼ Bread

* Primarily unsaturated fat
** If you request no added salt

Souplantation.

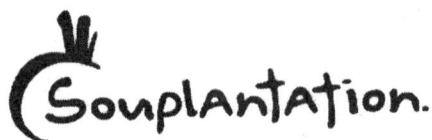

Souplantaion is the biggest, the best, the PREMIER, salad experience restaurant. All of our soups, chilies, muffins, and prepared salads are made from scratch. We serve fresh, healthful and wholesome food, which is perfect for everyday family dining. At Souplantation, there's LOTS TO FEEL GOOD ABOUT! Complete nutrition information available at www.souplantation.com. $

Souplantation Locations:

Alhambra: 2131 W. Commonwealth Av.	(626) 458-1173	Lakewood: 4720 Candlewood St.	(562) 531-6778
Arcadia: 301 E. Huntington Dr.	(626) 446-4248	Marina Del Rey: 13455 Maxella Av.	(310) 305-7669
Beverly: 8491 West 3rd St.	(323) 655-0381	Northridge: 19801 Rinaldi St.	(818) 363-3027
Brentwood: 11911 San Vicente Blvd.	(310) 476-7080	Pasadena: 201 S. Lake Ave.	(626) 577-4798
Camarillo:375 W. Ventura Blvd.	(805) 389-3500	Torrance: 21309 S. Hawthorne Blvd.	(310) 540-4998
City of Industry: 17411 Colima Rd.	(626) 810-5756	Valencia: 24303 Town Cntr. Dr..#150	(661) 286-1260

FRESH TOSSED SALADS (1 CUP)†

California Cobb, Won Ton Chicken Happiness, Strawberry Fields with Caramelized Walnuts, Watercress & Orange.

✓ CALORIES: Good Choice (130 to 180)   ✓✓ CHOLESTEROL: Excellent Choice (10 to 25 mg)
✓ FAT: Good Choice (4 to 8 g), some *   SODIUM: Strawberry Fields (75 mg), others (190-220)
PROTEIN: 3 to 6 g, CARBOHYDRATE: 4 to 15 g, FIBER: 2 to 3 g

SIGNATURE PREPARED SALADS (½ CUP)†

*Carrot Raisin, German Potato, Southern Dill Potato, Summer Barley with Black Beans,
Mandarin Noodle with Broccoli, Mandarin Shells with Almonds, Marinated Summer Vegetables,
Moroccan Marinated Vegetable, Oriental Ginger Slaw, Spicy Southwestern Pasta.*

✓✓ CALORIES: Excellent Choice (70 to 130)   ✓✓ CHOLESTEROL: Excellent Choice (0 to 5 mg)
✓✓ FAT: Excellent Choice (3 g)*   SODIUM: Carrot Raisin 80 mg; others 280 to 380 mg
PROTEIN: 2 to 5 g, CARBOHYDRATE: 8 to 21 g, Fiber: 2 to 4 g

SOUPS & CHILI (1 CUP)†

Soups: Big Chunk Chicken Noodle, French Onion, Garden Fresh Veg., Hungarian Veg., Living on the Veg., Old Fashioned Veg., Spicy 4 Bean Minestrone, Sweet Tomato Onion, Tomato Parmesan & Veg., Veg. Medley, Vegetarian, Veg. Lentils & Brown Rice, Veggie Jackson. Chilis: 3 Bean Turkey, Deep Kettle House, Santa Fe Black Bean.

✓ CALORIES: Good Choice (80 to 160, House Ch. 230)   ✓✓ CHOLESTEROL: Excellent Choice (0 to 20 mg)
✓✓ FAT: Excellent Choice (1 to 3 g), some *   SODIUM: High (460 to 990 mg)
PROTEIN: 2 to 15 g, CARBOHYDRATE: 11 to 26 g, FIBER: 1 to 7 g

FRESH BAKED MUFFINS & BREADS†

*Muffins: Apple Cinnamon Bran, Cranberry Orange Bran, Fruit Medley Bran , Buttermilk Corn Bread;
Breads (1 piece): Big Hearth Focaccia, Garlic Parmesan Focaccia, Sourdough Bread.*

✓✓ CALORIES: Excellent Choice (80 to 150)   ✓✓ CHOLESTEROL: Excellent Choice (0 to 10 mg)
✓✓ FAT: Excellent Choice (½ to 3 g)*   SODIUM: Muffins and Focaccia (110-170 mg)
                                           Corn Bread, Sourdough (240-270 mg)
PROTEIN: 2 to 9 g, CARBOHYDRATE: 15 to 27 g, FIBER: 0 to 2 g

DESSERTS & YOGURT BAR (½ CUP)†

*Banana Royale, Butterscotch Pudding, Nutty Waldorf Salad, Apple Medley,
Ghirardelli Chocolate Frozen Yogurt, Tapioca or Rice Pudding.*

✓✓ CALORIES: Excellent Choice (70 to 140)   ✓✓ CHOLESTEROL: Excellent Choice (0 to 20 mg)
✓✓ FAT: Excellent Choice (0 to 4 g)   SODIUM: (5 to 80 mg); Tapioca (160 mg)
PROTEIN: 1 to 4 g, CARBOHYDRATE: 12 to 24 g, FIBER: 0 to 3 g

Nutrition information supplied by Souplantation.

† Side dish guidelines are 1/3 of entree guidelines
☿ at least 2 fruit/vegetable servings

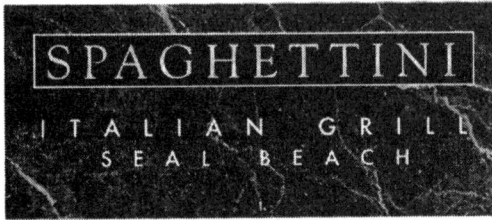

Spaghettini, a Northern Italian inspired grill, offers a variety of homemade pasta, pizza, fresh fish, meats and foul. To compliment your meal, Spaghettini offers an extensive wine list featuring both California and Italian wines (many available by the glass). The full cocktail lounge offers one of the largest back bars in Southern California with Happy Hour Monday through Friday 4-7 pm.

Six nights of the week (Tuesday - Sunday), Spaghettini showcases live jazz, featuring top name groups, as well as up-and-coming talent, ranging from traditional to contemporary styles. Conveniently located at the 405 Freeway & Seal Beach Blvd. $$

Spaghettini Italian Grill

3005 Old Ranch Parkway, Seal Beach, CA 90740   (562) 596-2199 or (714) 960-6002
Web site and email reservations: www.spaghettini.com

ANGEL HAIR PASTA AL FRESCA - SPECIAL REQUEST
Angel hair pasta tossed with roma tomatoes, sweet basil and garlic. Request less oil (½ oz).
✓✓ CALORIES: Excellent Choice (435)   ✓✓ CHOLESTEROL: Excellent Choice (0 mg)
✓✓ FAT: Excellent Choice (15 g)*   ✓✓ SODIUM: Excellent Choice (10 mg)**
EXCHANGES: 3¼ Bread, 1½ Veg, 2¾ Fat
PROTEIN: 9 g, CARBOHYDRATE: 64 g, FIBER: 4 g

BOW TIE PASTA WITH SPICY GRILLED CHICKEN - SPECIAL REQUEST ♨
Broccoli, tomatoes, capers, basil and artichoke hearts in a garlic butter sauce. Request less butter (¼ oz).
✓ CALORIES: Good Choice (620)   ✓ CHOLESTEROL: Good Choice (145 mg)
✓ FAT: Good Choice (17 g)   SODIUM: High (1675 mg)
EXCHANGES: 6¾ Meat (extra lean), 3¼ Bread, 1¾ Veg, 2 Fat
PROTEIN: 58 g, CARBOHYDRATE: 59 g, FIBER: 7 g

SHRIMP ARTICHOKE LINGUINI - SPECIAL REQUEST ♨
Garlic, basil, artichoke hearts and sun dried tomatoes with extra virgin olive oil. Request less oil (¼ oz).
✓ CALORIES: Good Choice (660)   CHOLESTEROL: High (445 mg)
✓✓ FAT: Excellent Choice (15 g)*   SODIUM: High (1265 mg)
EXCHANGES: 6¾ Meat (extra lean), 3¼ Bread, 2¾ Veg, 2¼ Fat
PROTEIN: 61 g, CARBOHYDRATE: 73 g, FIBER: 5 g

LINGUINE WITH CLAM SAUCE - SPECIAL REQUEST
Linguini tossed with fresh garlic, parsley and a rich clam broth with steamed Manila clams.
Request less butter (½ oz).
✓ CALORIES: Good Choice (480)   ✓✓ CHOLESTEROL: Excellent Choice (65 mg)
✓✓ FAT: Excellent Choice (14 g)   ✓ SODIUM: Good Choice (595 mg)**
EXCHANGES: 1¾ Meat (extra lean), 3¼ Bread, ½ Veg, 2¼ Fat
PROTEIN: 21 g, CARBOHYDRATE: 61 g, FIBER: 3 g

* Primarily unsaturated fat
** If you request no added salt

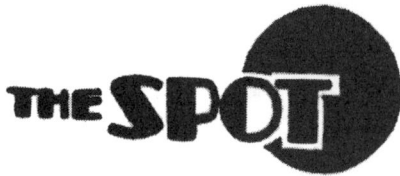

LA's oldest natural health food restaurant! Most of our menu is available fat free and non-dairy. We always serve organic whole grains and legumes. We use seasonal organic produce when available, and serve and cook with purified water. Our homemade bread and desserts are honey or maple syrup sweetened, and our fat free soups never contain any oils or dairy products! Located in beautiful Hermosa Beach, just 1 block from the beach on 2nd Street, the atmosphere is warm and casual. Open everyday from 11am-10pm. $

The Spot Natural Food Restaurant

110 Second St., Hermosa Beach, CA 90254   (310) 301-7074

SAVORY STEAMERS WITH BAKED TOFU – SPECIAL REQUEST ☺

Seasonal steamed veggies and baked tofu served on a bed of organic brown rice.
Request Savory sauce on the side (sauce not included in analysis, 2 Tbs. = 50 cal, 5 g fat).

✓ CALORIES: Good Choice (465)   ✓✓ CHOLESTEROL: Excellent Choice (0 mg)
✓✓ FAT: Excellent Choice (9 g)*   ✓✓ SODIUM: Excellent Choice (145 mg)**
EXCHANGES: 1½ Meat, 3¼ Bread, 3¾ Veg, ½ Fat
PROTEIN: 22 g, CARBOHYDRATE: 77 g, FIBER: 11 g

HOMEMADE CHILI

A big bowl of kidney beans, onions and tomatoes, topped with green onions and cheese.
Served with cornbread (not included in analysis).

✓✓ CALORIES: Excellent Choice (445)   ✓✓ CHOLESTEROL: Excellent Choice (30 mg)
✓✓ FAT: Excellent Choice (11 g)   SODIUM: Moderate (955 mg)**
EXCHANGES: 2 Meat, 3¼ Bread, 1¼ Veg, 1¼ Fat
PROTEIN: 28 g, CARBOHYDRATE: 61 g, FIBER: 14 g

SPOT CHEF SALAD ☺

Lettuce, shredded carrots, broccoli, seasonal veggies, sprouts, sunflower seeds, tofu and cheese. Served with your choice of dressing (not included in analysis). Creamy avocado dressing: 2 Tbs. = 20 cal, 1 g fat.

✓✓ CALORIES: Excellent Choice (325)   ✓✓ CHOLESTEROL: Excellent Choice (30 mg)
✓ FAT: Good Choice (19 g)   ✓✓ SODIUM: Excellent Choice (235 mg)**
EXCHANGES: 2 Meat, ¼ Bread, 2¼ Veg, 2½ Fat
PROTEIN: 22 g, CARBOHYDRATE: 20 g, FIBER: 7 g

NEPTUNE LOAF – SPECIAL REQUEST ☺

Fettucine pasta, veggies, tofu and cheese and smothered in our Savory Sauce. Served with vegetable of the day. Request Savory Sauce on the side (not included in analysis, 2 Tbs. = 50 cal, 5 g fat).

✓✓ CALORIES: Excellent Choice (300)   ✓✓ CHOLESTEROL: Excellent Choice (65 mg)
✓✓ FAT: Excellent Choice (13 g)   ✓ SODIUM: Good Choice (330 mg)**
EXCHANGES: 1½ Meat, 1¼ Bread, 2 Veg, 1½ Fat
PROTEIN: 20 g, CARBOHYDRATE: 31 g, FIBER: 8 g

VEGETABLE LENTIL SOUP *(cup size, 8 oz.)*†

✓✓ CALORIES: Excellent Choice (115)   ✓✓ CHOLESTEROL: Excellent Choice (0 mg)
✓✓ FAT: Excellent Choice (<1 g)*   SODIUM: High (695 mg)**
EXCHANGES: 1¼ Bread, ½ Veg; PROTEIN: 8 g, CARBOHYDRATE: 21 g, FIBER: 1 g

SPOT OATMEAL COOKIES *(½ large cookie)*†

✓✓ CALORIES: Excellent Choice (115)   ✓✓ CHOLESTEROL: Excellent Choice (0 mg)
✓ FAT: Good Choice (6 g)*   ✓✓ SODIUM: Excellent Choice (5 mg)
EXCHANGES: ½ Bread, 1¼ Fat; PROTEIN: 2 g, CARBOHYDRATE: 14 g, FIBER: 1 g

† Side dish guidelines are 1/3 of entree guidelines
☺ at least 2 fruit/vegetable servings

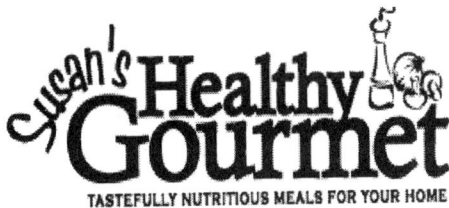

Healthy Gourmet is a one-of-a-kind service that provides delicious, fresh meals for the home that free you of shopping, cooking and clean up. Award winning bakery goods made from scratch and extensive a la carte selections supplement a complete weekly menu of low-fat, low-sodium, and low-cholesterol items offered in three daily calorie levels. All meals are prepared for pick-up or delivery every Monday and Friday. $

Susan's Healthy Gourmet - Meals for the Home and Office

For information & to order call: (949) 833-2929, (562) 630-2900, 1-888-EZ-MEALS (396-3257)
17851 Sky Park Circle, Suite G, Irvine, CA 92614   www.healthygourmetmeals.com

HONEY THYME PORK

Roasted pork loin glazed with honey and seasoned with garlic, dijon, and thyme.
- ✓✓ CALORIES: Excellent Choice (325)
- ✓✓ FAT: Excellent Choice (5 g)
- ✓✓ CHOLESTEROL: Excellent Choice (55 mg)
- ✓✓ SODIUM: Excellent Choice (220 mg)

PROTEIN: 21 g, CARBOHYDRATE: 51 g, Fiber: 0g

CRANBERRY BARBECUE CHICKEN

A boneless, skinless chicken breast topped with a tangy yet sweet sauce made from a combination of cranberry sauce and barbecue sauce, served with a side of sweet potato wedges.
- ✓✓ CALORIES: Excellent Choice (345)
- ✓✓ FAT: Excellent Choice (4 g)
- ✓ CHOLESTEROL: Good Choice (85 mg)
- ✓✓ SODIUM: Excellent Choice (275 mg)

PROTEIN: 33 g, CARBOHYDRATE: 42 g, Fiber: 4g

BEEF MEDALLIONS

A tender grilled beef filet, topped with a sauce of red wine, shallots, portobello, shitaki & crimini mushrooms.
- ✓✓ CALORIES: Excellent Choice (275)
- ✓✓ FAT: Excellent Choice (11 g)
- ✓✓ CHOLESTEROL: Excellent Choice (70 mg)
- ✓✓ SODIUM: Excellent Choice (80 mg)

PROTEIN: 30 g, CARBOHYDRATE: 15 g, Fiber: 4g

LINGUINI WITH CILANTRO PESTO SAUCE

Durum wheat semolina pasta tossed with a cilantro pesto sauce & topped with diced tomatoes and fresh garlic.
- ✓✓ CALORIES: Excellent Choice (285)
- ✓✓ FAT: Excellent Choice (7 g)
- ✓✓ CHOLESTEROL: Excellent Choice (5 mg)
- ✓✓ SODIUM: Excellent Choice (95 mg)

PROTEIN: 11 g, CARBOHYDRATE: 48 g, Fiber: 7 g

APRICOT CHICKEN SALAD ☕

A creamy combination of soy-marinated, grilled chicken breasts, apricots, walnuts and raisins, served on a bed of romaine lettuce.
- ✓✓ CALORIES: Excellent Choice (152)
- ✓✓ FAT: Excellent Choice (4 g)
- ✓✓ CHOLESTEROL: Excellent Choice (49 mg)
- ✓✓ SODIUM: Excellent Choice (281 mg)

PROTEIN: 21 g, CARBOHYDRATE: 8 g, Fiber: 1 g

TROPICAL SALMON

Citrus–marinated baked Atlantic Salmon, topped with pineapple jalapeño salsa, served over organic brown rice.
- ✓✓ CALORIES: Excellent Choice (312)
- ✓✓ FAT: Excellent Choice (10 g)
- ✓✓ CHOLESTEROL: Excellent Choice (52 mg)
- ✓✓ SODIUM: Excellent Choice (55 mg)

PROTEIN: 18 g, CARBOHYDRATE: 30 g, Fiber: 2 g

COQ AU VIN

Tender chicken breast cooked in a red wine, shallot and mushroom sauce, seasoned with paprika and thyme.
- ✓✓ CALORIES: Excellent Choice (348)
- ✓✓ FAT: Excellent Choice (6 g)
- ✓✓ CHOLESTEROL: Excellent Choice (85 mg)
- ✓✓ SODIUM: Excellent Choice (295 mg)

PROTEIN: 46 g, CARBOHYDRATE: 24, Fiber: 4 g

Nutrition analysis provided by Healthy Gourmet

* Primarily unsaturated fat

** If you request no added salt

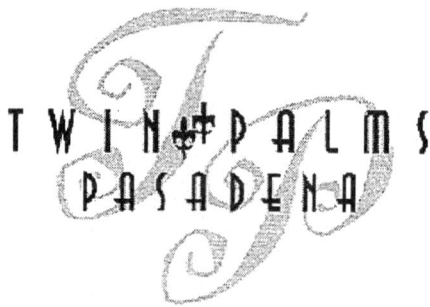

Twin Palms' menu is inspired by the simple, fresh foods of the California coast and America's affinity for the region's climate and healthy, casual lifestyle. Central to this cuisine are freshness, a light touch and clear flavors. Essentially Californian, however, means the culinary heritage of over a century of pioneers, visionaries and immigrants. Inspired by these diverse cuisines, Chef Tony Zidar has added his interpretations of multicultural dishes to the menu, expanding the concept of coastal cuisine from California to the Mediterranean, to Asia and beyond. $$

Twin Palms 101 West Green St., Pasadena 91105 (626) 577-2567

HAWAIIAN TUNA SUSHI ROLL
on a bed of fresh Haas avocado, golden beets, masago and wasabi-soy dressing.
✓✓ CALORIES: Excellent Choice (235)   ✓✓ CHOLESTEROL: Excellent Choice (35 mg)
✓✓ FAT: Excellent Choice (10 g)*   SODIUM: High (2315 mg)**
EXCHANGES: 1½ Meat (extra lean), 3 Bread, ¾ Veg, 1¾ Fat
PROTEIN: 15 g, CARBOHYDRATE: 23 g, FIBER: 3 g

PACIFIC SEAFOOD HOT POT
A generous heap of fish and shellfish, bathed in a fragrant tomato-lemongrass broth.
✓ CALORIES: Good Choice (645)   CHOLESTEROL: Moderate (235 mg)
✓✓ FAT: Excellent Choice (7 g)*   ✓ SODIUM: Good Choice (575 mg)**
EXCHANGES: 6¾ Meat (extra lean), 5¼ Bread, ¾ Veg
PROTEIN: 50 g, CARBOHYDRATE: 90 g, FIBER: 2g

SEAFOOD LINGUINE
with shrimp, clams and fresh fish in a white wine tomato-herb sauce.
✓ CALORIES: Good Choice (745)   CHOLESTEROL: Moderate (170 mg)
✓ FAT: Good Choice (16 g)*   ✓ SODIUM: Good Choice (405 mg)**
EXCHANGES: 4¾ Meat (extra lean), 5¼ Bread, 1¼ Veg, 1¾ Fat
PROTEIN: 51 g, CARBOHYDRATE: 90 g, FIBER: 6g

LEMON SCENTED PAPPARDELLE– SPECIAL REQUEST
a wide ribbon pasta, with fresh mozzarella, basil leaves and marinara. Request less cheese (1 oz.).
✓ CALORIES: Good Choice (720)   ✓ CHOLESTEROL: Good Choice (145 mg)
✓ FAT: Good Choice (19 g)   SODIUM: High (1065 mg)
EXCHANGES: ¾ Meat, 5½ Bread, 1½ Veg, 2½ Fat
PROTEIN: 26 g, CARBOHYDRATE: 107 g, FIBER: 1g

SEARED RARE AHI NICOISE SALAD – SPECIAL REQUEST ☙
with shrimp, green beans, black olives, tomatoes, chick peas and tomato-tarragon vinaigrette.
Request dressing on the side (60 calories & 7 grams of fat per Tbs.).
✓✓ CALORIES: Excellent Choice (385)   CHOLESTEROL: High (360 mg)
✓ FAT: Excellent Choice (11 g)   ✓ SODIUM: Good Choice (465 mg)**
EXCHANGES: 5½ Meat, 1 Bread, 1¼ Veg, ¾ Fat
PROTEIN: 45 g, CARBOHYDRATE: 25 g, FIBER: 3g

SEA BASS VERA CRUZ ☙
on a bed of new potatoes with cilantro-lime salsa.
✓✓ CALORIES: Excellent Choice (395)   ✓ CHOLESTEROL: Good Choice (80 mg)
✓✓ FAT: Excellent Choice (11 g)*   SODIUM: High (1065 mg)**
EXCHANGES: 3½ Meat (extra lean), 1½ Bread, 1½ Veg, 1½ Fat
PROTEIN: 41 g, CARBOHYDRATE: 35 g, FIBER: 5 g

☙ at least 2 fruit/vegetable servings

✓ Good Choice   ✓✓ Excellent Choice

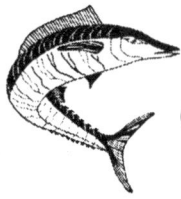

Wahoo's Fish Taco

FUELING THE FORCES SINCE 1988

Wahoo's Fish Taco serves a unique menu featuring Mexican dishes with a Brazilian twist in a beach-casual atmosphere. Known for our charbroiled fish tacos and Banzai burritos, we also serve chicken, steak, pork and veggie dishes. All ingredients are prepared fresh daily. $

Wahoo's Fish Taco Locations:

Manhattan Beach: 1129 Manhattan Ave. (310) 796-1044
Mid-Wilshire: 6258 Wilshire Blvd. (323) 933-2480
Torrance: 3556 Torrance Blvd., Ste. E (310) 540-7725
West Los Angeles: 11911 Wilshire Blvd. (310) 445-5990
Pasadena: 264 S. Lake Ave. (626) 449-2005
Santa Monica: 418 Wilshire Blvd.

Visit www.wahoos.com for other locations.

CHARBROILED FISH TACO

✓✓ CALORIES: Excellent Choice (225) ✓✓ CHOLESTEROL: Excellent Choice (50 mg)
✓✓ FAT: Excellent Choice (4 g) ✓ SODIUM: Good Choice (395 mg)**
EXCHANGES: 1¼ Meat, 1¾ Bread, ¼ Veg, ¾ Fat
PROTEIN: 15 g, CARBOHYDRATE: 27 g, FIBER 3 g

CHARBROILED CHICKEN TACO

✓✓ CALORIES: Excellent Choice (260) ✓✓ CHOLESTEROL: Excellent Choice (50 mg)
✓✓ FAT: Excellent Choice (6 g) ✓ SODIUM: Good Choice (380 mg)**
EXCHANGES: 2½ Meat, 1¾ Bread, ¼ Veg, ¾ Fat
PROTEIN: 20 g, CARBOHYDRATE: 27 g, FIBER 3 g

½ RICE & ½ BEAN COMBO BOWL

✓ CALORIES: Good Choice (475) ✓✓ CHOLESTEROL: Excellent Choice (10 mg)
✓✓ FAT: Excellent Choice (5 g) SODIUM: High (1030 mg)
EXCHANGES: 1 Meat, 5¾ Bread, ¼ Veg, 1 Fat
PROTEIN: 20 g, CARBOHYDRATE: 88 g, FIBER 16 g

CHARBROILED CHICKEN BURRITO

✓ CALORIES: Good Choice (510) ✓ CHOLESTEROL: Good Choice (115 mg)
✓✓ FAT: Excellent Choice (15 g) SODIUM: High (1205 mg)
EXCHANGES: 5½ Meat, 2½ Bread, ¾ Veg, 2 Fat
PROTEIN: 47 g, CARBOHYDRATE: 43 g, FIBER 3 g

VEGETARIAN BURRITO

✓ CALORIES: Good Choice (580) ✓✓ CHOLESTEROL: Excellent Choice (20 mg)
✓✓ FAT: Excellent Choice (13 g) SODIUM: High (1370 mg)
EXCHANGES: 1¼ Meat, 6 Bread, ¾ Veg, 2 Fat
PROTEIN: 24 g, CARBOHYDRATE: 93 g, FIBER 13 g

CHARBROILED FISH BURRITO

✓✓ CALORIES: Excellent Choice (430) ✓ CHOLESTEROL: Good Choice (110 mg)
✓✓ FAT: Excellent Choice (12 g) SODIUM: High (1235 mg)
EXCHANGES: 2½ Meat, 2½ Bread, ¾ Veg, 2 Fat
PROTEIN: 35 g, CARBOHYDRATE: 44 g, FIBER 3 g

* Primarily unsaturated fat
** If you request no added salt

WASABI LB わさび

Japanese Restaurant

With its rock'n'roll atmosphere, Wasabi is a Japanese style restaurant featuring sushi and teppan-yaki. Serving lunch and dinner. Enjoy karaoke on Wednesday and Thursday evenings. It's definitely the place to be in Long Beach for a serious good time. $$

Wasabi Japanese Restaurant
200 Pine Ave., Long Beach 90802 (562) 901-0300

SALMON TERIYAKI ☺
Salmon grilled with teriyaki sauce. Served with white rice and vegetables.
- ✓ CALORIES: Good Choice (745)
- ✓✓ FAT: Excellent Choice (12 g)*
- ✓ CHOLESTEROL: Good Choice (90 mg)
- SODIUM: High (3290 mg)**

EXCHANGES: 4¼ Meat, 6¼ Bread, 1 Veg, ¾ Fruit, ¼ Fat
PROTEIN: 45 g, CARBOHYDRATE: 113 g, FIBER: 5 g

WASABI CHICKEN ☺
Tender chicken breast rubbed with wasabi powder and shredded daikon root, pan seared and served with rice and veggies.
- ✓ CALORIES: Good Choice (730)
- ✓ FAT: Good Choice (17 g)
- CHOLESTEROL: Moderate (160 mg)
- SODIUM: High (1600 mg)**

EXCHANGES: 6¾ Meat (extra lean), 5 Bread, 1 Veg, 2¼ Fat
PROTEIN: 58 g, CARBOHYDRATE: 82 g, FIBER: 4 g

SAUTÉED SCALLOPS ☺
Large scallops sautéed and served with rice and veggies.
- ✓ CALORIES: Good Choice (610)
- ✓✓ FAT: Excellent Choice (4 g)*
- ✓ CHOLESTEROL: Good Choice (95 mg)
- SODIUM: High (1885 mg)**

EXCHANGES: 3¾ Meat (extra lean), 5½ Bread, 1 Veg, ¼ Fat
PROTEIN: 52 g, CARBOHYDRATE: 92 g, FIBER: 4 g

CHICKEN TERIYAKI ☺
Chicken breast grilled with teriyaki sauce. Served with white rice and veggies.
- ✓ CALORIES: Good Choice (725)
- ✓✓ FAT: Excellent Choice (6 g)
- ✓ CHOLESTEROL: Good Choice (130 mg)
- SODIUM: High (3330 mg)**

EXCHANGES: 6¾ Meat (extra lean), 5¾ Bread, 1 Veg, ¾ Fruit, ¼ Fat
PROTEIN: 59 g, CARBOHYDRATE: 105 g, FIBER: 4 g

CAJUN SEARED AHI
Ahi dusted in Cajun spices and pan seared, placed on a bed of soba noodles tossed in a Vietnamese vinaigrette.
- ✓✓ CALORIES: Excellent Choice (420)
- ✓ FAT: Good Choice (16 g)
- ✓✓ CHOLESTEROL: Excellent Choice (50 mg)
- SODIUM: Moderate (995 mg)**

EXCHANGES: 3¾ Meat, 2 Bread, ½ Veg, 2¾ Fat
PROTEIN: 34 g, CARBOHYDRATE: 38 g, FIBER: 3 g

☺ at least 2 fruit/vegetable servings
✓ Good Choice ✓✓ Excellent Choice

WHOLE FOODS MARKET

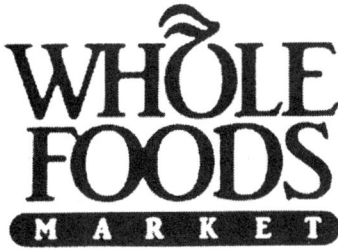

Whole Foods Markets are dedicated to supplying the finest, most natural, wholesome foods available, including an ever-increasing selection of organically grown ingredients. Our savory salads, delectable dressings, steamy soups, enticing entrees and many of our delicious baked goods are prepared in our own kitchen, using time honored recipes with no artificial flavors, artificial colors, artificial sweeteners or preservatives. $

Whole Foods Market

3rd & Fairfax: 6350 W. Third St.	(323) 964-6800
Beverly Hills: 239 N. Crescent Dr.	(310) 274-3360
Brentwood: 11737 San Vicente Blvd.	(310) 826-4433
Glendale: 826 N. Glendale Ave.	(818) 240-9350
Pasadena: 3751 East Foothill Blvd.	(626) 351-5994
Porter Ranch: 19340 Rinaldi	(818) 363-3933
Redondo Beach: 405 N. PCH	(310) 376-6931
Sherman Oaks East: 12905 Riverside Dr.	(818) 762-5548
Sherman Oaks West: 4520 Sepulveda Blvd.	(818) 382-3700
Thousand Oaks: 451 Avenida de los Arboles	(805) 492-5340
Torrance: 2655 Pacific Coast Hwy.	(310) 257-8700
Tustin: 14945 Holt Ave.	(714) 731-3400
West Hollywood: 7871 W. Santa Monica Blvd.	(323) 848-4200
West LA: 11666 National Blvd.	(310) 996-8840
Woodland Hills: 21347 Ventura Blvd.	(818) 610-0000

Analyses below are for ½ lb. serving

BUTTERNUT SQUASH WITH CARAMELIZED ONIONS

✓✓ CALORIES: Excellent Choice (130)
✓✓ FAT: Excellent Choice (2 g)*
✓✓ CHOLESTEROL: Excellent Choice (0 mg)
✓✓ SODIUM: Excellent Choice (35 mg)**
EXCHANGES: 1½ Bread, ¼ Veg, ¼ Fruit, ¼ Fat
PROTEIN: 2 g, CARBOHYDRATE: 31 g, FIBER: 4 g

EMERALD SESAME KALE

✓✓ CALORIES: Excellent Choice (215)
✓✓ FAT: Excellent Choice (14 g)*
✓✓ CHOLESTEROL: Excellent Choice (0 mg)
✓ SODIUM: Good Choice (450 mg)**
EXCHANGES: 3½ Veg, 2 Fat
PROTEIN: 7 g, CARBOHYDRATE: 18 g, FIBER: 9 g

HOT & SWEET CORN SALAD

✓✓ CALORIES: Excellent Choice (255)
✓✓ FAT: Excellent Choice (15 g)
✓✓ CHOLESTEROL: Excellent Choice (20 mg)
✓ SODIUM: Good Choice (500 mg)**
EXCHANGES: ½ Meat, 1¼ Bread, 1 Veg, 2½ Fat
PROTEIN: 7 g, CARBOHYDRATE: 27 g, FIBER: 5 g

GRILLED MANGO WITH RASPBERRY COULIS

✓✓ CALORIES: Excellent Choice (190)
✓✓ FAT: Excellent Choice (1 g)*
✓✓ CHOLESTEROL: Excellent Choice (0 mg)
✓✓ SODIUM: Excellent Choice (10 mg)**
EXCHANGES: 2 Fruit
PROTEIN: 1 g, CARBOHYDRATE: 50 g, FIBER: 5 g

* Primarily unsaturated fat
** If you request no added salt

zax
restaurant

Natural hues and rich textures lend warmth to the charming dining room which boasts high ceilings, exposed brick walls, white linen-covered tables, and an exhibition kitchen with a gorgeous brass hood, achieving a sophisticated bistro-style atmosphere. Linen-covered menus and fresh flower arrangements from the nearby Veteran's Garden add to the inviting eatery's refined ambiance. We serve seasonally inspired, Contemporary American food. $$-$$$

Zax Restaurant   11604 San Vicente Blvd., Brentwood 90049 (310) 571-3800

BUTTERNUT SQUASH SOUP †
with pumpkin seed oil.
- ✓ CALORIES: Good Choice (240)
- ✓✓ CHOLESTEROL: Excellent Choice (0 mg)
- ✓✓ FAT: Excellent Choice (5 g)*
- SODIUM: High (1625 mg)

EXCHANGES: 2¾ Bread, 1 Veg, 1 Fat
PROTEIN: 4 g, CARBOHYDRATE: 51 g, FIBER: 7 g

AHI TUNA NICOISE SALAD ☺
- ✓✓ CALORIES: Excellent Choice (395)
- CHOLESTEROL: Moderate (270 mg)
- ✓ FAT: Good Choice (18 g)
- SODIUM: Moderate (650 mg)**

EXCHANGES: 2¼ Meat (extra lean), 1½ Bread, 1¾ Veg, 2¼ Fat
PROTEIN: 24 g, CARBOHYDRATE: 37 g, FIBER: 5 g

MAINE STERLING SALMON – SPECIAL REQUEST ☺
with rapini, leeks, asparagus, and tomato vinaigrette.
Request pesto sauce on the side (not included in analysis).
- ✓ CALORIES: Good Choice (460)
- ✓ CHOLESTEROL: Good Choice (90 mg)
- ✓ FAT: Good Choice (25 g)*
- ✓ SODIUM: Good Choice (375 mg)**

EXCHANGES: 4¼ Meat, 3½ Veg, 2¾ Fat
PROTEIN: 39 g, CARBOHYDRATE: 22 g, FIBER: 7 g

PUMPKIN & SAGE GNOCCHI – SPECIAL REQUEST ☺
Served with roasted onions, pea tendrils and sugar snap peas. Request no butter.
- ✓ CALORIES: Good Choice (480)
- ✓ CHOLESTEROL: Good Choice (80 mg)
- ✓ FAT: Good Choice (20 g)
- SODIUM: Moderate (810 mg)**

EXCHANGES: 1¼ Meat, 2½ Bread, 2½ Veg, 3¼ Fat
PROTEIN: 17 g, CARBOHYDRATE: 62 g, FIBER: 6 g

GRILLED ALASKAN HALIBUT – SPECIAL REQUEST ☺
with roasted fingerling potatoes, baby turnips, and haricots verts. Request less oil (1 Tbs.) and no cream.
- ✓ CALORIES: Good Choice (510)
- ✓✓ CHOLESTEROL: Excellent Choice (55 mg)
- ✓ FAT: Good Choice (18 g)*
- ✓✓ SODIUM: Excellent Choice (235 mg)**

EXCHANGES: 3¼ Meat (extra lean), 1¾ Bread, 3 Veg, 2¾ Fat
PROTEIN: 41 g, CARBOHYDRATE: 47 g, FIBER: 7 g

OVEN ROASTED CHICKEN BREAST – SPECIAL REQUEST ☺
with sautéed spinach, grilled escarole & red wine-braised onions. Request sautéed spinach & skinless chicken.
- ✓ CALORIES: Good Choice (605)
- CHOLESTEROL: Moderate (225 mg)
- ✓ FAT: Good Choice (25 g)
- ✓ SODIUM: Good Choice (410 mg)**

EXCHANGES: 10 Meat, 2½ Veg, 2¾ Fat
PROTEIN: 83 g, CARBOHYDRATE: 15 g, FIBER: 4 g

† Side dish guidelines are 1/3 of entree guidelines
☺ at least 2 fruit/vegetable servings, 1 for side dishes

Health Resource Guide

It's probably easier to live a more healthful lifestyle in Southern California than anywhere in the country. The agreeable climate, gentle pace, health-conscious mindset, and accessibility to health-oriented products and services all promote a healthier way of life.

Healthful living includes more than healthy dining. So in the Health Resource Guide that follows, you'll find an array of "tools" to further support your healthful lifestyle. We think you'll find this guide useful, informative and interesting. The *Healthy Dining* team recognizes the Health Resource Guide companies and organizations for their contribution to a healthier community.

Index

AMERICAN CANCER SOCIETY

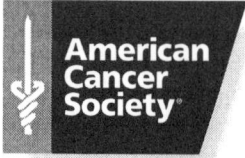

American Cancer Society

1-800-ACS-2345
www.cancer.org

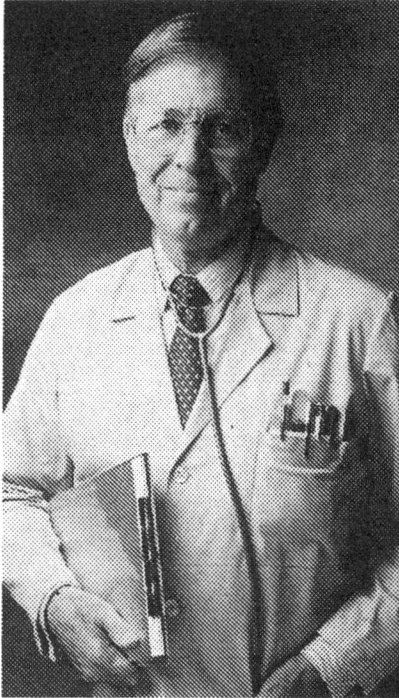

**FOR THE BEST
DEFENSE AGAINST
CANCER, SEE HIM
ONCE A YEAR.**

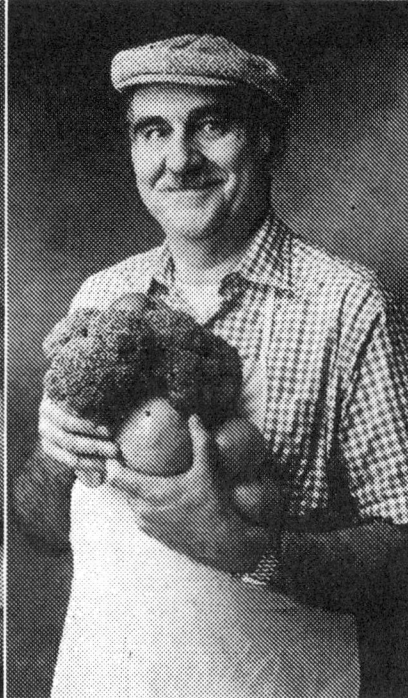

**AND HIM ONCE
A DAY.**

He may not look like a cancer specialist, but there's strong evidence that your neighborhood grocer has access to cancer protection you won't find in any doctor's office.

Broccoli, peaches, cantaloupes, spinach, sweet potatoes, carrots, pumpkin, tomatoes, citrus fruits and other sources of vitamin A are related to lowering the risk of cancer of the larynx and esophagus.

Vegetables such as cabbage, broccoli, Brussels sprouts, kohlrabi and cauliflower may help reduce the risk of cancers of the colon, rectum, lung and bronchus. Fruits, vegetables and whole grains such as bran, whole wheat and oatmeal may also help reduce the risk of colorectal cancer.

In short, make sure you do what your mother always told you. Eat your vegetables!
And if you're worried about cancer, remember this: Wherever you are, we are here. Just call the American Cancer Society at 1-800-ACS-2345 or visit our website at www.cancer.org.

AMERICAN DIABETES ASSOCIATION

1-800-DIABETES
(1-800-342-2383)

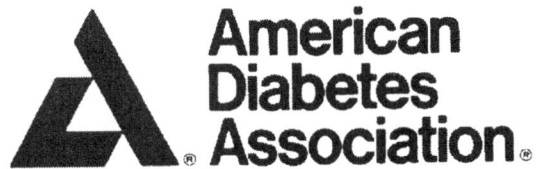

American Diabetes Association.

Western Region
Serving California and Nevada

The American Diabetes Association is the nation's leading nonprofit health organization providing diabetes research, information and advocacy. The mission of the organization is to "prevent and cure diabetes, and to improve the lives of all people affected by diabetes." To fulfill this mission, the American Diabetes Association funds research, publishes scientific findings, and provides information, education programs and other services to people with diabetes, their families, health care professionals, and the public.

The Diabetes Information and Action Line (D.I.A.L.) program is the cornerstone of the Association's information programs. D.I.A.L. is a toll-free help line for people who have questions and concerns about diabetes. Through D.I.A.L., people can request information and literature about diabetes-related topics, including exercise, nutrition and self-management.

AMERICAN HEART ASSOCIATION

Western States Affiliate
1055 Wilshire Blvd., Ninth Floor
Los Angeles, CA 90017
(213) 580-1408

Heart disease is the leading cause of death in America, claiming almost one million lives a year. Stroke is the third leading cause of death and the number one cause of disability. The American Heart Association is the nation's oldest and largest voluntary health agency fighting these diseases. Through lifesaving research and preventive education, together we can reduce disability and death from heart disease and stroke.

The soul of the American Heart Association is its people – especially the tireless local volunteers who devote their skills, time and energy for a cause that is "close to their hearts." Donations come from individuals and businesses who understand the need for research and appreciate the value of the work we are doing in the community.

For more information, call (213) 580-1408 or reach us online at www.heartsource.org.

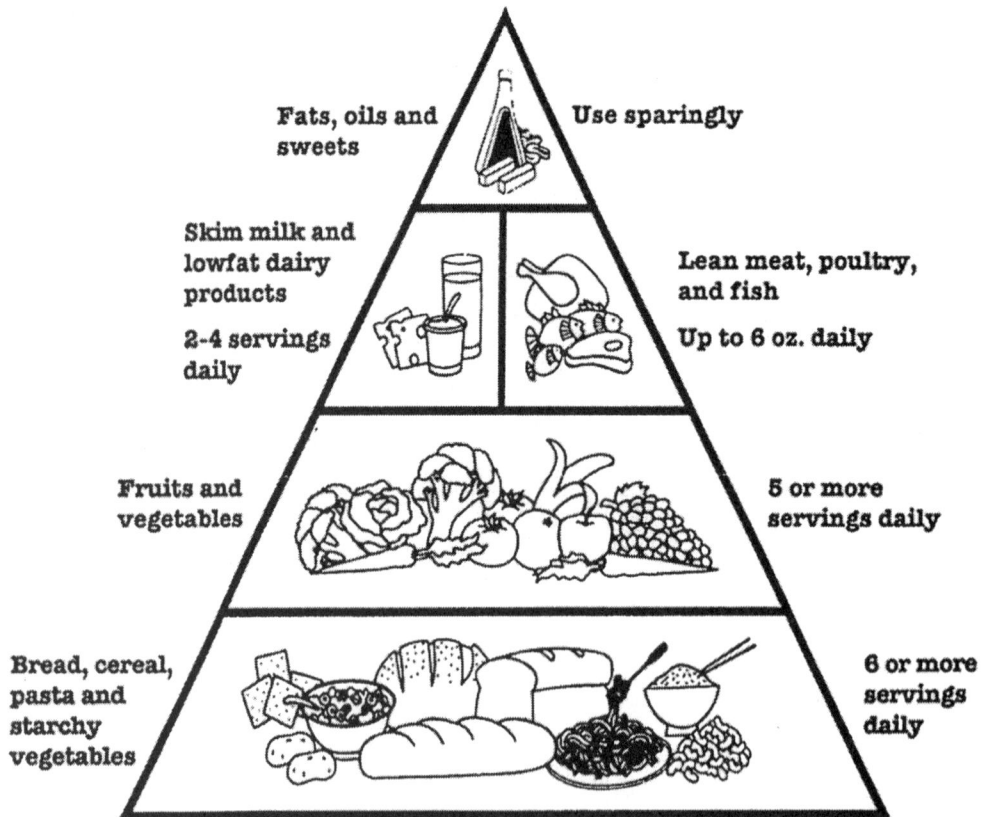

Fats, oils and sweets — Use sparingly

Skim milk and lowfat dairy products — 2-4 servings daily

Lean meat, poultry, and fish — Up to 6 oz. daily

Fruits and vegetables — 5 or more servings daily

Bread, cereal, pasta and starchy vegetables — 6 or more servings daily

California Dietetic Association

For further information contact:
California Dietetic Association
7740 Manchester Blvd., Suite 102, Playa del Rey, CA 90293-8499
tel: 310.822.0177, fax: 310.823.0264

Our Mission:

The California Dietetic Association is the advocate of the dietetic profession, benefiting the public through the promotion of optimal nutrition, health and well-being.

What is a Registered Dietitian?

In California, the Registered Dietitian (RD) is the health care professional legally recognized and trained to provide nutrition counseling to promote optimal health as well as medical nutrition therapy. The California Dietetic Association is a professional organization with approximately 7,000 members.

How Can I Find a Registered Dietitian in my Area?

The American Dietetic Association (ADA) has a national referral service "Find a Dietitian." All registered dietitians in the referral service are professionals who provide reliable, objective nutrition information. They can help you develop an eating plan specifically for your nutrition and health goals. Registered dietitians are experts in separating facts from fads and translating the latest scientific findings into easy-to-understand nutrition information.

To Find a Registered Dietitian and Answers to Nutrition Questions, Visit
www.eatright.org

California 5 A Day Campaign

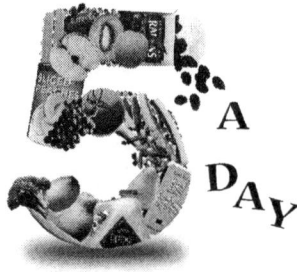

CANCER PREVENTION and NUTRITION
California Department of Health Services
601 N. 7th Street, P.O. Box 942732, MS-662
Sacramento, CA 94234-7320

Did you know that eating at least 5 servings of fruits and vegetables every day is one of the most important choices you can make to improve your health? Fruits and vegetables can help reduce the risk of diet-related chronic diseases, especially cancer, heart disease, diabetes, and obesity. They are low in fat and rich in vitamin A, vitamin C, fiber and other nutrients important to good health.

The *Cancer Prevention and Nutrition Section (CPNS)* works in cooperation with the expanded National 5 a Day Partnership to encourage Californians to consume five or more servings of fruits and vegetables and be physically active at least 30 minutes a day for adults and 60 minutes a day for children. CPNS operates large-scale social marketing campaigns including the *California Children's 5 A Day – Power Play! Campaign, Latino 5 A Day Campaign,* and *California Nutrition Network*, all of which offer a variety of materials to help reach the 5 A Day goal. CPNS partners with a consortium of state, local and private partners, including California agriculture, major supermarket retailers, and a wide variety of social, service, civic and faith organizations, as well as government agencies.

Go to the web site for more information
www.ca5aday.com
or call 1-888-EAT-FIVE

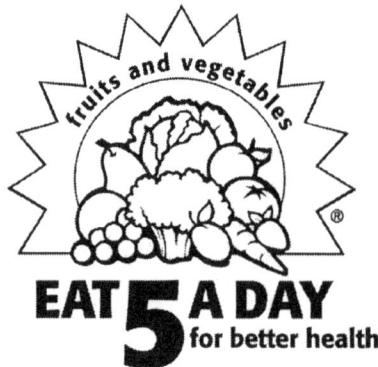

SOUTHLAND FARMERS' MARKET ASSOCIATION

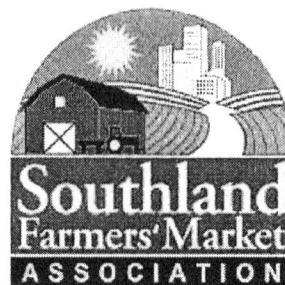

We're farm fresh and friendly! The freshest produce, fish, breads, herbs and other items, all locally grown. Available every week at a market near you. For more information about Farmers' Markets in your area, visit our website at www.sfma.net.

Market Locations & Hours:

Beverly Hills- Sundays, 9:00 am - 1:00 pm
200 block of North Canon Drive

Calabasas- Saturdays: 8 am to 12 Noon
23504 Calabasas Road, at the intersection of Calabasas Road & El Canon Avenue

Claremont- Sundays: 8 am to 12 Noon
235 Yale Ave. at Bonita Ave.

Covina- Fridays; 4 pm to 9 pm
Citrus Ave. in front of City Civic Center

Gardena- Saturdays, 6:30 am to 12:00 Noon
13000 Van Ness Ave., South of El Segundo Blvd.

La Cienega- Thurdays 3 pm to 7 pm
Corner of La Cienega and 18th St.

Los Angeles- Wednesdays: 1 pm to 6 pm
(2 PM to 5:00 PM Sept.-May). 1432 W. Adams Blvd., near Vermont (St. Agnes Church)

Monrovia- Fridays: 5 pm to 9 pm
Myrtle Avenue, between Olive & Lime Avenues, at Library Park

Montrose – Thursdays: 5 pm to 9 pm
2200 block of Honolulu Avenue, between Mountain View and Verdugo

Oxnard- Thursdays: 9:30 am to 1 pm
Plaza Park, corner of Fifth and "C" Street

Pomona -- Saturdays: 7:30 am to 11:30 am
North west corner of Garey Avenue and Pearl, one block North of Holt Avenue

Redondo Beach-- Thursdays: 8 am to 1 pm
End of Torrance Blvd., at the Redondo Pier

San Dimas- Wednesdays: 5 pm to 9 pm
(4 PM to 7 PM October - March) Bonita Ave. between Monte Vista Ave.

Santa Monica - Saturdays: 8:30 am to 1 pm
Intersection of Arizona Ave. & Second Street

Santa Monica - Saturdays: 8 am to 1 PM
Corner of Cloverfield and Pico Boulevards

Santa Monica - Wednesdays: 9 am to 2 pm
Intersection of Arizona Ave. & Second Street

Silverlake - Saturdays: 8 am to 12 Noon
3700 Sunset Blvd. (between Edgefliff Ave. & Maltman Ave.)

Studio City - Sundays: 8 am to 1 pm
Ventura Place between Ventura Blvd. and Laurel

West Hollywood-- Mondays: 9 AM to 2
7377 Santa Monica Blvd. in Plummer Park

Westwood- Thursdays, 2:00 pm - 7:00 pm
on Weyburn Ave., at Westwood Blvd

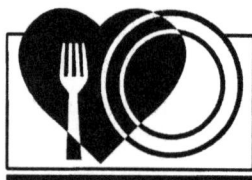

Part IV

Chefs' Recipes

Healthy Dining in Los Angeles is pleased to present a diverse selection of recipes created by chefs of restaurants featured in this book. We are delighted that so many restaurants have elected to participate in this section of *Healthy Dining*, sharing some of their culinary "trade secrets" with *Healthy Dining* readers. The recipes include a wide range of selections --- varying ethnic and regional origins, combinations of flavors, preparation time required, preparation difficulty, and types of dishes (soups, entrees, salads, etc.)

The Recipe Index

On pages 132 through 134 you'll find the Recipe Indexes, first arranged by the type of dish, then by the name of the restaurant that submitted the recipe. Many recipes could easily fall into more than one category within the Recipe Index. For example, a seafood salad could be under either the salads or seafood category. We suggest that you scan the entire Recipe Index to identify dishes that may appeal to you.

Nutritional analysis and modification of the recipes

With few exceptions, the recipes represent dishes that appear on the restaurant's menu page in *Healthy Dining*. We've stated on each recipe page that "This nutritional analysis corresponds to the recipe below. The restaurant version may differ." This notice indicates: (1) The recipe originally submitted to us for nutrition analysis was in bulk quantity and was adjusted to make 4 to 6 servings. In the process, we may have reformulated the recipe slightly so that amounts are expressed in convenient units – for example, ½ cup and not 7 /12 of a cup; (2) We may have substituted more common ingredients; or (3) We may have adjusted the quantities of some ingredients to further improve the nutrition profile.

Unfamiliar ingredients

When an ingredient is included that might be unfamiliar to the "average" cook, we've given some explanation and direction for finding it. If you need further explanation, please call the restaurant, a cooking school, or a specialty market. Or use your creativity and try your own substitutions!

Talk to us!

We wish you enjoyment and satisfaction, challenge and variety in experimenting with the recipes included. We're eager to get your feedback on the recipes included -- please return the questionnaire at the back of your book.

Recipe Index
by Type of Cuisine

Recipe Index by Restaurant Name

ANASTASIA'S NICOISE SALAD ☙

Albacore tuna, tomatoes, red onions,
artichoke hearts and kalamata olives.

Nutrition Information per Serving:

✓✓ CALORIES: Excellent Choice (285)   ✓✓ CHOLESTEROL: Excellent Choice (45 mg)
✓✓ FAT: Excellent Choice (11 g)*   SODIUM: Moderate (630 mg)
EXCHANGES: 4¼ Meat (extra lean), 2 Veg, 1¼ Fat
PROTEIN: 34 g, CARBOHYDRATE: 13 g, FIBER: 5 g

This nutrition analysis corresponds to the recipe below. The restaurant version may differ.

*Primarily unsaturated fat

Ingredients (4 servings):

¼ cup balsamic vinegar
2 Tbs. olive oil
4 cups mixed greens
¼ cup red onion, diced
2 oz. kalamata olives, quartered

½ cup tomato, chopped
8 oz. artichoke hearts, packed
   in water, quartered
16 oz. Albacore Tuna, packed in water

Directions:

1. In a small bowl, whisk together the balsamic vinegar and olive oil.
2. In a medium bowl, toss the mixed greens with the vinegar and oil mixture.
3. Add the onion, olives, tomatoes and artichoke hearts to greens and toss.
4. Place tuna on top of salad.
5. Serve and enjoy!

Recipe supplied by:

ANASTASIA'S

ASYLUM

SANCTUARY
of FINE FOOD & COFFEE

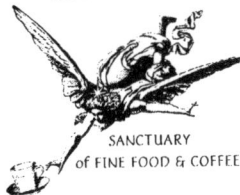

Anastasia's Asylum
SANCTUARY OF FINE FOOD AND COFFEE
1028 Wilshire Boulevard, Santa Monica 90401
(310) 394-7113

BeauRivage Salade Exotique 🍎

Hearts of palm, Belgian endive, watercress and tomatoes with Chutney Vinaigrette.

Nutrition Information per Serving:

✓✓ CALORIES: Excellent Choice (185)   ✓✓ CHOLESTEROL: Excellent Choice (0 mg)

✓✓ FAT: Excellent Choice (14 g)*   ✓✓ SODIUM: Excellent Choice (155 mg)

EXCHANGES: ¾ Veg, ¾ Fruit, 2¾ Fat

PROTEIN: 1 g, CARBOHYDRATE: 15 g

This nutrition analysis corresponds to the recipe below. The restaurant version may differ.

*Primarily unsaturated fat

Ingredients (8 servings):

Salad Exotique:
- 4 hearts of palm, quartered
- 4 Belgian endives
- 2 bunches watercress, chopped
- 4 large tomatoes, sliced medium
- 1 Tbs. fresh chives, chopped

Chutney Vinaigrette:
- 1 lemon, juiced
- ¼ tsp. <u>each</u> curry powder & white pepper
- 1 tsp. red wine vinegar
- ½ tsp. <u>each</u> English dry mustard & salt
- ½ cup virgin olive oil
- ½ cup Major Grey Chutney, chopped

Directions:

Chutney Vinaigrette:
1. Place all ingredients in a small bowl except olive oil and chutney. Mix well.
2. Add olive oil and whisk in well.
3. Add the chopped chutney and mix in.
4. Chill the dressing in the refrigerator.

Salade Exotique:
1. On a large serving platter arrange the hearts of palm, Belgian endives, watercress and tomato slices in an attractive way.
2. Spoon the Chutney Vinaigrette dressing over the salad.
3. Sprinkle on the chives.

Recipe supplied by:

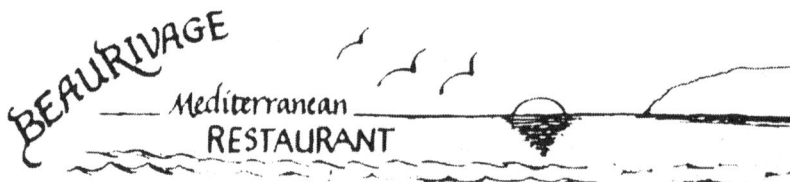

BeauRivage
Mediterranean
RESTAURANT

BeauRivage

🍎 at least 2 fruit/vegetable servings

BROWN RICE SALAD

with kidney beans, grilled corn, pumpkin seeds, feta cheese, turkey and seasonings.

Nutrition Information per Serving:

✓✓ CALORIES: Excellent Choice (225)   ✓✓ CHOLESTEROL: Excellent Choice (30 mg)
✓✓ FAT: Excellent Choice (7 g)   SODIUM: Moderate (640 mg)
EXCHANGES: 1 Meat, 1½ Bread, ¼ Veg, 2 Fat
PROTEIN: 12 g, CARBOHYDRATE: 29 g

This nutrition analysis corresponds to the recipe below. The restaurant version may differ.

Ingredients (8 servings):

1 cup brown rice
2 small ears corn
¼ cup pumpkin seeds
¼ cup kidney beans, rinsed
½ red onion, diced
½ cup diced jicama
2 Tbs. finely diced jalapenos
2½ oz. feta cheese, crumbled
½ lb. turkey breast, deli style, diced

½ cup salsa
2 Tbs. lime juice
1 Tbs. olive oil
¾ tsp. cumin
1 Tbs. fresh oregano
¾ tsp. garlic, minced
⅓ tsp. black pepper

Directions:

1. Cook rice according to package directions and chill.
2. Grill corn and cut off cob. Toast pumpkin seeds.
3. Place rice, corn and toasted pumpkin seeds in a large bowl and add kidney beans, red onions, jicama, jalapeno, feta cheese, and diced turkey. Toss gently.
4. In another bowl, mix salsa, lime juice, olive oil, oregano, cumin and garlic to make a dressing. Mix well.
5. Add dressing to the rice mixture and toss. Season with salt and pepper to taste if desired (not included in analysis).

Recipe supplied by:

Bristol's Café

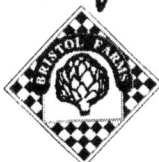

Bristol Farms' Deli

1570 Rosecrans Ave., Manhattan Beach   (310) 643-5229
837 Silver Spur Rd., Rolling Hills Estates   (310) 541-9157
606 Fair Oaks Ave., South Pasadena   (626) 441-5450
6227 Topanga Canyon Bl., Woodland Hills   (818) 227-8400
140 Promenade Way, West Lake Village   (805) 370-9193
2080 Bellflower Blvd., Long Beach   (562) 430-4134

CHARBROILED AHI TUNA SALAD
WITH FRESH MANGO KIWI SALSA ☙

Nutrition Information per Serving:

✓✓ CALORIES: Excellent Choice (290)   ✓✓ CHOLESTEROL: Excellent Choice (50 mg)
✓✓ FAT: Excellent Choice (2 g)*   SODIUM: High (1095 mg)
EXCHANGES: 3½ Meat (extra lean), 3 Veg, 1¼ Fruit
PROTEIN: 29 g, CARBOHYDRATE: 40 g

This nutrition analysis corresponds to the recipe below. The restaurant version may differ.

*Primarily unsaturated fat

Ingredients (4 servings):

Ahi Tuna Salad
1 lb. ahi tuna
2 cups shredded jicama
5 cups salad greens
1½ cups shredded cabbage
1½ carrots, shredded
1 red pepper, roasted
10 oz. fat-free roasted
    bell pepper dressing

Mango Kiwi Salsa
⅔ mango
1 kiwi
1 small serrano chili
¼ red sweet pepper, roasted
3 Tbs. each lemon juice & lime juice
pinch fresh mint
2 cloves garlic
½ tsp. each salt & black pepper
1½ tsp. sugar

Directions:

Mango Kiwi Salsa:
1. Chop fruit and vegetables into small-to-medium sized chunks.
2. Add remaining ingredients and let flavors mix for at least 2 hours.

Ahi Tuna Salad:
1. Roast red peppers. Cut into thin strips.
2. Season tuna with ground white pepper and salt (optional, not included in analysis).
3. Broil tuna on both sides for at least two minutes. Slice into thin slices.
4. Mix greens, cabbage and carrots in salad bowl. Pour dressing on top and mix well.
5. Arrange salad mix on plates. Place cooked, sliced ahi tuna in the middle top of each salad plate. Add shredded jicama and mango kiwi salsa on top.
6. Arrange roasted red pepper strips around the tuna.

Recipe supplied by:

JACK SPRAT'S
— G R I L L E —

Jack Sprat's Grille
10668 W. Pico Blvd. (at Overland)
Los Angeles, CA 90064
(310) 837-6662

☙ at least 2 fruit/vegetable servings

CHICKEN AND SHRIMP SALAD WITH PAPAYA ☙
and honey-poppy seed dressing.

Nutrition Information per Serving:

✓ CALORIES: Good Choice (560)   CHOLESTEROL: Moderate (275 mg)
✓✓ FAT: Excellent Choice (12 g)   ✓ SODIUM: Good Choice (555 mg)
EXCHANGES: 8¼ Meat, ¾ Veg, ¼ Milk, 2 Fruit, 1 Fat
PROTEIN: 64 g, CARBOHYDRATE: 47 g, FIBER: 6 g

This nutrition analysis corresponds to the recipe below. The restaurant version may differ.

Ingredients (2 servings):

Dressing:

½ tsp. shallots, finely chopped
1 tsp. fresh parsley
1 tsp. fresh chives
1 Tbs. honey
1 Tbs. rice vinegar

½ cup non-fat plain yogurt
1½ tsp. poppy seeds
1 pinch salt
1 pinch pepper

Salad:

2 tsp. olive oil for chicken
1 pinch salt
2 – 5 oz. skinless chicken breasts
1 Tbs. parsley, chopped
1 Tbs. tarragon, chopped
2 cups salad greens, chopped

½ head butter lettuce, chopped
6 large shrimp
1 papaya, sliced
2 oz. teardrop or cherry
  tomatoes, halved
2 sprigs chervil (French parsley)

Directions:

Dressing:

1. In a small sauté pan, cook shallots in vinegar until soft. Allow to cool.
2. Put the remaining ingredients in a bowl and whisk together.
3. Cover and refrigerate until needed.

Salad:

1. Heat olive oil in a sauté pan. Season chicken with salt and cook until cooked through. Cut each chicken breast into 5 pieces. Remove chicken from pan and set aside. Put shrimp in same pan and stir fry until done. Chill cooked chicken and shrimp.
2. Toss parsley, tarragon and salad greens together. Place ½ of the salad in the center of each large, cold dinner plate.
3. Drizzle half of the dressing over greens. Reserve half of the dressing for use later.
4. Arrange 3 shrimp and 3 pieces of papaya on the top of each salad.
5. Place 5 pieces of chicken around each salad.
6. Drizzle the remaining dressing around each salad and chicken.
7. Garnish with the halved tomatoes and sprigs of chervil.

Recipe supplied by:

HOTEL *Bel-Air*

LOS ANGELES

The Restaurant at Hotel Bel Air
701 Stone Canyon Road, Los Angeles 90077
(310) 472-1211

Healthy Dining in Los Angeles **139**

GRILLED SALMON SALAD ☙

with Star Anise dressing, Asian spicy mix, cucumber, tomatoes and onion.
Available at the Calabasas location only.

Nutrition Information per Serving:

✓✓ CALORIES: Excellent Choice (300)   ✓✓ CHOLESTEROL: Excellent (60 mg)
✓ FAT: Good Choice (18 g)   ✓✓ SODIUM: Excellent Choice (60 mg)
EXCHANGES: 3½ Meat, 1Veg, 3 Fat
PROTEIN: 25 g, CARBOHYDRATE: 11 g, FIBER: 3 g

This nutrition analysis corresponds to the recipe below. The restaurant version may differ.

Ingredients (4 servings):

Star Anise Dressing:
¾ tsp. star anise
¾ tsp. honey
¾ Tbs. white wine vinegar
1 tsp. balsamic apple cider

¼ tsp. sugar
2 Tbs. olive oil
salt and pepper to taste (not
   included in analysis)

Salmon Salad:
1 Tbs. olive oil
1 lb. Salmon, cut into 4 pieces
12 oz. Asian spicy lettuce mix
1 cucumber, sliced
1 small onion, diced

2 medium organic tomatoes,
   peeled and sliced
1 tsp. chives, diced
½ tsp. balsamic vinegar

Directions:
1. Combine all dressing ingredients and allow to sit for several hours
   in the refrigerator to allow flavors to mix.
2. Heat sauté pan. Add olive oil.
3. Grill salmon until done.
4. Toss Asian lettuce mix with cucumber, onion, tomato and chives.
5. Toss with star anise dressing.
6. Drizzle with balsamic vinegar.

Recipe supplied by:

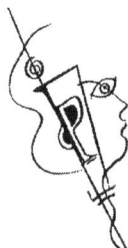

Mi Piace
25 E. Colorado Blvd., Old Town Pasadena
(626) 795-3131
801 N. San Fernando Rd., Burbank
(818) 843-1111
4799 Commons Way, Calabasas
(818) 591-8822

☙ at least 2 fruit/vegetable servings

INSALATE MALVASIA 👌

Mixed baby greens, chicken breast, sliced red onions, fire roasted
red peppers, fresh mozzarella, kalamata olives, roma tomatoes, capers and artichoke hearts.

Nutrition Information per Serving:

✓✓ CALORIES: Excellent Choice (430)   ✓ CHOLESTEROL: Good Choice (145 mg)
✓✓ FAT: Excellent Choice (13 g)*   SODIUM: High (1046 mg)
EXCHANGES: 7¾ Meat, 2 Veg, ¼ Fat
PROTEIN: 58 g, CARBOHYDRATE: 16 g, FIBER: 5 g

This nutrition analysis corresponds to the recipe below. The restaurant version may differ.

*Primarily unsaturated fat

Ingredients (2 servings):

3 cups mixed baby greens
2 6-oz. chicken breasts, skinless
½ red onion, chopped
½ cup red bell peppers, chopped
12 kalamata olives, chopped

4 roma tomatoes, chopped
2 Tbs. capers
½ cup artichoke hearts (not marinated)
½ cup mozzarella cheese, shredded

Directions:
1. Grill or bake chicken breasts until done. Slice into strips.
2. Toss together greens, red onion, roasted peppers, olives, capers and artichoke hearts.
3. Place tossed salad on dinner plates. Arrange chicken breasts strips over greens.
4. Sprinkle with cheese.
5. Serve with your choice of dressing (not included in analysis).

Recipe supplied by:

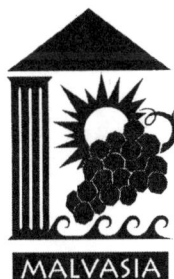

Malvasia
5316 E. 2nd Street, Long Beach 90803
(562) 433-5005

PAPAYA GRILLED CHICKEN SALAD ᪥

Field greens, sliced avocado and ripe papaya
with charbroiled chicken breast and mango vinaigrette.

Nutrition Information per Serving:

✓✓ CALORIES: Excellent Choice (340) ✓ CHOLESTEROL: Good Choice (85 mg)
✓ FAT: Good Choice (17 g) ✓✓ SODIUM: Excellent Choice (140 mg)**
EXCHANGES: 4½ Meat, ¼ Veg, ½ Fruit, 2¾ Fat
PROTEIN: 34 g, CARBOHYDRATE: 13 g, FIBER: 3 g

This nutrition analysis corresponds to the recipe below. The restaurant version may differ.

Ingredients (4 servings):

Dressing:
2 oz. pureed mango
2 Tbs. white vinegar
1 tsp. honey
2 Tbs. olive oil
1 tsp. black pepper

Chicken Marinade:
½ tsp. black pepper
⅓ tsp. paprika
½ tsp. chili powder
½ tsp. garlic
½ tsp. salt
¼ cup vegetable oil
1 Tbs. white wine

Salad:
1 lb. chicken, skinless breast sliced
  into 1 inch strips
8 oz. baby field greens salad mix

½ avocado, cut into 4 slices
1 cup fresh papaya, diced

Directions:

1. Mix together all marinate ingredients and pour over chicken. Refrigerate for 1-2 hours. Pour off and discard excess marinate.
2. Puree dressing ingredients together.
3. Grill or bake marinated chicken until done.
4. Place greens on 4 plates. Place chicken slices over greens. Add diced papaya and sliced avocado.
5. Drizzle dressing over salad.

Recipe supplied by:

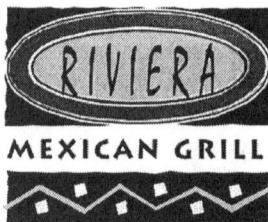

Riviera Mexican Grill
1615 Pacific Coast Hwy Redondo Beach 90277
(310) 540-2501

᪥ at least 2 fruit/vegetable servings

SHRIMP & CRAB LOUIE COMBO ♍

Bay shrimp and King crab meat with onion, cucumber, tomato, carrot, celery and avocado.

Nutrition Information per Serving:

✓✓ CALORIES: Excellent Choice (340)   CHOLESTEROL: Moderate (155 mg)
✓✓ FAT: Excellent Choice (13 g)*   SODIUM: High (1070 mg)
EXCHANGES: 4½ Meat (extra lean), 6 Veg, 4½ Fat
PROTEIN: 40 g, CARBOHYDRATE: 19 g, FIBER: 8 g

This nutrition analysis corresponds to the recipe below. The restaurant version may differ.

*Primarily unsaturated fat

Ingredients (2 servings):

2 slices red onion
4 cucumber slices
4 tomato wedges
1 hard boiled egg
8 carrot sticks
8 celery sticks
6 black olives

½ medium avocado, cut into wedges
6 oz. shrimp
6 oz. crab
7 cups lettuce mix
1 cup cabbage, shredded
salad dressing (not included in analysis)

Directions:

1. Place 3½ cups lettuce and ½ cup cabbage in each of 2 large bowls.
2. Add red onion slices to one side of each bowl.
3. Place cucumber slices, tomato and egg wedges on each side of both bowls.
4. Place the carrot sticks beside the egg wedges.
5. Place the celery sticks beside the carrots.
6. Place the whole black olives beside the celery sticks.
7. Add shrimp and crab meat to the top of each salad.
8. Place avocado slices on each side.
9. Serve with your choice of dressing on the side (not included in analysis).

Recipe supplied by:

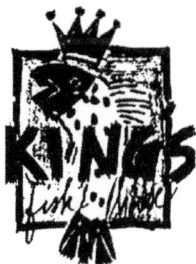

PINE AVENUE

King's Fish House
100 W. Broadway
 Long Beach 90802
(562) 432-7463

4798 Commons Way
The Commons at Calabasas 91302
(818) 225-1979

WARM POACHED SALMON, TOMATO & HERB SALAD
with dill dressing.

Nutrition Information per Serving:

✓✓ CALORIES: Excellent Choice (330)   ✓ CHOLESTEROL: Good Choice (110 mg)
✓✓ FAT: Excellent Choice (13 g)*   ✓✓ SODIUM: Excellent Choice (115 mg)
EXCHANGES: 5 Meat, ½ Veg
PROTEIN: 42 g, CARBOHYDRATE: 9 g

This nutrition analysis corresponds to the recipe below. The restaurant version may differ.

*Primarily unsaturated fat

Ingredients (4 servings):

Salad:
2 tomatoes
½ cup chopped fresh basil leaves
½ cup chopped watercress
½ cup chopped chervil
½ cup chopped chives
½ cup chopped fresh dill
1½ Tbs. white wine
1½ Tbs. chicken stock

Salmon:
4 salmon filets (7 oz. each)

Dill Dressing:
¼ cup rice wine vinegar
¼ cup white wine
¼ cup chicken stock
½ cup chopped shallots
¼ cup chopped fresh dill

Directions:

1. Mix Dill Dressing ingredients together and set aside.
2. Cut tomatoes into wedges. Add basil leaves, watercress, chervil, chives and dill.   Toss together. Add part of Dill Dressing and arrange tomato-herb salad on plates.
3. Poach salmon in mixture of white wine and chicken stock until medium rare (or desired cooking time).
4. Place salmon on plates next to salad and spoon dill dressing over salmon.

Recipe supplied by:

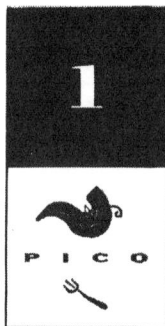

1
PICO

One Pico
at Shutters On The Beach
One Pico Blvd.
Santa Monica, CA 90405
(310) 587-1717

BROILED HALIBUT WITH TROPICAL FRUIT SALSA

Ingredients (6 servings):

½ cup red onion, diced
1 cup mango, chopped
1 cup papaya, chopped
1-2 jalapeños, seeded, diced
juice of ½ fresh lime
juice of ½ fresh orange

⅓ cup seasoned rice vinegar
1 Tbs. fresh cilantro, chopped
¼ tsp. white pepper
½ tsp. salt (optional, not included in analysis)

6 halibut steaks, 8 oz. each

Directions:

1. Combine all ingredients except fish in bowl. Chill for 30 minutes.
2. Barbecue or broil halibut steaks.
3. Serve salsa on top of fish steaks.

Recipe supplied by:

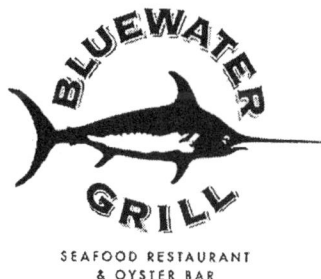

Bluewater Grill

665 N. Harbor Dr., Redondo Beach, CA 90277
(310) 318-3474

CEVICHE

Ingredients (for 5 servings of approx. 8 oz. each):

1¼ lb. Pacific red snapper
2 oz. Atlantic salmon
1 cup lemon juice
⅔ cup lime juice
½ tsp. salt
⅓ tsp. white pepper

⅔ tsp. Tabasco sauce
¼ tomato, chopped
½ Tbs. jalapenos, chopped
¾ cup cilantro, chopped
10 green onions, chopped
⅓ tsp. oregano

Directions:

1. Rinse and drain fish. Cut into small cubes.
2. Mix lemon juice, lime juice, salt, pepper, and Tabasco sauce. Marinate fish in this mixture overnight to "cure" the fish.
3. Drain fish. Toss together with tomatoes, jalapenos, cilantro, green onions & oregano.

Recipe supplied by:

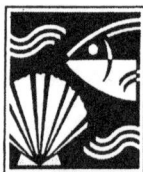

Santa Monica Seafood
1205 Colorado Ave., Santa Monica, 90404
(310) 393-5244

424 South Main Street, Suite F, Orange, 92868
(714) 921-2632

154 East 17th St., Costa Mesa, 92627
(949) 574-8862

SANTA MONICA
SEAFOOD

CHARBROILED FISH TACO

Nutrition Information per Serving:

✓✓ CALORIES: Excellent Choice (220)   ✓✓ CHOLESTEROL: Excellent Choice (50 mg)

✓✓ FAT: Excellent Choice (4 g)   ✓ SODIUM: Good Choice (340 mg)

EXCHANGES: 1¼ Meat, 1¾ Bread, ¼ Veg, ½ Fat

PROTEIN: 15 g, CARBOHYDRATE: 27 g, Fiber: 3g

This nutrition analysis corresponds to the recipe below. The restaurant version may differ.

Ingredients (4 servings):

½ lb. fresh mahi mahi fillets (¾-1 inch thick)

pinch of garlic salt

8 corn tortillas

1 oz. shredded cheese (Jack and/or cheddar)

2 oz. cabbage, shredded

4 oz. salsa

2 limes, quartered

cilantro (optional)

Directions:

1. Season fish with pinch of garlic salt.
2. Grill each side over medium heat until done. Divide into 4 portions.
3. Heat tortillas in pan and keep warm.
4. Fill tortillas with fish and top with cheese, cabbage, and salsa. In the restaurant the tacos are made using a double layer of corn tortillas. Alternatively, you can divide the filling evenly between all 8 tortillas to make 2 tacos per serving that contain less filling per taco.
5. Garnish with lime and cilantro.

Recipe supplied by:

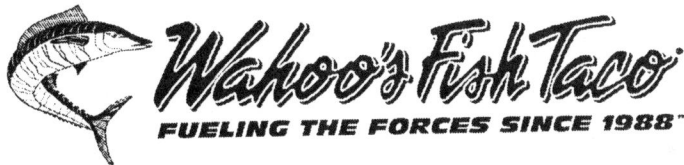

Wahoo's Fish Taco locations:

Visit www.wahoos.com for a list of all southern California locations!

Manhattan Beach: 1129 Manhattan Ave.   (310) 796-1044

Mid-Wilshire: 6258 Wilshire Blvd.   (323) 933-2480

Torrance: 3556 Torrance Blvd., Ste. E   (310) 540-7725

West Los Angeles: 11911 Wilshire Blvd.   (310) 445-5990

Pasadena: 264 S. Lake Ave.   (626) 449-2005

Santa Monica: 418 Wilshire Blvd.

PESCADO VERACRUZANA

This is one of the most popular dishes at Border Grill, where we use the freshest fish available. Our Favorite is sea bass as it sears well in the pan, cooks evenly without flaking or overcooking easily, which makes it a good choice for a party. The key is to get the searing pan very hot to caramelize the fish, then quick fry the vegetable garnish and finish it all with a short simmer.

Nutrition Information per Serving:

✓✓ CALORIES: Excellent Choice (320)   ✓✓ CHOLESTEROL: Excellent Choice (70 mg)
✓ FAT: Good Choice (16 g)*   SODIUM: Moderate (805 mg)
EXCHANGES: 3 Meat (extra lean), ¾ Veg, ¼ Fruit, 2½ Fat
PROTEIN: 33 g, CARBOHYDRATE: 8 g

This nutrition analysis corresponds to the recipe below. The restaurant version may differ.

*Primarily unsaturated fat

Ingredients (4 servings):

1½ lb. skinless, boneless sea bass,
   cut into 4 portions
salt & freshly ground black pepper
   to taste (not included in analysis)
3 Tbs. olive oil
1 small yellow onion, peeled & sliced
2 cloves garlic, peeled & minced

2 jalepenos, stemmed & sliced
1 lime, cut into eight pieces
1 tomato, cored, seeded & cut in strips
½ cup Spanish green olives, sliced
½ bunch fresh oregano leaves
½ cup white wine
¾ cup fish stock or clam juice

Directions:

1. Season fish with salt and pepper if desired.
2. Heat one very large or two medium sized sauté pans over medium high heat for a minute, then add olive oil.
3. When oil is sizzling, add fish filets, flesh side down and turn heat to very high. Sear the filets until golden brown and flip to sear the other side.
4. Remove filets from pan and reserve on a rack over a plate to catch juices.
5. Return the pan(s) to heat. Add onions and cook, stirring often over high heat 2 - 3 minutes.
6. Add garlic, jalepeno, lime wedges, tomatoes, oregano & olives. Sauté briskly 1 minute more.
7. Add white wine and reduce to half. Add fish stock and bring to a boil. Reduce to a simmer and return fish filets along the juices to pan to finish cooking, covered, about 1 - 3 minutes, depending on the thickness of filets.
8. Taste broth and adjust seasoning. Serve immediately in soup plates with a generous puddle of broth. Garnish with vegetables. Use new potatoes or rice as accompaniment (not included in analysis).

Recipe supplied by:

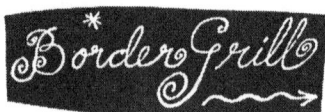

Border Grill
1445 Fourth Street
Santa Monica, CA 90401
(310) 451-1655

PRADEEP'S SALMON

*Marinated salmon served over turmeric
and cilantro flavored mashed potatoes with organic greens.*

Nutrition Information per Serving:

✓✓ CALORIES: Excellent Choice (350)   ✓ CHOLESTEROL: Good Choice (90 mg)
✓✓ FAT: Excellent Choice (12 g)*   ✓✓ SODIUM: Excellent Choice (190 mg)
EXCHANGES: 4⅓ Meat, ¾ Bread, ¼ Veg, ¾ Fat, ½ Milk
PROTEIN: 40 g, CARBOHYDRATE: 21 g, FIBER: 3 g

This nutrition analysis corresponds to the recipe below. The restaurant version may differ.

Ingredients (4 servings):

¼ tsp. each of clove powder, cinnamon, cumin, mace, and chili powder
1 tsp. each of fresh ginger, garlic and lemon juice
¼ Tbs. olive oil
1.5 lbs. salmon
1 cup non-fat plain yogurt
3 tsp. cilantro, finely diced

1½ tsp. brown sugar
1½ tsp. lime juice
8 oz. potatoes
½ tsp. turmeric
pinch salt
½ tsp. mustard seeds
8 oz. organic greens, washed

Directions:

1. Mix together clove powder, cinnamon, cumin, mace, and chili powder. Add fresh ginger, garlic and lemon juice.
2. Add salmon to the above marinate. Cover and marinate for 3 hours in refrigerator.
3. Mix the yogurt and cilantro together. Cover and set aside in refrigerator.
4. Mix brown sugar and lime juice together. Cover and set aside.
5. Bake salmon in 400° oven until done and tender.
6. While salmon is baking, boil potatoes with turmeric and a pinch of salt.
7. Heat oil in sauté pan. Add mustard seeds and toast lightly. Add mustard seeds to potatoes. Mash potatoes lightly with a fork.
8. Toss organic greens with the lime juice and brown sugar mixture.
9. Place potatoes in the center of plate. Place greens on top of potatoes. Drizzle yogurt dressing over greens. Place salmon on top of greens. Serve and enjoy.

Recipe supplied by:

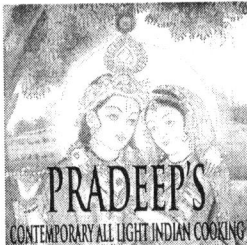

Pradeep's
Contemporary All Light Indian Cooking
www.pradeepsindiancuisine.com

1405 Montana Avenue, Santa Monica 90403
(310) 393-1467

SAN FRANCISCO SWORDFISH

Marinated in soy, Dijon, lemon and garlic and charbroiled.

Nutrition Information per Serving:

✓✓ CALORIES: Excellent Choice (370)   ✓ CHOLESTEROL: Good Choice (90 mg)
  ✓ FAT: Good Choice (16 g)*   ✓ SODIUM: Good Choice (560 mg)
EXCHANGES: 5 Meat, 1¼ Veg, 1¼ Fat
PROTEIN: 49 g, CARBOHYDRATE: 7 g

This nutrition analysis corresponds to the recipe below. The restaurant version may differ.
*Primarily unsaturated fat

Ingredients (4 servings):

1¼ Tbs. soy sauce
¼ tsp. garlic, minced
¼ tsp. grated lemon peel
1 Tbs. lemon juice

½ tsp. Dijon mustard
2 Tbs. olive oil
2 lbs. swordfish (4 filets 8 oz. each)
1 lb. vegetables of your choice

Directions:

1. Mix first six ingredients together in a blender until emulsified. Reserve half in a bowl.
2. Pour remaining liquid into baking pan. Add fish and marinate for 15 - 20 minutes.
3. Broil or grill swordfish using reserved liquid to baste.
4. Served with steamed vegetables.

Recipe supplied by:

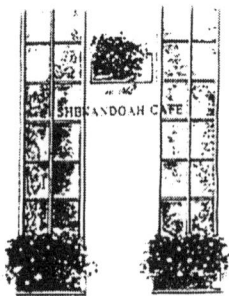

Shenandoah Cafe
4722 East 2nd Street,
Long Beach, CA 90803
(562) 434-3469

SEARED BLACKENED AHI

Served rare with Cajun spices, pickled ginger and wasabi.

Nutrition Information per Serving:

✓✓ CALORIES: Excellent Choice (175)   ✓✓ CHOLESTEROL: Excellent Choice (50 mg)
✓✓ FAT: Excellent Choice (2 g)*   SODIUM: High (1680 mg)
EXCHANGES: 3½ Meat, ¼ Veg, ¾ Fruit
PROTEIN: 31 g, CARBOHYDRATE: 9 g, FIBER: 1 g

This nutrition analysis corresponds to the recipe below. The restaurant version may differ.
*Primarily unsaturated fat

Ingredients (4 servings):

1 Tbs. paprika
1¼ tsp. onion powder
1¼ tsp. garlic powder
¼ Tbs. white pepper
¼ Tbs. black pepper
1¼ Tbs. thyme
½ Tbs. oregano
1¼ tsp. cayenne pepper

½ tsp. salt
1 lb. ahi tuna, sashimi quality
cooking spray
4 tsp. ginger root, grated
1 oz. pickled ginger
1 oz. wasabi
½ cup soy sauce, reduced sodium

Directions:

1. Combine dry seasonings (first 9 ingredients) and mix thoroughly.
2. Coat both sides of tuna with seasoning mix, shaking off excess.
3. Heat a cast-iron skillet over high heat with exhaust fan on.
4. Spray tuna with nonstick spray and place in super-hot pan.
5. Sear fish about 1 minute on all sides. Do not overcook. Fish should be rare or medium-rare.
6. Slice thinly and fan on plate.
7. Serve with soy sauce mixed with grated ginger in a small bowl, pickled ginger and wasabi.

Recipe supplied by:

MᶜCORMICK&SCHMICK'S
S E A F O O D   R E S T A U R A N T

McCormick & Schmick's Seafood Restaurant

111 N. Los Robles, Pasadena, CA 91101   (626) 405-0064
633 West 5th St. 4th Level, Los Angeles, CA 90071   (213) 629-1929
206 North Rodeo Drive, Beverly Hills, CA 90210   (310) 859-0434
2101 Rosecrans Ave., El Segundo, CA 90245   (310) 416-1123

STEAMED SALMON FILLET WITH SOY-LEMON SAUCE

Served with grilled artichoke hearts, black shiitake mushrooms and asparagus.

Nutrition Information per Serving:

✓✓ CALORIES: Excellent Choice (425) ✓ CHOLESTEROL: Good Choice (125 mg)
  ✓ FAT: Excellent Choice (17 g)*   SODIUM: Moderate (720 mg)
EXCHANGES: 5¾ Meat, ½ Bread, 1½ Veg, ½ Fat
PROTEIN: 50 g, CARBOHYDRATE: 19 g, Fiber: 7 g

This nutrition analysis corresponds to the recipe below. The restaurant version may differ.

Ingredients (2 servings):

1 lb. salmon   4 each artichoke hearts
4 each shiitake mushrooms   1 tsp. peanut oil
1 green onion stalk   2 Tbs. lite soy sauce
3 slices ginger   ½ tsp. sugar
1 cup chicken stock   2½ Tbs. lemon juice, divided
6 spears asparagus

Directions:

1. Clean artichoke hearts and cook in boiling water. Drain and let cool. Pour 2 tablespoons of lemon juice over artichoke hearts. Grill artichoke hearts until grill marks appear.
2. Cut green onions into 3 sections. Place green onions and ginger over salmon.
3. Steam salmon and shitake mushrooms in chicken stock until salmon is cooked through and mushrooms are tender, about 8 minutes.
4. Steam asparagus (may be steamed with salmon for three minutes).
5. Place artichoke hearts and mushrooms on plate. Place salmon over vegetables. Save juices.
6. Heat oil until almost smoking (do not let oil smoke or catch on fire). Immediately drizzle oil over salmon.
7. Sprinkle a pinch of sugar and soy sauce and then finish with ½ tsp. of lemon juice.
8. Place asparagus on side of plate.
9. Pour some of the saved juices over the salmon and serve.

Recipe supplied by:

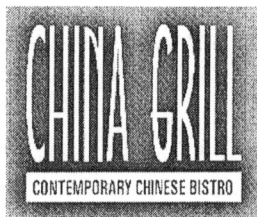
CHINA GRILL
CONTEMPORARY CHINESE BISTRO

China Grill

3282 Sepulveda Blvd., Manhattan Beach 90266
(310) 546-7284

GARLIC SHRIMP

Stir fry shrimp with garlic, black pepper and cilantro.

Nutrition Information per Serving:

✓✓ CALORIES: Excellent Choice (300)   CHOLESTEROL: High (350 mg)
✓✓ FAT: Excellent Choice (13 g)*   SODIUM: High (2345 mg)
EXCHANGES: 5 Meat(extra lean), ¼ Bread, ¼ Veg, 1¾ Fat
PROTEIN: 40 g, CARBOHYDRATE: 7 g

This nutrition analysis corresponds to the recipe below. The restaurant version may differ.
*Primarily unsaturated fat

Ingredients (4 servings):

1½ lb. medium shrimp
2 Tbs. vegetable oil
2 Tbs. plus 2 tsp. oyster sauce
3½ Tbs. soy sauce
2½ tsp. sugar

3 cloves garlic, minced
¼ cup chopped fresh cilantro
1½ tsp. black pepper
2 cups chicken broth, reduced
   sodium

Directions:

1. Sauté shrimp in oil.
2. Mix together all remaining ingredients (except sautéed shrimp) in a sauce pan. Heat over medium-high heat and bring to a boil.
3. Reduce heat and simmer until sauce is reduced by half.
4. Add shrimp to sauce and cook for a few additional minutes.
5. Serve over rice (not included in analysis).

Recipe supplied by:

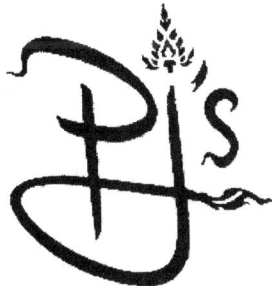

PJ's
5372 East 2nd Street, Long Beach, CA 90803
(562) 434-3565

PAN SEARED SCALLOPS ✆

Tender scallops pan-seared with a sweet Cabernet
reduction and garnished with toasted macadamia nuts.

Nutrition Information per Serving:

✓✓ CALORIES: Excellent Choice (415)   ✓ CHOLESTEROL: Good Choice (120 mg)
✓ FAT: Good Choice (16 g)   SODIUM: Moderate (625 mg)
EXCHANGES: 7¼ Meat, ½ Bread, 1 Veg, 2½ Fat
PROTEIN: 56 g, CARBOHYDRATE: 16 g, FIBER: 3 g

This nutrition analysis corresponds to the recipe below. The restaurant version may differ.

Ingredients (2 servings):

5 fl. oz. cabernet wine   1 lb. scallops
5 tsp sugar   salt and pepper to taste (not
¼ tsp lime juice   included in analysis)
2 cups seasonal vegetables, chopped   1 Tbs. macadamia nuts
1 Tbs. oil

Directions:

1. Combine cabernet wine and sugar in a very small, shallow heavy saucepan.
2. Heat over medium heat, bringing ingredients to a simmer. Once simmering, turn heat down to low.
3. Continue simmering over low heat until a syrup consistency is achieved (about 40-60 minutes). Do not allow the mixture to scorch.
4. Remove reduction from heat and add lime juice. Set aside reduction and keep warm.
5. Steam vegetables.
6. Heat oil in sauté pan over medium-high heat.
7. Season scallops with salt and pepper.
8. Place scallops in pan and sear until golden brown. Turn scallops over and continue to sear until done.
9. Transfer and arrange scallops on plate.
10. Drizzle warm cabernet reduction over the scallops.
11. Garnish scallops with nuts and serve with vegetables.

Recipe supplied by:

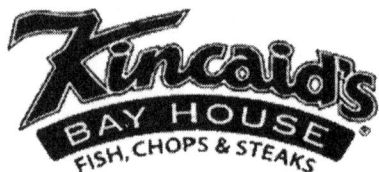

Kincaid's Bay House
500 The Pier, Redondo Beach 90277
(310) 318-6080

SEAFOOD LINGUINE

with shrimp, clams and fresh fish in a white wine tomato-herb sauce.

Nutrition Information per Serving:

✓ CALORIES: Good Choice (645)   CHOLESTEROL: MODERATE (170 mg)
✓ FAT: Good Choice (16 g)*   ✓ SODIUM: Good Choice (405 mg)
EXCHANGES: 4¾ Meat (extra lean), 5¼ Bread, 1¼ Veg, 1¾ Fat
PROTEIN: 51 g, CARBOHYDRATE: 90 g, FIBER: 6 g

This nutrition analysis corresponds to the recipe below. The restaurant version may differ.

*Primarily unsaturated fat

Ingredients (4 servings):

12 oz. linguini
4 tsp olive oil
24 manilla clams (¼ lb. meat)
4 tsp. shallots, minced
4 tsp. garlic, minced
½ lb. rock shrimp
½ lb. salmon

¼ lb snapper
1 cup white wine
1 cup tomato puree
4 tsp. parsley
½ tsp. red chile flakes
½ tsp. salt

Directions:

1. Pre-cook pasta according to package directions. Once al dente, shock in an ice bath to stop the cooking process. Drain and reserve pasta at room temperature.
2. Heat a medium sauté pan over high heat.
3. Add olive oil, clams and shallots to hot pan. Sauté 1 to 2 minutes.
4. In quick succession, add garlic, shrimp, salmon and snapper. (Note: It is important to add the garlic with the seafood – otherwise the garlic may burn and taste bitter.)
5. Add white wine and cover.
6. When the clams have opened, (usually takes between 3 to 4 minutes) add the tomato puree, parsley, chile flakes and salt.
7. Add the pasta and toss until hot.
8. Serve and enjoy!

Recipe supplied by:

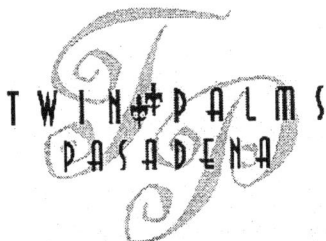

Twin Palms
101 West Green St., Pasadena 91105
(626) 577-2567

SHRIMP IN SPICY TOMATO SAUCE

Penne in a light spicy tomato sauce with shrimp.

Nutrition Information per Serving:

✓ CALORIES: Good Choice (610)   CHOLESTEROL: Moderate (277 mg)
✓ FAT: Good Choice (17 g)*   SODIUM: Moderate (920 mg)
EXCHANGES: 4¼ Meat, 4 Bread, 1½ Veg, 2¾ Fat
PROTEIN: 41 g, CARBOHYDRATE: 67 g, Fiber: 17 g

This nutrition analysis corresponds to the recipe below. The restaurant version may differ.

*Primarily unsaturated fat

Ingredients (4 servings):

1 lb. tomatoes
1 Tbs. basil, chopped
¼ tsp salt
¼ cup olive oil
8 cloves garlic, minced
1 pinch red pepper

1½ lb. shrimp, cleaned and de-veined
1 pinch black pepper
¼ cup white wine
1 cup clam juice
12 oz. pasta, dry weight
4 tsp. parsley

Directions:

1. Prepare tomato sauce by mixing tomatoes, basil and salt in saucepan.
2. Cook for approximately one hour on medium heat, stirring occasionally. While sauce is cooking, begin preparing pasta and other ingredients.
3. Cook penne in a separate large pot of water until almost done. Pasta will finish cooking after mixed with other ingredients. Drain and set aside.
4. Mix olive oil, garlic and chili pepper in a large pan over high heat until garlic is browned.
5. Add shrimp, pepper and white wine. Cook for approximately 3 minutes until wine has evaporated.
6. Combine tomato sauce, clam juice, cooked penne and shrimp. Cook for approximately 5-6 minutes. Serve on 12" oval plate and garnish with parsley.

Recipe supplied by:

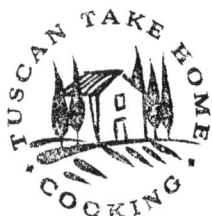

TUSCAN TAKE HOME COOKING

Rosti

160 Promenade Way, Ste A, Westlake 91362   (805) 370-1939
16403 Ventura Blvd., Encino 91436   (818) 995-7179
233 S. Beverly Drive, Beverly Hills 90212   (310) 275-3285
931 Montana Ave., Santa Monica 90403   (310) 393-3236

GRILLED CHICKEN BREAST WITH APRICOT SAUCE ☙

With fresh ginger, onion and plum tomatoes.

Nutrition Information per Serving:

✓✓ CALORIES: Excellent Choice (445)   ✓ CHOLESTEROL: Good Choice (130 mg)
✓✓ FAT: Excellent Choice (12 g)   ✓ SODIUM: Good Choice (485 mg)**
                    EXCHANGES: 6¾ Meat, 1¾ Veg, ¼ Fruit, 1 Fat
                    PROTEIN: 52 g, CARBOHYDRATE: 33 g, FIBER: 6 g

This nutrition analysis corresponds to the recipe below. The restaurant version may differ.

Ingredients (4 servings):

Marinade & Chicken:

1½ Tbs. Dijon mustard	1½ Tbs. white wine	4 each 6 oz. chicken
1 pinch cayenne pepper	1¼ Tbs. lemon juice	breasts, skinless
½ tsp. pepper	¾ tsp. thyme	4 cups seasonal
½ tsp. salt	¼ cup olive oil	vegetables

Apricot Sauce:

½ cup dried apricots	2 Tbs. fresh cilantro,	⅓ cup apricot preserves
¾ Tbs. canola oil	chopped	1 tsp. lemon juice
2 Tbs. onion, minced	1 pinch cloves	¼ tsp. kosher salt
1½ Tbs. ginger, minced	⅓ tsp. white pepper	¼ tsp. pepper
⅓ tsp. ground coriander	1½ cups tomatoes, chopped	

Directions:

Prepare Marinade:
1. In a food processor, combine mustard, cayenne, pepper, salt and white wine. Pour in lemon juice and thyme. Blend for 10 seconds.
2. While processor is running, slowly pour in oil until sauce emulsifies.
3. Coat chicken with marinade. Cover and marinate at least 3 hours in refrigerator.

Prepare Apricot Sauce:
1. Place dried apricots in a bowl with boiling water. Let soak for 30 minutes.
2. Drain water from apricots. Coarsely chop with a knife until pieces are about ½ inch.
3. Heat oil in a sauce pot over medium-high heat. Add the onions and ginger; sauté until the onions are tender and translucent.
4. Add the remaining ingredients. Bring to a simmer and let cook for an additional 20-30 minutes, stirring occasionally.

Prepare Chicken & Vegetables:
1. While sauce is simmering, grill chicken breasts until done.
2. Steam vegetables.
3. To serve, place chicken breasts on plates. Top chicken with sauce. Serve with steamed vegetables.

Recipe supplied by:

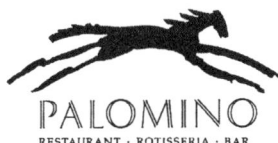

Palomino
10877 Wilshire Blvd., Los Angeles 90024
(310) 208-1960

PALOMINO
RESTAURANT · ROTISSERIA · BAR

☙ at least 2 fruit/vegetable servings

HONEY THYME PORK LOIN

Roasted pork loin glazed with honey and seasoned with garlic, dijon, and thyme.

Nutrition Information per Serving:

✓✓ CALORIES: Excellent Choice (270)   ✓✓ CHOLESTEROL: Excellent Choice (55 mg)

✓✓ FAT: Excellent Choice (5 g)   ✓✓ SODIUM: Excellent Choice (220 mg)

PROTEIN: 21 g, CARBOHYDRATE: 51 g, Fiber 0 g

This nutrition analysis corresponds to the recipe below. The restaurant version may differ.

Ingredients (9 servings):

2 lb. pork loin

1 Tbs. canola oil

1 Tbs. shallots, chopped

2 cloves garlic, minced

2 Tbs. tomato paste

1 Tbs. dijon mustard

5 Tbs. red wine vinegar

1 cup honey

1 tsp. thyme leaves

1 tsp. cracked black peppercorns

1 ⅔ cup beef stock

3 Tbs. cornstarch

½ tsp. salt

⅓ cup water

½ cup chicken stock

Directions:

1. Heat oil and brown pork tenderloin in a medium size pan.
2. Remove pork and pour off excess oil.
3. Add chopped shallots, minced garlic, tomato paste, and mustard. Sauté for one to two minutes. Add the red wine vinegar and deglaze (cook until the mixture thickens as the vinegar evaporates).
4. Add honey, thyme, and cracked peppercorns.
5. Generously spoon glaze on the pork; put in a roasting pan. Set remaining glaze aside for later use.
6. Roast at medium heat (300°) until pork reaches an internal temperature of 160° (about 1 hour). Don't overcook the pork or it will be dry.
7. Add beef stock to remaining glaze in sauté pan and simmer for one minute. Stir in mixture of cornstarch, salt, water, and chicken stock. Let mixture cook until sauce coats a spoon.
8. Serve pork with thickened sauce spooned over the top.

Recipe supplied by:

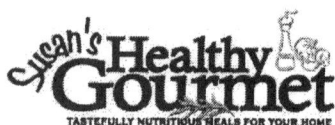

Susan's Healthy Gourmet
1-888-EZ-MEALS (396-3257)
Conveniently located pick-up around Los Angeles County

POBLANO TURKEY CHILI

The creative blending of mild poblano and pasilla peppers enriches the character of this healthy, substantive chili reminiscent of Mexican mole. Analysis for 8oz. (cup) serving.

Nutrition Information per Serving:

✓✓ CALORIES: Excellent Choice (215) ✓ CHOLESTEROL: Good Choice (95 mg)
✓✓ FAT: Excellent Choice (4 g) ✓ SODIUM: GOOD CHOICE (410 mg)
EXCHANGES: 5 Meat, 1¼ Veg, ½ Fat
PROTEIN: 36 g, CARBOHYDRATE: 9 g, FIBER: 2 g

This nutrition analysis corresponds to the recipe below. The restaurant version may differ.

Ingredients (12 servings):

2 Tbs. vegetable oil
2 large yellow onions, coarsely chopped
3 lbs. ground white meat turkey (no skin)
4 Tbs. ground Pasilla chili powder
2 whole poblano chile peppers, seeded & coarsely chopped
4 cloves garlic, minced
1 Tbs. ground cumin
1 can (28oz.) chopped tomatoes with liquid
1 tsp each salt and pepper

Directions:
For best results, use heavy sauce pan or dutch oven with lid.

1. Sauté the chopped onions in vegetable oil until slightly softened (excess oil will be removed later in process).
2. Add ground turkey and Poblano chile and continue to cook with onions while stirring frequently until turkey is "crumbly".
3. Cover with water and bring to a low boil.
4. Add Pasilla chile powder, garlic, salt and pepper.
5. Reduce heat to simmer, partially cover with lid and continue to simmer for about one hour.
6. Skim any residual fat from surface, stir and continue to cook for 10 minutes*.
7. Serve with fresh scallions and cilantro.

* For a slightly "thicker chili, after defatting, add 3 Tbs. corn masa flour or 2 Tbs. cornstarch diluted with warm water. Masa flour or cornstarch not included in analysis.

Recipe supplied by:

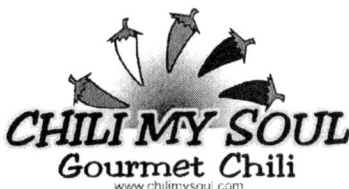

CHILI MY SOUL
Gourmet Chili
www.chilimysoul.com

Chili My Soul
4928 Balboa Blvd., Encino 91316
(818) 981-SOUL (7685)

POLLO PRIMAVERA ☙

Chicken sautéed with vegetables and served with spaghetti in a marinara sauce.

Nutrition Information per Serving:

✓ CALORIES: Good Choice (675)　　✓ CHOLESTEROL: Good Choice (85 mg)
✓✓ FAT: Excellent Choice (14 g)　　　SODIUM: Moderate (685 mg)
EXCHANGES: 4½ Meat, 4 Bread, 5¼ Veg, 1½ Fat
PROTEIN: 49 g, CARBOHYDRATE: 91 g, FIBER: 12 g

This nutrition analysis corresponds to the recipe below. The restaurant version may differ.

Ingredients (4 servings):

4 - 4oz. chicken breasts
2 Tbs. olive oil
2 Tbs. garlic, minced
3 cups carrots, diced
1 lb fresh broccoli, chopped

½ lb. eggplant, chopped
1 medium zucchini, chopped
2 tsp. black pepper
12 oz. spaghetti (dry wt.)
marinara sauce (see recipe below)

Marinara Sauce:
3 lbs. fresh tomatoes
1 Tbs. fresh basil, diced
½ tsp salt

¼ tsp. sugar
¼ Tbs. oil

Directions:

1. Skin, seed and dice tomatoes. Place diced tomatoes in a large saucepan and heat over low-medium heat.
2. Heat olive oil and garlic in a large pan until garlic is golden brown.
3. Brown chicken in oil and garlic.
4. While chicken is cooking, add basil, salt, sugar and oil to tomatoes. Simmer approximately two minutes.
5. Add the raw, chopped vegetables and pepper to the chicken and sauté until vegetables are cooked but still firm.
6. Cook spaghetti according to package directions. Once cooked, keep warm and set aside.
7. Add the marinara sauce to chicken and vegetables and cook until heated through (about one minute).
8. Pour sauce over the cooked spaghetti and serve!

Recipe supplied by:

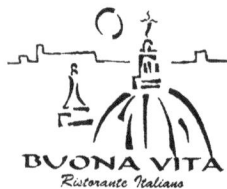

Buona Vita

Buona Vita Pizzeria 425 Pier Avenue,
Hermosa Beach 90254 (310) 372-2233

Buona Vita Trattoria 439 Pier Avenue,
Hermosa Beach 90254 (310) 379-7626

Buona Vita On Main 427 Main Street,
Park City Utah 84060 (435) 658-0999

　　　　　　☙at least 2 fruit/vegetable servings

RIGATONI AL POLLO

Pasta tubes, grilled chicken breast, broccoli, sun-dried tomatoes, olive oil & garlic.

Nutrition Information per Serving:

✓ CALORIES: Good Choice (570) ✓✓ CHOLESTEROL: Excellent Choice (65 mg)
✓✓ FAT: Excellent Choice (12 g) SODIUM: Moderate (665 mg)
EXCHANGES: 3½ Meat (extra lean), 4 Bread, 1¾ Veg, 1½ Fat
PROTEIN: 40 g, CARBOHYDRATE: 79 g

This nutrition analysis corresponds to the recipe below. The restaurant version may differ.

Ingredients (4 servings):

12 oz. tube pasta (dry weight) 4 oz. sun-dried tomatoes
12 oz. chicken breast, skinless, boneless 2 Tbs. extra virgin olive oil
½ lb. broccoli 1 clove garlic, minced

Directions:

1. Cook rigatoni in salted boiling water. Drain.
2. Grill the chicken until done. Cut into cubes.
3. Sauté the chicken, oil, broccoli, sun-dried tomatoes and garlic for 1 to 2 minutes. Chicken broth may be substituted for oil, if desired.
4. Toss the sautéed chicken-vegetable mix with the pasta.
5. Serve with grated parmesan cheese if desired (not included in analysis above).

Recipe supplied by:

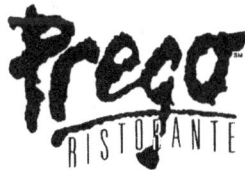

Prego Ristorante
362 N. Camden Drive
Beverly Hills, CA 90210
(310) 277-7346

SPICY CHICKEN SICILLIANO ♉

Sautéed chicken breast topped with a red spicy garlic sauce, capers, black olives and mushrooms.

Nutrition Information per Serving:

✓ CALORIES: Good Choice (480)   ✓ CHOLESTEROL: Good Choice (130 mg)
✓ FAT: Good Choice (20 g)   SODIUM: High (1340 mg)
EXCHANGES: 6¾ Meat, 3¾ Veg, 3 Fat
PROTEIN: 52 g, CARBOHYDRATE: 22 g, FIBER: 1 g

This nutrition analysis corresponds to the recipe below. The restaurant version may differ.

Ingredients (4 servings):

4 6-oz. chicken breast, skinless   ½ tsp. chili peppers
2 Tbs. olive oil   ½ tsp. pepper
¾ lb. mushrooms, fresh   ¾ cup white wine
4 tsp. capers   3 cups marinara sauce
1 oz. olives

Directions:
1. Heat olive oil in large sauté pan. Add mushrooms and sauté until browned.
2. Add remaining ingredients except chicken. Bring to a boil and then turn heat to low and let simmer.
3. While sauce is simmering, grill or bake chicken breasts until done.
4. Place chicken breasts on plates. Cover with marinara sauce.

Recipe supplied by:

Café Luna
1870 W. Carson St., Torrance 90501   (310) 787-1223
8383 Wilshire Blvd. Beverly Hills, 90210 (323) 658-6080

♉ at least 2 fruit/vegetable servings

ALLA BUON GUSTO ✿

Pasta with zucchini, mushrooms, fresh tomato sauce and garlic.

Nutrition Information per Serving:

✓ CALORIES: Good Choice (485)   ✓✓ CHOLESTEROL: Excellent Choice (0 mg)
✓✓ FAT: Excellent Choice (15 g)   ✓✓ SODIUM: Excellent Choice (280 mg)
EXCHANGES: 4¼ Bread, 1½ Veg, 2¾ Fat
PROTEIN: 13 g, CARBOHYDRATE: 75 g, FIBER: 6 g

This nutrition analysis corresponds to the recipe below. The restaurant version may differ.
*Primarily unsaturated fat

Ingredients (4 servings):

¼ cup olive oil
4 tsp. garlic
¼ cup onions, chopped
2 cups zucchini, sliced
2 cups fresh tomatoes, chopped
½ cup mushrooms, chopped

2 tsp. parsley
1 cup white wine
12 oz. pasta, uncooked
½ tsp salt
½ tsp. pepper

Directions:

1. Prepare pasta as directed on package.
2. Heat olive oil in a large sauté pan. Add garlic and onions.
3. When onions are soft, add zucchini, tomatoes and mushrooms.
4. Add white wine and reduce.
5. Add salt, pepper and parsley.
6. Toss with pasta and serve.
7. Sprinkle with Parmesan cheese if desired (not included in analysis).

Recipe supplied by:

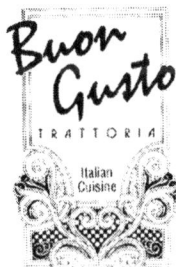

Buon Gusto
5755 East Pacific Coast Highway
Long Beach 90803
(562) 498-1135

LASAGNA POMODORO ♉

Spinach lasagna with layers of sautéed vegetables and herbed tomato sauce.

Nutrition Information per Serving:

✓✓ CALORIES: Excellent Choice (405) ✓✓ CHOLESTEROL: Excellent Choice (35mg)
✓✓ FAT: Excellent Choice (13 g)   SODIUM: High (1,000 mg)
EXCHANGES: 1¾ Meat, ¾ Bread, 6 Veg, 1¼ Fat
PROTEIN: 24 g, CARBOHYDRATE: 54 g, FIBER: 10 g

This nutrition analysis corresponds to the recipe below. The restaurant version may differ.

Ingredients (9 servings):

1 lb. spinach, washed   48 oz. herbed pasta sauce**
1 Tbs. olive oil (for sautéing)   1 Tbs. garlic, minced
6 cups onions, julienned   1 Tbs. basil, dried
6 cups carrots (cut into rounds)   1 Tbs. dried oregano
6 cups zucchini (cut into rounds)   ½ Tbs. sea salt
6 cups mushrooms, thinly sliced   ½ tsp. black pepper
1 tsp. olive oil (for oiling pan)   4 cups skim ricotta or soft tofu cheese***
6 spinach dry lasagna noodles, eggless*

*   Real Food Daily recommends Westbrae Natural Organic Spinach Lasagna noodles.
**   Real Food Daily recommends Muir Glen Organic Italian Herb Pasta Sauce (used for analysis).
*** Real Food Daily recommends that you use a soft tofu cheese.

Directions:

1. Steam the spinach until it just wilts. Cool with cold running water and press out any excess liquid. Set aside.
2. Heat 1 Tbs. olive oil in a large stockpot. Add onions and carrots and sauté until the onions are translucent and begin to soften.
3. Add the zucchini and mushrooms and sauté until all of the vegetables start to soften. Add the garlic, basil, oregano, salt and pepper. Sauté a few minutes more.
4. Strain any excess water off of the vegetables. Set vegetables aside.
5. Soak the spinach noodles until soft and flexible.
6. Coat a 2-inch deep lasagna pan with 1 tsp. oil. Layer the ingredients in pan in this order: ½ cup tomato sauce, 3 noodles, 2 cups ricotta or tofu cheese, sautéed vegetable mixture, steamed spinach, ½ cup tomato sauce, 3 noodles, 2 cups ricotta or tofu cheese, ½ cup tomato sauce.
7. Cover lasagna with aluminum foil. The lasagna can be refrigerated or baked immediately.
8. Bake in a 350° oven for 1 hour and 15 minutes.
9. Remove from oven and let rest for 5-10 minutes before cutting. Cut lasagna into 9 pieces.
10. Heat remaining pasta sauce. Spoon ½ cup sauce over each piece of lasagna.

Recipe supplied by:

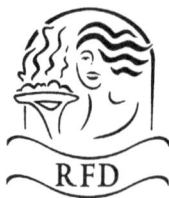

REAL FOOD DAILY
ORGANIC VEGETARIAN COOKING

514 Santa Monica Blvd., Santa Monica 90401 (310) 451-7544
414 N. La Cienega Blvd., Los Angeles 90048 (310) 289-9910

♉ at least 2 fruit/vegetable servings

LINGUINE ALLA TREVI

Linguine pasta with eggplant, basil, garlic, fresh tomatoes and extra virgin olive oil.

Nutrition Information per Serving:

✓✓ CALORIES: Excellent Choice (390)   ✓✓ CHOLESTEROL: Excellent Choice (0 mg)
✓✓ FAT: Excellent Choice (7 g)   ✓✓ SODIUM: Excellent Choice (15 mg)**
EXCHANGES: 5½ Bread, ¾ Veg, 1 Fat
PROTEIN: 15 g, CARBOHYDRATE: 91 g, FIBER: 6 g

This nutrition analysis corresponds to the recipe below. The restaurant version may differ.

Ingredients (4 servings):

1 large eggplant
12 oz. pasta, dry weight
4 tsp. olive oil
3 medium tomatoes, chopped

4 cloves garlic, minced
16 fresh basil leaves, chopped
½ tsp. pepper
salt to taste (not included in analysis)

Directions:

1. Chop eggplant. Spread out eggplant pieces on a cookie sheet and bake at 350° until soft (10 – 15 minutes).
2. Boil water and cook pasta as directed on package.
3. Add oil to sauté pan, and sauté eggplant, tomato, garlic, basil, salt and pepper.
4. Drain pasta and add to tomato/eggplant mix. Sauté until hot.

Recipe supplied by:

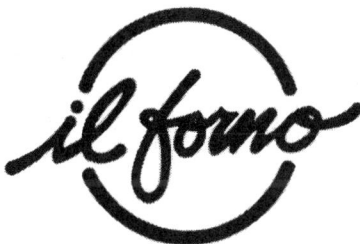

il Forno

2901 Ocean Park Blvd., Santa Monica 90405   (310) 450-1241

LINGUINI DEL MAR

Assorted seafood with marinara sauce over pasta.

Nutrition Information per Serving:

✓ CALORIES: Good Choice (690)   CHOLESTEROL: Moderate (275 mg)

✓ FAT: Good Choice (19 g)*   SODIUM: Moderate (850 mg)

EXCHANGES: 4½ Meat (extra lean),4¼ Bread, 1¼ Veg, 3 Fat

PROTEIN: 49 g, CARBOHYDRATE: 76 g, Fiber: 5 g

This nutrition analysis corresponds to the recipe below. The restaurant version may differ.

* primarily unsaturated fat

Ingredients (4 servings):

12 oz. linguini (dry weight)	½ lb. halibut
2 Tbs. olive oil	½ lb. shrimp
1¼ lb. (about 20) small clams	½ lb. calimari
2 tsp. minced garlic	1 cup clam juice
pinch red pepper flakes	2 cups (16 oz) marinara sauce

Directions:

1. Cook the linguini according to directions. Rinse and drain.
2. Heat oil in sauté pan. Add the clams and sauté until they begin to open.
3. Add garlic and chili flakes and cook until garlic starts to brown.
4. Add the halibut, shrimp and calamari. Cook until shrimp starts to turn pink.
5. Add the clam juice and marinara and cook until the seafood is fully cooked.
6. Toss the pasta into the sauce and serve.

Recipe supplied by:

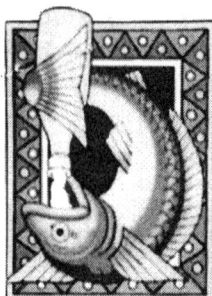

Rock'N Fish
120 Manhattan Beach Boulevard
Manhattan Beach, CA 90266
(310) 379-9900

NEPTUNE LOAF ☯

Fettucine pasta, veggies, tofu & cheese, smothered in Savory Sauce.

Nutrition Information per Serving:

✓✓ CALORIES: Excellent Choice (250)   ✓✓ CHOLESTEROL: Excellent Choice (65 mg)
✓✓ FAT: Excellent Choice (12 g)   ✓✓ SODIUM: Excellent Choice (285 mg)
EXCHANGES: 1½ Meat, 1¼ Bread, ½ Veg, 1½ Fat
PROTEIN: 15 g, CARBOHYDRATE: 22 g

This nutrition analysis corresponds to the recipe below. The restaurant version may differ.

Ingredients (12 servings):

12 oz. whole wheat noodles (dry weight)
½ bell pepper
1½ stalks celery
½ cup chopped onion
2 cups assorted vegetables of your choice
3 cups shredded cheddar cheese

1 lb. tofu, chopped into
   small cubes
2 eggs
½ tsp. minced garlic
1 Tbs. Bragg liquid aminos
1 tsp. tamari sauce

Directions:

1. Cook noodles as directed on package. Drain and rinse.
2. Steam bell pepper, celery, onion and assorted vegetables for 3 to 5 minutes.
3. Mix 2 cups of cheese and remaining ingredients in a large bowl. Add pasta and vegetables and stir until well combined.
4. Press into a lightly oiled 9x12-inch pan. Sprinkle with remaining cheese and bake 40 to 45 minutes in a 400° oven.

Recipe from: *Recipes from the Heart* book by Tonya Beaudet, owner of :

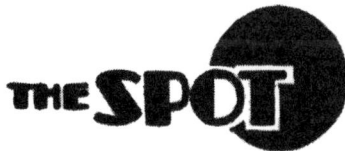

THE SPOT

The Spot
Natural Food Restaurant
110 Second Street
Hermosa Beach, CA 90254
(310) 301-7074

PASTA MARE E MONTI

Pasta with Italian porcini mushrooms, shrimp, garlic, white wine & light tomato sauce.

Nutrition Information per Serving:

✓ CALORIES: Good Choice (500)   CHOLESTEROL: Moderate (220 mg)
✓✓ FAT: Excellent Choice (10)*   SODIUM: High (1560 mg)**
     EXCHANGES: 3½ Meat (extra lean), 2½ Bread, ¼ Veg, 1¼ Fat
          PROTEIN: 38 g, CARBOHYDRATE: 62 g

This nutrition analysis corresponds to the recipe below. The restaurant version may differ.

* Primarily unsaturated fat
** Sodium may be reduced by using low-sodium marinara sauce

Ingredients (4 servings):

8 oz. dry pasta

2 Tbs. olive oil

4 tsp. garlic, minced

4 oz. dried porcini mushrooms, thinly sliced

10 oz. white shrimp

¾ cup white wine

3½ cups marinara sauce

4 tsp. parsley

1 tsp. black pepper

1 tsp. red pepper

Directions:

1. Cook pasta al dente and set aside.
2. Rehydrate porcini mushrooms in water for a few minutes.
3. Heat olive oil in a saucepan.
4. Add garlic, shrimp and mushrooms and sauté.
5. Add white wine to shrimp mix and allow to fully evaporate (approx. 2 min.).
6. Add tomato sauce, parsley, pepper (and salt to taste if desired - not included in analysis above).
7. Simmer 10 to 20 minutes.
8. Drain pasta and add to sauce. Sauté together until heated.

Recipe supplied by:

IL MORO
RISTORANTE • CAFÉ

Il Moro
11400 W. Olympic Blvd.
Los Angeles, CA 90064
(310) 575-3530

SPAGHETTI WITH MUSHROOM SAUCE ☙

Fresh tender mushrooms, swimming in authentic Italian tomato sauce.

Nutrition Information per Serving:

✓✓ CALORIES: Excellent Choice (440) ✓✓ CHOLESTEROL: Excellent Choice (0 mg)
✓✓ FAT: Excellent Choice (4 g)   ✓ SODIUM: Good Choice (580 mg)
EXCHANGES: 2¼ Veg, 5¼ Bread, ½ Fat,
PROTEIN: 12 g, CARBOHYDRATE: 91 g, FIBER: 5 g

This nutrition analysis corresponds to the recipe below.   The restaurant version may differ.

Ingredients (6 servings):

1 Tbs. vegetable oil, divided
⅓ cup onion, chopped fine
3 cloves garlic, minced
1 28 oz. can diced tomatoes in juice
6 oz tomato puree
1 tsp. salt
¾ Tbs. sugar
1 pinch black pepper

½ Tbs. crushed oregano
½ Tbs. fresh parsley (chopped fine)
1 Tbs. red wine
⅓ cup water
½ Tbs. corn starch
½ lb. large mushrooms, sliced
16 oz. spaghetti, uncooked

Directions:

1. Place a large saucepan on stove over medium heat.
2. Add ½ Tablespoon oil, onions and garlic. Cook the garlic and onions until tender; stir frequently (add a little water to prevent scorching if needed).
3. Add the diced tomatoes and tomato puree. Mix thoroughly.
4. Add spices, parsley, and wine. Mix thoroughly.
5. Bring all ingredients to a boil. Simmer for 30 minutes.
6. While sauce simmers, cook pasta according to package directions.
7. Mix cornstarch with water and stir into sauce. Continue simmering while preparing mushrooms.
8. In a separate sauté pan, heat the remaining ½ tablespoon oil.
9. Add mushrooms and sauté until they start to "sweat".
10. Stir the mushrooms into the sauce.
11. Portion spaghetti into dishes. Spoon sauce over pasta.

Recipe supplied by:

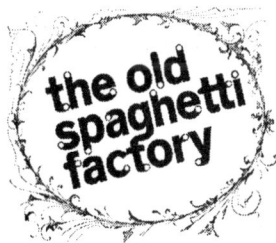

The Old Spaghetti Factory

5939 Sunset Blvd.
Hollywood 90028 (323) 469-7149

1431 Buena Vista
Duarte 91010 (626) 358-2115

☙ at least 2 fruit/vegetable servings

ZITI ALLA PUTTANESCA

Short tube pasta, capers, olives, oregano, and tomato sauce.

Nutrition Information per Serving:

✓ CALORIES: Good Choice (475)   ✓✓ CHOLESTEROL: Excellent Choice (0 mg)
✓ FAT: Good Choice (16 g)*   SODIUM: Moderate (835 mg)
EXCHANGES: 4 Bread, 1¼ Veg, 2¼ Fat
PROTEIN: 12 g, CARBOHYDRATE: 67 g

This nutrition analysis corresponds to the recipe below. The restaurant version may differ.

*Primarily unsaturated fat

Ingredients (4 servings):

12 oz. ziti (short tube pasta), dry weight

Tomato Sauce:
5 cloves garlic
3 Tbs. olive oil
32 oz. canned tomatoes (chopped) with juice
½ tsp. salt
½ tsp. white pepper
10 leaves basil, coarsely chopped

Topping:
2 tsp. oil
4 garlic cloves, crushed
4 tsp. capers
¾ cup chopped black olives
¼ tsp. oregano
4 oz. white wine

Directions:

Pasta:
Cook pasta according to directions on package. Drain.

Tomato sauce:
1. In saucepan, sauté garlic in olive oil at medium high heat until almost black.
2. Discard the garlic (flavor remains in the oil). Add chopped tomatoes and juice.
3. Add salt, pepper and coarsely chopped basil. Stir.
4. Simmer 20 minutes or until desired consistency. (Sauce can be frozen).

Topping:
1. Sauté olive oil, garlic, capers, olives and oregano.
2. Add white wine and simmer until wine evaporates.
3. Add tomato sauce.
4. Simmer for several minutes, add to cooked pasta and serve.

Recipe supplied by:

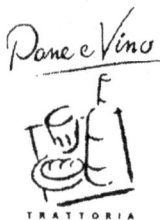

Pane e Vino

Pane e Vino
8265 Beverly Boulevard
Los Angeles, CA   90048
(323) 651-4600

TRATTORIA

BRUSCHETTA

A great dip! Serve with toasted bread slices or crackers.

Nutrition Information per Serving †:
(2 Tablespoons)

✓✓ CALORIES: Excellent Choice (30)   ✓✓ CHOLESTEROL: Excellent Choice (0 mg)
✓✓ FAT: Excellent Choice (3 g)   ✓✓ SODIUM: Excellent Choice (2 mg)
EXCHANGES: ¼ Veg, 1 Fat
PROTEIN: 0 g, CARBOHYDRATE: 1 g, FIBER: 0 g

This nutrition analysis corresponds to the recipe below. The restaurant version may differ.
† Side dish guidelines are 1/3 of entrée guidelines

Ingredients (20 servings):

2 cups (1 lb.) Roma tomatoes, chopped
2 tsp. garlic, chopped
½ cup basil, chopped
¼ cup olive oil
Squeeze of lemon

Directions:

1. Mix together chopped tomatoes, garlic and chopped basil.
2. Drizzle olive oil over mixture and stir lightly.
3. Finish with a squeeze of lemon and serve.

Recipe supplied by:

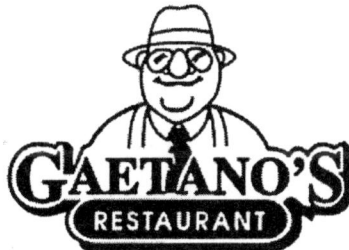

Gaetano's Restaurant
25345 Crenshaw Blvd., Torrance 90505 (310) 326-0266

CLAM AND MUSHROOM MISO SOUP

Ingredients (4 servings):

2 lbs. marina clams
2 oz. oyster mushrooms, chopped
2 oz. shiitake mushrooms, chopped
2 oz. white mushrooms, chopped
1½ cups spinach

4 cups water
5 oz. white miso soy pesto (soy bean paste)
2 green onion stems, chopped
½ bunch chives, chopped

Directions:

1. In a medium saucepan add clams, chopped mushrooms, spinach and water.
2. Heat at medium-high heat until clamshells open.
3. Next, add miso soy pesto, stir, and cook for approximately 2½ minutes.
4. To serve – Pour in soup bowls and garnish with chopped green onions and chives.

Recipe supplied by:

CHAYA
BRASSERIE

8741 Alden Dr., Los Angeles 90048
(310) 859-883

CHAYA
VENICE

110 Navy St., Venice 90291
(310) 396-1179

GARLIC MASHED POTATOES

Ingredients (4 servings):

1½ lb red potatoes   ¼ tsp kosher salt
8-10 garlic cloves, peeled $^1/_3$ tsp black pepper
½ cup non-fat sour cream

Directions:

1. Clean and peel potatoes. It is okay to leave some of the potato skin on.
2. Boil potatoes and garlic until fork-tender in a large pot.
3. Drain water.
4. Add non-fat sour cream, salt and black pepper to cooked potatoes and garlic.
5. Hand mash ingredients together, creating a smooth and lumpy texture.

Recipe supplied by·

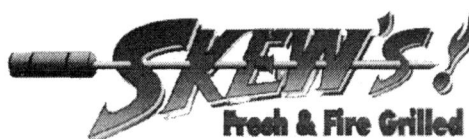

Skew's Fresh and Fire Grilled
300 South Grand Ave., Los Angeles 90036 (213) 613-0300

MISTICANZA DI VERDURE GRIGLIATE ♂

Zucchini, yellow squash, mushrooms, eggplant, carrots, red onions, bell peppers, vine-ripened tomatoes, and asparagus grilled to perfection. Dressing is not included in analysis.

Nutrition Information per Serving:

✓✓ CALORIES: Excellent Choice (205)   ✓✓ CHOLESTEROL: Excellent Choice (0 mg)
✓✓ FAT: Excellent Choice (14 g)*   ✓✓ SODIUM: Excellent Choice (10 mg)
EXCHANGES: ¾ Bread, 2 Veg, 2¾ Fat
PROTEIN: 4 g, CARBOHYDRATE: 21 g

This nutrition analysis corresponds to the recipe below. The restaurant version may differ.

*Primarily unsaturated fat

Ingredients (4 servings):

½ zucchini   ½ lb. shiitake mushrooms
½ yellow squash   ½ red onion
1 Japanese eggplant   1 large tomato
¼ lb. asparagus   1 carrot
¼ green bell pepper   3 Tbs. olive oil
¼ red or yellow bell pepper

Directions:

1. Cut the vegetables into slices.
2. Heat a large cast iron skillet to medium high. Pour oil into skillet, evenly coating it.
3. Grill each vegetable on each side for about 2 minutes, and arrange on 3 to 4 large plates as vegetables are grilled.
4. Finish (coat lightly) with remaining oil and serve with dressing on the side (not included in analysis).

Recipe supplied by:

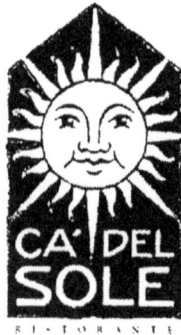

Ca' Del Sole
4100 Cahuenga Blvd.
North Hollywood, CA 91602
(818) 985-4669

♂ at least 2 fruit/vegetable servings

RED BEET CARPACCIO ♨

red onions, ricotta salata & tangerine emulsion.

Nutrition Information per Serving †:

✓ CALORIES: Good Choice (175)   ✓✓ CHOLESTEROL: Excellent Choice (5 mg)
   FAT: Moderate (9 g)   SODIUM: Moderate (210 mg)
   EXCHANGES: ½ Meat, 1½ Veg, 1½ Fat, ½ Fruit
   PROTEIN: 5 g, CARBOHYDRATE: 20 g, FIBER: 4 g

This nutrition analysis corresponds to the recipe below. The restaurant version may differ.

† Side dish guidelines are ⅓ of entrée guidelines

Ingredients (4 servings):

½ cup orange juice
2 Tbs. sherry vinegar
1 medium shallot, chopped
2 Tbs. extra virgin olive oil
1 pinch each salt and pepper
2 medium beets, peeled, roasted or
  boiled until soft

3 tangerines
½ medium red onion, chopped
1 bunch watercress, rinsed & chopped
1 oz. ricotta salata or
  parmesan (shaved)

Directions:

1. In a small saucepan heat the orange juice and simmer until reduced by half.
2. Once orange juice is reduced, whisk in sherry vinegar, shallots, olive oil, salt and pepper. Set aside and allow to cool.
3. Slice one beet thinly and arrange disks to cover the bottom of a large plate. Cover with ¾ of the shaved cheese.
4. Dice the remaining beet into ½ inch cubes.
5. Zest the tangerine peels. Segment the inner fruit.
6. Toss the zest, tangerines, diced beets, onion and watercress with the cooled dressing.
7. Place this mixture in the center of the sliced beets and top with the remaining cheese.

Recipe supplied by:

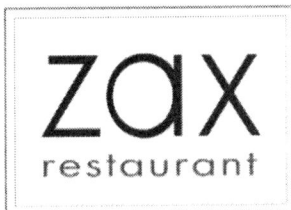

zax
restaurant

Zax Restaurant
11604 San Vicente Blvd.,
Brentwood 90049 (310) 571-3800

SEMOLINA GRIDDLE CAKES
WITH COCONUT CHUTNEY (UTTAPAMS)

Uttapams are delicious griddle cakes, fragrant with onions, cilantro, or whatever flavoring strikes your fancy, topped with spicy coconut chutney. They are frequently served for brunch in southern India.

Nutrition Information per Serving:

✓✓ CALORIES: Excellent Choice (415)   ✓✓ CHOLESTEROL: Excellent Choice (10 mg)
✓ FAT: Good Choice (19 g)   ✓ SODIUM: Good Choice (570 mg)
EXCHANGES: 2¾ Bread , ½ Veg, ¼ Milk, 3¾ Fat
PROTEIN: 10 g, CARBOHYDRATE: 49 g

This nutrition analysis corresponds to the recipe below. The restaurant version may differ.

Ingredients (6 servings of 2 cakes each):

Griddle Cakes:
2 cups semolina flour†
1¼ cups plain yogurt
1 cup water
1 tsp. salt
¼ cup corn oil
1 cup toppings of your choice
  (onion, cilantro, serrano
  chilies, tomatoes, etc.)

Coconut Chutney:
½ coconut, peeled & grated
1 Tbs. sour cream
1½ Tbs. plain yogurt
½ tsp. salt   1 Tbs. corn oil
½ tsp. mustard seeds†   ¼ tsp. urid dal†
½ tsp. cumin seeds†   2-3 kari leaves†
1-2 dried red chiles, broken in small pieces
1-2 green Serrano chiles, coarsely chopped

†Available in Indian or specialty markets. Cream of Wheat can be substituted for semolina flour.

Directions:

Semolina Griddle Cakes:
1. Combine semolina flour, yogurt, water, and salt, stirring until smooth. Cover bowl with plastic wrap and set aside at room temp. for 2 hours.
2. Heat a non-stick griddle or skillet until droplets of water dance, as for pancakes. Pour ¼ cup of batter onto griddle and spread to ¼ inch thick. Quickly sprinkle the desired toppings onto batter and press into batter with the back of a spoon. Drizzle a tsp. oil around edges of pancake and cook 1 min. Flip over, drizzle more oil. Cook 1-2 min. more, until lightly browned. Continue until batter is used, keeping the uttapams under foil in a warm oven as they are made.
3. To serve, place on a warm platter with a Tbs. of chutney beside each uttapam.

Coconut Chutney:
1. Place grated coconut, sour cream, and yogurt in a blender and process, with a little water as needed, to make a smooth paste. Add salt, transfer to a small serving bowl, and set side.
2. Heat oil in a small saucepan with a lid over high heat. Add remaining ingredients and cover to avoid splattering. After the popping has subsided (30 - 45 sec.), lift the lid and sauté until the spices have finished sizzling (1-2 min.). Stir into the coconut mixture and serve with uttapams.

Recipe supplied by:

BOMBAY
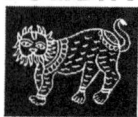
C A F E

Bombay Cafe
12021 W. Pico Blvd.
West Los Angeles
(310) 473-3388

SOFT TOFU AND BROCCOLI ✣

Soft cubes of tofu with broccoli, black mushrooms, garlic and special sauce.

Nutrition Information per Serving:

✓✓ CALORIES: Excellent Choice (315)   ✓✓ CHOLESTEROL: Excellent Choice (<1 mg)
✓✓ FAT: Excellent Choice (6 g)*   SODIUM: High (3585 mg)
EXCHANGES: 1¼ Meat, 1 Bread, 2½ Veg, 2¾ Fat
PROTEIN: 19 g, CARBOHYDRATE: 47 g

This nutrition analysis corresponds to the recipe below. The restaurant version may differ.
*Primarily unsaturated fat

Ingredients (4 servings):

Brown sauce:

1⅓ cup hot water
2½ tsp. chicken powder
1½ Tbs. corn syrup
¾ cup soy sauce
2½ Tbs. sugar
¼ cup rice wine
1¼ Tbs. sherry
¼ tsp. Gravy Master or Kitchen Bouquet
1½ Tbs. oyster sauce

Tofu & Broccoli:

3 to 4 oz. black mushrooms (dry)
24 oz. soft tofu, cut in ¾ inch cubes
2 tsp. garlic, minced
2 lbs. broccoli, steamed until
    just crunchy
¼ cup cornstarch
5 Tbs. hot water

Directions:

Brown sauce:
1. Mix chicken granules and corn syrup in hot water with a wire whip.
2. Add soy sauce, sugar, gravy master, rice wine, sherry, and oyster sauce.
3. Blend again with wire whip and set aside.

Tofu & Broccoli:
1. Quickly rinse black mushroom halves. Place mushrooms in medium sauté pan with 2 cups boiling water and cook 5 to 10 seconds until mushrooms change from dull to shiny in appearance. Drain, reserving the water and hold mushrooms.
2. Blanch soft tofu cubes in hot water approx. 10 seconds. Drain water from tofu cubes.
3. Add garlic to wok and stir fry for 5 seconds on medium heat.
4. Add black mushrooms and stir fry for approximately 15 - 20 seconds on medium heat.
5. Add brown sauce & broccoli. Stir fry for 10 - 15 sec. on high until sauce boils.
6. Add 2 Tbs. warm water to cornstarch and stir. Add 3 Tbs. more water and stir again. Then add mixture to the garlic-broccoli-mushroom mixture and cook until thickened.
7. Add soft tofu cubes and gently toss for approx. 5 seconds (so tofu doesn't break up but is evenly distributed and coated with sauce).

Recipe supplied by:

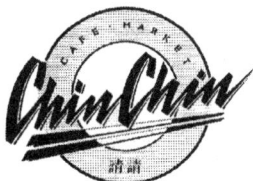

Chin Chin

West Hollywood: 8618 Sunset Blvd.	(310) 652-1818
Brentwood: 11740 San Vicente Blvd.	(310) 826-2525
Beverly Hills: 206 So. Beverly Dr.	(310) 248-5252
Studio City: 12215 Ventura Blvd.	(818) 985-9090
Marina Del Rey: 13455 Maxella Ave.	(310) 823-9999
Encino: 16101 Ventura Boulevard	(818) 783-1717
Las Vegas: New York, NY Hotel & Casino	(702) 240-6300

FRESH PEACH COBBLER 🍎

Nutrition Information per Serving†:

CALORIES: Moderate (355) ✓ CHOLESTEROL: Good Choice (45 mg)
✓✓ FAT: Excellent Choice (3 g) ✓✓ SODIUM: Excellent Choice (100 mg)
EXCHANGES: ¼ Meat, 4¼ Bread, 1 Fruit, ½ Fat
PROTEIN: 4 g, CARBOHYDRATE: 81 g

This nutrition analysis corresponds to the recipe below. The restaurant version may differ.

† Side dish guidelines are ⅓ of entrée guidelines

Ingredients (8 servings):

2¾ lbs. fresh peaches
¾ cups sugar
½ cup brown sugar
¾ tsp. cinnamon
½ Tbs. flour
¼ tsp. salt
½ Tbs. orange juice

¼ Tbs. lemon juice
1 Tbs. butter
½ Tbs. vanilla extract
1 cup flour
¾ cup sugar
½ Tbs. baking powder
1½ eggs

Directions:

1. Peel peaches and cut into thin slices.
2. Combine peaches, sugar, cinnamon, flour, salt, orange juice, lemon juice, butter and vanilla extract. Mix well and place in baking dish.
3. In a bowl, mix together flour, sugar, and baking powder. Add eggs and mix well.
4. Spread topping over peach mixture. Bake at 350 for about 30 minutes, until topping rises and is golden brown. Enjoy!

Recipe supplied by:

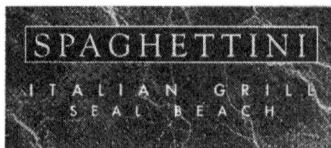

Spaghettini Italian Grill
3005 Old Ranch Parkway
Seal Beach, CA 90740
(562) 596-2199 or
(714) 960- 6002

GRILLED MANGO WITH RASPBERRY COULIS ♉

Ingredients (4 servings):

2 mangos
3 Tbs. lime juice

3 Tbs. brown sugar
½ cup fresh raspberries

1. Peel mangos and slice them into "filets".
2. In a medium bowl, mix brown sugar and lime juice.
3. Marinate mangos in the brown sugar and lime juice mixture.
4. Grill mangoes flat side down to caramelize the brown sugar. Once done, remove from heat.
5. Reserve marinade and blend with raspberries in a blender or food processor (to create raspberry coulis).
6. Cut grilled mangoes into spears and divide equally among four dessert dishes.
7. Pour sauce over mangos. Serve and enjoy!

Recipe supplied by:

Whole Foods Market

3rd & Fairfax: 6350 W. Third St.   (323) 964-6800
Beverly Hills: 239 N. Crescent Dr.   (310) 274-3360
Brentwood: 11737 San Vicente Blvd.   (310) 826-4433
Glendale: 826 N. Glendale Ave.   (818) 240-9350
Porter Ranch: 19340 Rinaldi   (818) 363-3933
Pasadena: 3751 East Foothill Blvd.   (626) 351-5994
Redondo Beach: 405 N. PCH   (310) 376-6931
Sherman Oaks East: 12905 Riverside Dr.   (818) 762-5548
Sherman Oaks West: 4520 Sepulveda Blvd.   (818) 382-3700
Thousand Oaks: 451 Avenida de los Arboles   (805) 492-5340
Torrance: 2655 Pacific Coast Hwy.   (310) 257-8700
Tustin: 14945 Holt Ave.   (714) 731-3400
W. Hollywood: 7871 W. Santa Monica Blvd.   (323) 848-4200
W. LA: 11666 National Blvd.   (310) 996-8840
Woodland Hills: 21347 Ventura Blvd.   (818) 610-0000

SPARKLING FRUIT ♨

A light and refreshing dessert of fresh fruit served in champagne or sparking juice.

Nutrition Information per Serving †:

✓ CALORIES: Good Choice (155)   ✓✓ CHOLESTEROL: Excellent Choice (0 mg)
✓✓ FAT: Excellent Choice (<1 g)   ✓✓ SODIUM: Excellent Choice (10 mg)
EXCHANGES: 1¾ Bread, 1 Fruit
PROTEIN: 1 g, CARBOHYDRATE: 39 g, FIBER: 1 g

This nutrition analysis corresponds to the recipe below. The restaurant version may differ.

† Side dish guidelines are ⅓ of entrée guidelines

Ingredients (2 servings):

2 cups fresh fruit seeded and cut into bite-size pieces*
½ cup sugar
1 cup champagne, white wine or sparkling juice
½ tsp. fresh mint, chopped

*Recommended fruits are melon balls, strawberries (hulled and sliced lengthwise), plums, peaches, pears, nectarines (peeled, quartered and seeded).

Directions:

1. In a shallow serving bowl, mix the fruit gently so it is not crushed.
2. Evenly sprinkle with sugar and gently mix again.
3. Pour cold champagne, wine or sparkling juice over fruit.
4. Chill in refrigerator for 1-2 hours.
5. Serve in chilled champagne glasses.

Serving suggestion! Serve with low-fat cookies that will not dissolve quickly in liquid. (not included in analysis).

Recipe supplied by: www.redlobster.com

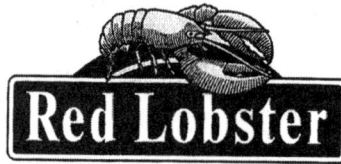

Red Lobster

1041 W. Avenue "P", Palmdale	(661) 538-9707	27524 The Old Road, Valencia	(661) 257-8900
8501 Wilshire Blvd., Beverly Hills	(310) 657-2090	250 Brea Mall, Brea	(714) 529-0632
1740 Venture Blvd., Oxnard	(805) 981-9595		

Part V

Other Editions in the *Healthy Dining* Book Series,

Response Forms,

and

Restaurant Discount Coupons

Healthy Dining in San Diego
Participating Restaurants:

Acapulco Mexican Restaurant Y Cantina
Andiamo! Italian Restaurant
Anthony's Fish Grotto
Bandar Fine Persian Cuisine
Bernard'O Restaurant
Bistro Yang
Brasserie La Costa
Bully's
Café India
Café Japengo
Casa de Bandini
Casa de Pico
Casa Guadalajara
Chili's Grill & Bar
Chin's Szechwan Cuisine
Claim Jumper Restaurant
Coco's Bakery Restaurant
Daily's Restaurant
El Callejon
El Indio Mexican Restaurant
Eva's Cocina & Cantina
The Fish Market
The Fish Merchant
Fortune Cookie
French Gourmet
French Market Grille
Greek Palace
Healthy Gourmet
Il Fornaio
Jack in the Box
Jamba Juice
Jimbo's...Naturally!
Kabul West
KC's Tandoor
Ki's Restaurant & Juice Bar
Koo Koo Roo
La Costa Resort & Spa
Ladles
La Salsa

Leucadia Pizzeria
Lino's Italian Restaurant
Los Cabos
Montanas
Mucho Gusto
Nicolosi's Italian Restaurant
The Old Spaghetti Factory
Pacific Coast Grill
Pick Up Stix
Pisces
Pizza Nova
Prego Ristorante
Rainwater's On Kettner
Rancho el Nopal
Ranchos Cocina
Ristorante Figaro
Rock Bottom
Roppongi
Round Table Pizza
Royal Thai Cuisine
Ruby's Diner
St. Germain's Café
Sammy's Woodfired Pizza
SandCrab Café
Sbicca
Sizzler
Souplantation
Spices Thai Café
Star of India
Su Casa
Subway
Sushi On the Rock
Tio Leo's
Trattoria Acqua
Trellises Garden Grille
Tutto Mare
The Vegetarian Zone
Whole Foods Market

Healthy Dining in <u>Orange County</u>

Participating Restaurants:

A La Carte
Acapulco Mexican Restaurant
Antonello Ristorante
Au Lac Vegetarian Restaurant
Back Bay Rowing & Running Club
Bagels & Brew
The Beach House
Birraporetti's
Blueberry Hill
Bluewater Grill
Café Hidalgo
Caffé il Farro
California Pizza Kitchen
California Wok
Capistrano's Restaurant
Carrows
China West
Chin Chin
Chin's Chinese Kitchen
Ciao
The Cottage
Culinary Wraps
Disney's PCH Grill
Dolce Ristorante Italiano
El Torito Restaurants
El Torito Grill
Ferdussi Taste of Persia
Great Harvest Bread Co.
Haute Links
The Health Emporium
Healthy Gourmet
Ho Sum Bistro
Hyatt Newporter, Cantori
Hyatt Newporter, Jamboree Cafe
Inca Amazon Grill
Jamba Juice
Java City
JT Schmid's
JW's Calif. Grill, Newport Beach Marriott
Koo Koo Roo
La Fayette
La Salsa
Lotus Cafe
Luigi's D'Italia
Maggiano's Little Italy

McCormick & Schmick's
Mezzanine at the Towers
Mother's Market and Kitchen
The Old Spaghetti Factory
Peppino's Italian Family Restaurant
Pick Up Stix
Pinot Provence
The Quiet Woman
Red Lobster
Redberry Kaffe
Ristorante Rumari
Romeo Cucina
Round Table Pizza
Royal Thai
Ruby's Diner
Rutabegorz
Sagami Japanese Restaurant
Santa Monica Seafood
Sapori Ristorante, Sapori Trattoria
Scott's Seafood Grill & Bar
Sizzler
Souplantation
Spaghettini Italian Grill
Split Rock Tavern
Stix
Subway
SunFlour Natural Bakery
The Taco Company
Thai Spice
Todai Restaurant
Tustin Ranch Golf Club Restaurant
Tutto Mare
230 Forest Avenue
Vie de France
Villa Roma Ristorante Italiano
Villa Romana Trattoria
The Village Farmer
Wahoo's Fish Taco
Walt's Wharf
Waters Lakehouse
Wendy's
Whole Foods Market
Wild Oats Community Market
Your Personal Chef
Z Pizza

To order any of the *Healthy Dining* editions, see page 186 or call 1-800-DINE (3463)

Say "Thank You" to Restaurant Management

Restaurants that honor your special requests and take active steps to serve healthier meals need to hear from you, the consumer. Write a note of thanks on the restaurant's customer comment card. Or…you can photocopy and clip out this sample Thank You note and give it to management. Use your *Healthy Dining* book to select which restaurants to visit, order menu items featured in the book, and tell management whenever possible that you appreciate the restaurant's participation in *Healthy Dining,* that you use the book and recommend it to your friends and family.

You can also give these notes to restaurants that are not in the *Healthy Dining* book. Tell management about the program and encourage them to get involved. Call the *Healthy Dining* office with any names of potential restaurants for future publications.

Restaurants listen to you, the "Healthy Diner." <u>Together</u>, we can lead the way to a healthier community.

Dear Restaurant Owner/Manager:

THANK YOU…for serving such satisfying food that is lower in calories, fat, cholesterol, and sodium – and dishes that include fruits and vegetables. The top killers of Americans – heart disease, cancer, stroke and diabetes – are closely linked with diet. Your "healthy" leadership is helping improve – even save – lives in Southern California!

To learn more about *Healthy Dining*, call 1-800-953-DINE

Dear Restaurant Owner/Manager:

THANK YOU…for serving such satisfying food that is lower in calories, fat, cholesterol, and sodium – and dishes that include fruits and vegetables. The top killers of Americans – heart disease, cancer, stroke and diabetes – are closely linked with diet. Your "healthy" leadership is helping improve – even save – lives in Southern California!

To learn more about *Healthy Dining*, call 1-800-953-DINE

Dear Restaurant Owner/Manager:

THANK YOU…for serving such satisfying food that is lower in calories, fat, cholesterol, and sodium – and dishes that include fruits and vegetables. The top killers of Americans – heart disease, cancer, stroke and diabetes – are closely linked with diet. Your "healthy" leadership is helping improve – even save – lives in Southern California!

To learn more about *Healthy Dining*, call 1-800-953-DINE

Dear Restaurant Owner/Manager:

THANK YOU…for serving such satisfying food that is lower in calories, fat, cholesterol, and sodium – and dishes that include fruits and vegetables. The top killers of Americans – heart disease, cancer, stroke and diabetes – are closely linked with diet. Your "healthy" leadership is helping improve – even save – lives in Southern California!

To learn more about *Healthy Dining*, call 1-800-953-DINE

Thank You notes are also available at www.healthy-dining.com

$5.00 OFF
your next purchase of *Healthy Dining*

We want to know more about you and your thoughts about *Healthy Dining*. So we'll give you $5.00 off your next copy of *Healthy Dining* if you'll return this questionnaire (information is confidential). To thank you, we will contact you when new editions are published and offer $5.00 off the retail price. You may also order now at the discount price (see reverse side).

1. How did you learn about *Healthy Dining in Los Angeles*?

____ Newspaper	____ Family or friend	____ Dietitian
____ Radio	____ Restaurant	____ Personal Trainer/Fitness Ctr.
____ Television	____ Health Organization	____ Special Event _____
____ Store _____	____ Physician	____ TrEAT Yourself Well Campaign
____ Workplace	____ Internet	____ Other _____

2. Are you on any of these special diets?

____ Weight loss	____ Low-cholesterol	____ Diabetic	____ General health-conscious
____ Low-fat	____ Low-sodium	____ Vegetarian	____ Other _____

3. Please rate the following features of the book:

	Very helpful	Moderately helpful	Not needed
Chapters on general nutrition	____	____	____
List of restaurants offering healthier items	____	____	____
Specific menu items available at these restaurants	____	____	____
Numerical values of fat, calories, cholesterol, etc.	____	____	____
"Excellent Choice" (✓✓) and "Good Choice" (✓) categories	____	____	____
Restaurant coupons	____	____	____
Chefs' recipes section	____	____	____

4. Please list your favorite restaurants from this book:

5. What other restaurants would you like to see in the next edition?

6. Please list your favorite recipes from the Chefs' Recipes section:

7. On average, how many times <u>per month</u> do you dine out? _____ Do you use the coupons? _____

8. Is this book primarily used by: ___ female ___ male ___ both ____ how many?

9. What is the age of the primary user of this book?
   ____ Under 30 ____ 30 to 45 ____ 45 to 60 ____ over 60

10. What other food or health-related publications do you read? (Health Magazine, Berkeley Wellness, Nutrition Action Healthletter, Eating Well, Cooking Light, etc.)

11. Would you or any of your personal contacts like more information about: ____ fund-raising _____ seminars or community events _____ wholesale prices for *Healthy Dining* books?

   Other Comments?

Please complete name and address on reverse side, fold and mail. Photocopy acceptable. LA4

Fold on lines with address on outside.

Name: _____

Address:_____

_____

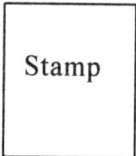

Healthy Dining
8305 Vickers Street, Suite 106
San Diego, CA 92111

Special $5.00 OFF *Healthy Dining* books.

Order as many as you want at the special discount! It's our thank-you for answering our questionnaire. You will also receive the $5.00 discount on future editions. Orders normally processed within 1 week.

Quantity		Price
_____ ***Healthy Dining in San Diego***	$19.95 - $5.00 discount = $14.95	_____
_____ ***Healthy Dining in Orange County***	$19.95 - $5.00 discount = $14.95	_____
_____ ***Healthy Dining in Los Angeles***	$19.95 - $5.00 discount = $14.95	_____

Call (800) 953-3463 for more information

Shipping & Handling ($2.50 for 1st book + 99¢ each for additional books)   _____

Subtotal   _____

Tax (8¼% in Los Angeles)   _____

_____ Check enclosed   Phone (   ) _____   Total   _____

_____ VISA/Mastercard # _____ exp._____ Signature_____

Please fill out questionnaire on reverse and your name & address above. If sending check, make to **Healthy Dining** and fasten your check securely to this sheet or use a separate envelope. Thanks.

Coupons

$5.00 OFF
your next purchase of *Healthy Dining*
See page 186 for details.

Coupon   *Healthy Dining in Los Angeles*   Coupon

Healthy Dining entrée for $2.49!

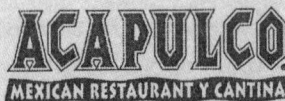

ACAPULCO
MEXICAN RESTAURANT Y CANTINA

Acapulco

Buy one Healthy Dining entrée at regular price and receive another Healthy Dining entrée of equal or lesser value for $2.49!

Valid at all Los Angeles
Acapulco locations.
Not valid with any other advertised special,
banquet or for carry out.

Coupon   *Healthy Dining in Los Angeles*   Coupon

FREE!
Burrito or Taco!

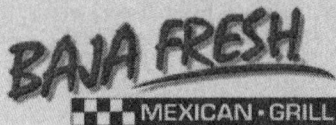

BAJA FRESH
MEXICAN · GRILL

Baja Fresh

Present this coupon and receive a
FREE Burrito or Taco with purchase
of a large drink! Up to a $5.45 value.
One coupon per customer. Not valid with any other offer or
discount. No product substitutes. Not valid if reproduced.

37 locations
throughout Los Angeles
Visit our website for a complete list
of all locations www.bajafresh.com.

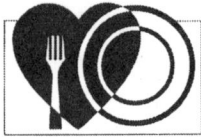 *Healthy Dining in Los Angeles*

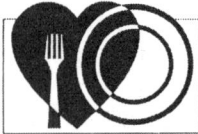 *Healthy Dining in Los Angeles*

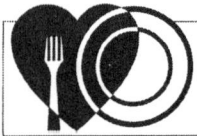 *Healthy Dining in Los Angeles*

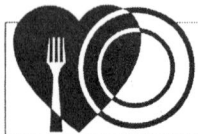 *Healthy Dining in Los Angeles*

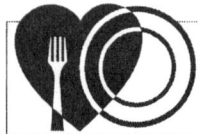 *Healthy Dining in Los Angeles*

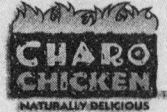

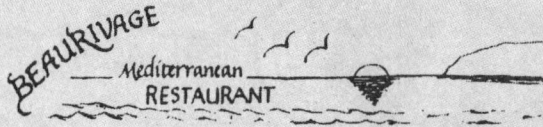

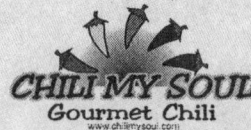

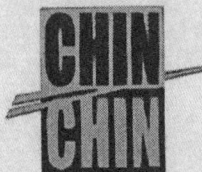

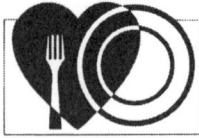 *Healthy Dining in Los Angeles*

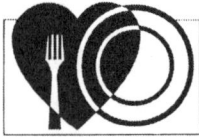 *Healthy Dining in Los Angeles*

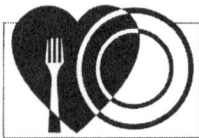 *Healthy Dining in Los Angeles*

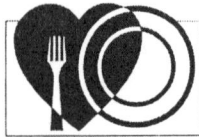 *Healthy Dining in Los Angeles*

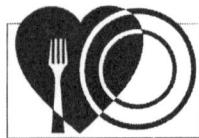 *Healthy Dining in Los Angeles*

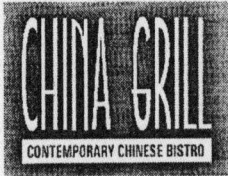

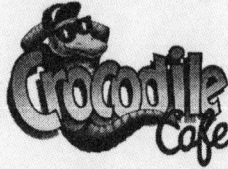

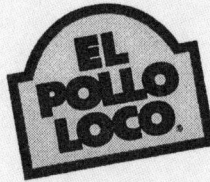

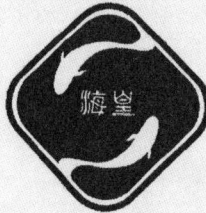

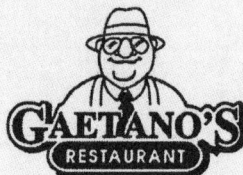

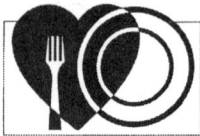

Healthy Dining in Los Angeles

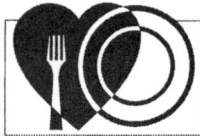

Healthy Dining in Los Angeles

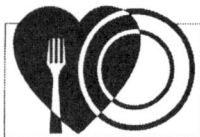

Healthy Dining in Los Angeles

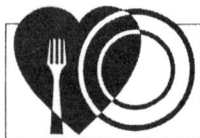

Healthy Dining in Los Angeles

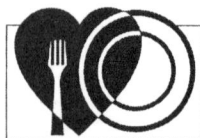

Healthy Dining in Los Angeles

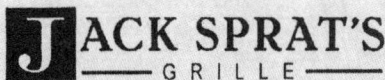

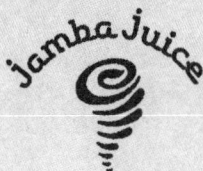

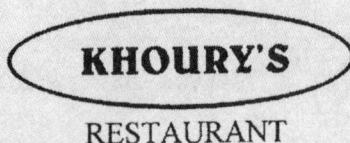

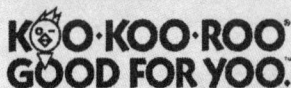

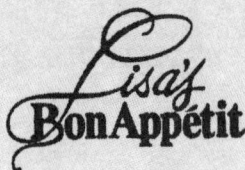

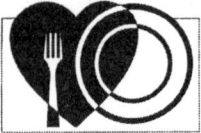

Healthy Dining in Los Angeles

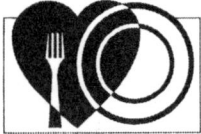

Healthy Dining in Los Angeles

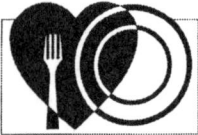

Healthy Dining in Los Angeles

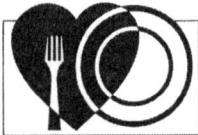

Healthy Dining in Los Angeles

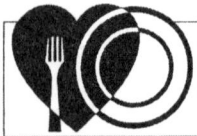

Healthy Dining in Los Angeles

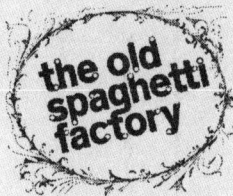

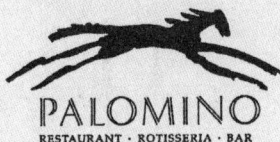

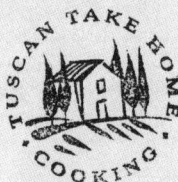

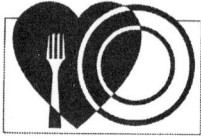

Healthy Dining in Los Angeles

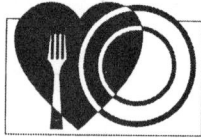

Healthy Dining in Los Angeles

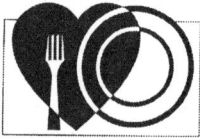

Healthy Dining in Los Angeles

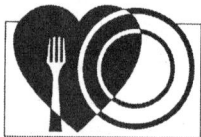

Healthy Dining in Los Angeles

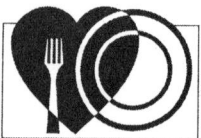

Healthy Dining in Los Angeles

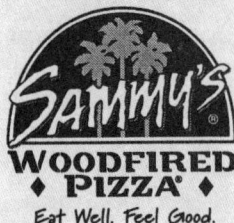

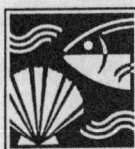

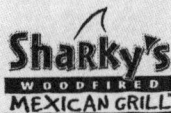

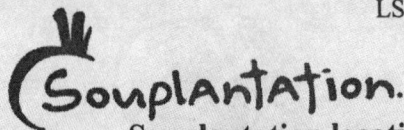

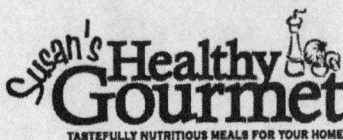

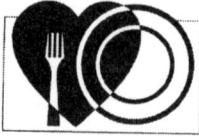 *Healthy Dining in Los Angeles*

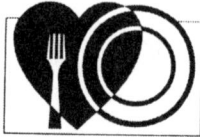 **Healthy Dining in Los Angeles**

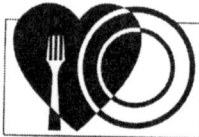 **Healthy Dining in Los Angeles**

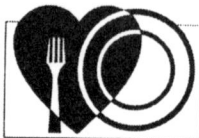 **Healthy Dining in Los Angeles**

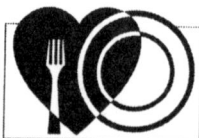 **Healthy Dining in Los Angeles**

Part VI

Indexes

Index by Location - Central and Western Locations

Index by Location - Coastal and South Bay Locations

Index by Location – North and Northwest Locations

Index by Location – East and Southeast Locations

Index by Cuisine

Italian

Allegria	47
Buon Gusto	55
Buona Vita On Main	56
Buona Vita Pizzeria	56
Buona Vita Trattoria	56
Ca'Brea	57
Ca' del Sole	58
Carmine's	62
Gaetano's Restaurant	75
il Forno	78
il Moro	79
Mi Piace	91
Old Spaghetti Factory	93
Pane e Vino	96
Prego Ristorante	102
Rosti	106
Sisley Italian Kitchen	112
Spaghettini	115

Japanese/American

Chaya Brasserie	65
Chaya Venice	65
Wasabi Japanese Restaurant	120

Juice Bar

Jamba Juice	81

Mediterranean

Beau Rivage	50
Café Santorini	60
Malvasia	89

Mexican/Southwest

Acapulco	46
Baja Fresh	49
Border Grill	53
El Pollo Loco	72
El Torito	73
La Salsa	87
Riviera Mexican Grill	104
Sharky's	110
Wahoo's Fish Taco	119

Pizza

Buona Vita Pizzeria	56
Sammy's Woodfired Pizza	108

Quick Serve

Baja Fresh	49
Charo Chicken	64
El Pollo Loco	72
Jamba Juice	81
Koo Koo Roo	86
La Salsa	87
Sharky's	110
Skew's Fresh & Fire Grilled	113
Wahoo's Fish Taco	119

Seafood

Bluewater Grill	51
Empress Harbor Seafood	74
Gaetano's Restaurant	75
Kincaid's Bay House	84
King's Fish House	85
McCormick & Schmick's	90
Ocean Avenue Seafood	92
Rock'N Fish	105
Santa Monica Seafood	109
Twin Palms	118

Thai

PJ's Thai Restaurant	100

Vietnamese/French Fusion

Crustacean	71

Vegetarian/Natural Foods

Anastasia's Asylum	48
Real Food Daily	103
The Spot Natural Food Restaurant	116
Whole Foods Market	121

Alphabetical Index